BUILDING RESILIENCE
into the Nation's
MEDICAL PRODUCT SUPPLY CHAINS

Wallace J. Hopp, Lisa Brown, and Carolyn Shore, *Editors*

Committee on Security of America's Medical Product Supply Chain

Board on Health Sciences Policy

Health and Medicine Division

A Consensus Study Report of

The National Academies of
SCIENCES • ENGINEERING • MEDICINE

THE NATIONAL ACADEMIES PRESS
Washington, DC
www.nap.edu

THE NATIONAL ACADEMIES PRESS   500 Fifth Street, NW   Washington, DC 20001

This activity was supported by a contract between the National Academy of Sciences and the Office of the Assistant Secretary for Preparedness and Response (75A50120C00129). Any opinions, findings, conclusions, or recommendations expressed in this publication do not necessarily reflect the views of any organization or agency that provided support for the project.

International Standard Book Number-13: 978-0-309-27469-2
International Standard Book Number-10: 0-309-27469-9
Digital Object Identifier: https://doi.org/10.17226/26420

Additional copies of this publication are available from the National Academies Press, 500 Fifth Street, NW, Keck 360, Washington, DC 20001; (800) 624-6242 or (202) 334-3313; http://www.nap.edu.

Copyright 2022 by the National Academy of Sciences. All rights reserved.

Printed in the United States of America

Suggested citation: National Academies of Sciences, Engineering, and Medicine. 2022. *Building resilience into the nation's medical product supply chains*. Washington, DC: The National Academies Press. https://doi.org/10.17226/26420.

The National Academies of
SCIENCES · ENGINEERING · MEDICINE

The **National Academy of Sciences** was established in 1863 by an Act of Congress, signed by President Lincoln, as a private, nongovernmental institution to advise the nation on issues related to science and technology. Members are elected by their peers for outstanding contributions to research. Dr. Marcia McNutt is president.

The **National Academy of Engineering** was established in 1964 under the charter of the National Academy of Sciences to bring the practices of engineering to advising the nation. Members are elected by their peers for extraordinary contributions to engineering. Dr. John L. Anderson is president.

The **National Academy of Medicine** (formerly the Institute of Medicine) was established in 1970 under the charter of the National Academy of Sciences to advise the nation on medical and health issues. Members are elected by their peers for distinguished contributions to medicine and health. Dr. Victor J. Dzau is president.

The three Academies work together as the **National Academies of Sciences, Engineering, and Medicine** to provide independent, objective analysis and advice to the nation and conduct other activities to solve complex problems and inform public policy decisions. The National Academies also encourage education and research, recognize outstanding contributions to knowledge, and increase public understanding in matters of science, engineering, and medicine.

Learn more about the National Academies of Sciences, Engineering, and Medicine at **www.nationalacademies.org**.

The National Academies of
SCIENCES • ENGINEERING • MEDICINE

Consensus Study Reports published by the National Academies of Sciences, Engineering, and Medicine document the evidence-based consensus on the study's statement of task by an authoring committee of experts. Reports typically include findings, conclusions, and recommendations based on information gathered by the committee and the committee's deliberations. Each report has been subjected to a rigorous and independent peer-review process and it represents the position of the National Academies on the statement of task.

Proceedings published by the National Academies of Sciences, Engineering, and Medicine chronicle the presentations and discussions at a workshop, symposium, or other event convened by the National Academies. The statements and opinions contained in proceedings are those of the participants and are not endorsed by other participants, the planning committee, or the National Academies.

For information about other products and activities of the National Academies, please visit www.nationalacademies.org/about/whatwedo.

COMMITTEE ON SECURITY OF AMERICA'S MEDICAL PRODUCT SUPPLY CHAIN[1]

WALLACE J. HOPP (*Chair*), Distinguished University Professor of Business and Engineering, Stephen M. Ross School of Business, University of Michigan

MAHSHID ABIR, Associate Professor, Department of Emergency Medicine, University of Michigan

GEORGE BALL, Associate Professor, Operations and Decision Technologies Department, Kelley School of Business, Indiana University Bloomington

RAQUEL C. BONO, Principal, RCB Consulting (resigned from the committee February 2021)

LEE BRANSTETTER, Professor of Economics and Public Policy, Carnegie Mellon University

ROBERT CALIFF, Former Medical Strategy and Senior Advisor at Alphabet Inc., Verily Life Sciences and Google Health (resigned from the committee November 2021)

ASHA DEVEREAUX, Physician, Sharp Healthcare System

OZLEM ERGUN, Professor and Associate Chair for Graduate Affairs, Department of Industrial and Mechanical Engineering, Northeastern University College of Engineering

ERIN R. FOX, Senior Pharmacy Director, Drug Information and Support Services, Department of Pharmacy Services, University of Utah Health

LARRY M. GLASSCOCK, Chief Operating Officer, NFH, Inc.

LEWIS GROSSMAN, Professor of Law, Washington College of Law, American University

W. CRAIG VANDERWAGEN, Partner, East West Protection, LLC

ALASTAIR WOOD, Emeritus Professor of Medicine and Pharmacology, Vanderbilt University

MARTA WOSIŃSKA, Former Deputy Director, Policy at the Duke-Margolis Center for Health Policy (resigned from the committee April 2021)

MATTHEW K. WYNIA, Director, Center for Bioethics and Humanities, University of Colorado

Study Staff

LISA BROWN, Study Co-Director
CAROLYN SHORE, Study Co-Director
LEAH CAIRNS, Program Officer (from June 2021)

---

[1] NOTE: See Appendix F, Disclosure of Unavoidable Conflict of Interest.

KELSEY R. BABIK, Associate Program Officer (from August 2021)
BEN KAHN, Associate Program Officer (until June 2021)
EESHAN KHANDEKAR, Associate Program Officer (until October 2020)
ANDREW MARCH, Associate Program Officer
SHALINI SINGARAVELU, Associate Program Officer (from August 2021)
REBECCA CHEVAT, Research Associate (until June 2021)
MARGARET MCCARTHY, Research Associate (from August 2021)
KIMBERLY SUTTON, Senior Program Assistant (from June 2021)
MELVIN JOPPY, Senior Program Assistant (until June 2021)
ANDREW M. POPE, Senior Director, Board on Health Sciences Policy

Science Writers

JOANNA LOCKE, Locke Public Health
ANNA NICHOLSON, Doxastic LLC
EVAN RANDALL, Doxastic LLC

Commissioned Paper Author

PHILIP ELLIS, Ellis Health Policy

Reviewers

This Consensus Study Report was reviewed in draft form by individuals chosen for their diverse perspectives and technical expertise. The purpose of this independent review is to provide candid and critical comments that will assist the National Academies of Sciences, Engineering, and Medicine in making each published report as sound as possible and to ensure that it meets the institutional standards for quality, objectivity, evidence, and responsiveness to the study charge. The review comments and draft manuscript remain confidential to protect the integrity of the deliberative process.

We thank the following individuals for their review of this report:

GE BAI, Johns Hopkins Carey Business School and Bloomberg School of Public Health
ILISA BERNSTEIN, American Pharmacists Association
MATTHEW GRENNAN, University of California, Berkeley
MARGARET A. HAMBURG, Nuclear Threat Initiative
JANE E. HENNEY, University of Kansas Medical Center
PINAR KESKINOCAK, Georgia Institute of Technology
NICOLETTE LOUISSAINT, Healthcare Ready
NICOLE LURIE, Coalition for Epidemic Preparedness Innovations (CEPI)
BILL MURRAY, Deloitte Consulting LLP
PAUL E. PETERSEN, Tennessee Department of Health
KATHERYN RUSS, University of California, Davis
STEPHEN W. SCHONDELMEYER, University of Minnesota
MARTIN VANTRIESTE, Civica Rx

Although the reviewers listed above provided many constructive comments and suggestions, they were not asked to endorse the conclusions or recommendations of this report nor did they see the final draft before its release. The review of this report was overseen by **DAVID R. CHALLONER,** University of Florida, and **VINOD K. SAHNEY,** Northeastern University. They were responsible for making certain that an independent examination of this report was carried out in accordance with the standards of the National Academies and that all review comments were carefully considered. Responsibility for the final content rests entirely with the authoring committee and the National Academies.

Preface

Supply chains have never had a higher profile than they do right now. Once the arcane purview of specialists and scholars, the field of supply chain management has been front page news throughout the COVID-19 pandemic. Unfortunately, the reason for this newfound notoriety is that everything, from cars to coffee, seems to be in irritatingly short supply. These shortages have awakened us all to the reality that the products we take for granted are delivered through complex, global supply chains, which can break down.

Not being able to buy toilet paper or a television set is certainly an inconvenience. But not being able to get a chemotherapy drug or mechanical ventilator is life threatening. Of the many supply chains whose fragility was exposed by the pandemic, none are more vital to public health and safety than those for medical products. Recognizing this, Congress, as part of the 2020 CARES Act, called for establishment of an ad hoc committee to examine the security and resilience of U.S. medical product supply chains. This report is the result of a year-long study by that committee.

To focus its work, the committee interpreted "resilience" to refer to the ability of medical product supply chains to match supply with demand under both normal and emergency conditions, so that patients and providers can count on access to medical products when they need them. But matching supply with demand is precisely the role of supply chain management. Why then have we experienced so many shortfalls in normal times, such as chronic shortages of generic injectable drugs for over a decade, and during emergencies, such as inadequate supplies of N95 masks to meet surging demand during the recent pandemic?

The kneejerk response in the media and elsewhere has been to blame globalization. And to be sure, long supply chains with many production stages spread over many locations with many transportation links between them have more failure modes than short domestic supply chains. However, there are also reasons supply chains have become increasingly globalized. Locating production of the various steps in places with cost or capability advantages can facilitate lower prices, higher quality, wider variety, and more innovation. On-shoring a global supply chain by moving all production stages to domestic sites would therefore have consequences. Most prominently, on-shoring could increase costs and reduce affordability of medical products. Indeed, affordability concerns are the reason domestic companies that stepped up to produce N95 masks at the beginning of the pandemic found themselves struggling to survive once international supplies resumed and health systems shifted back to them to reduce costs.

Beyond cost concerns, the resilience benefits of on-shoring depend on what stages are domesticated and how. Moving only the final assembly stage to the United States, as is often proposed in glib on-shoring proposals, will have a limited impact on resilience because it leaves the supply chain vulnerable to disruptions of component and raw material supplies. Even if all stages of a medical product supply chain could be on-shored, if this served to concentrate production of a key stage in a single location, it could leave the very supply chains we are trying to protect more vulnerable to disruption by local disasters like earthquakes or hurricanes.

Finally, even if we could overcome the economic obstacles and risks of supply concentration, it would be irresponsible to on-shore medical products if there were more cost-effective ways to achieve medical product supply chain resiliency. For example, if holding a vast stockpile of a critical medical product would provide more protection for less cost than on-shoring the product, why wouldn't we do it? As a country, we have many social priorities. Unnecessary spending on one means less funds will be available for another.

All this quickly led the committee to the realization that our focus could not be limited to assessing risks of globalization and finding ways to on-shore critical medical products. Nor could it be to simply enumerate ways to make medical product supply chains more resilient. To serve the overarching goal of making the American public safer and more secure, we had to create a framework for systematically enumerating, evaluating, and combining measures into a cost-effective medical product supply chain resiliency strategy.

Fortunately, the committee was comprised of experts in supply chain management, economics, and medicine. While this sometimes led to discussions that sounded like those of the five blind men describing an elephant, it allowed us to leverage our different disciplinary lenses to create a medical product supply chain resilience framework. We made use of this framework, which contains four tiers that address awareness, mitigation, preparedness, and response, to craft and motivate our recommendations. Under the awareness category, we propose measures to collect, compile, and disseminate information about medical product supply chain risks and vulnerabilities. Under the mitigation category, we advocate steps to reduce the likelihood and magnitude of supply disruptions. Under the preparedness category, we describe a range of options for preventing a supply shortage from impacting patients and medical personnel. Under the response category, we suggest policies for building organizational capabilities that protect health during emergency disruptions.

In the end, as our report makes abundantly clear, there is no single "silver bullet" for the medical product supply chain problem. Instead, we believe it is a case of the quote, "God is in the details." Slogans won't make us safer in the next crisis than we were in this one, but a host of coordinated activities by medical product supply chain managers, government agents, and medical providers will.

Lastly, I want to express my deepest gratitude to the committee members and the National Academies staff members who worked on this study. The volunteers on the committee devoted major amounts of time and energy on top of their regular professional responsibilities that were heightened by the added burden of dealing with a pandemic. In the case of the clinical members of the committee, this often meant rotating in and out of meetings to treat patients. It was truly an example of America at its best, with people helping people in every way they could. But the discussions, emails, snippets of text, and comments on drafts from these dedicated committee members could not have become a report without the writing and editing skills of the staff. In particular, Lisa Brown and Carolyn Shore organized both the activities of the committee and the writing of the report with exceptional vision and leadership, while Kelsey Babik, Leah Cairns, Andrew March, Margaret McCarthy, and Shalini Singaravelu skillfully bore the brunt of the writing responsibility. It was an honor and a delight to work with all of these wonderful people.

Wallace (Wally) Hopp, *Chair*
Committee on Security of America's
Medical Product Supply Chain

Abstract

During the coronavirus disease 2019 (COVID-19) pandemic, shortages of medical devices, supplies, and drugs have risked the lives of Americans and have compromised the ability to deliver care. However, medical product shortages are not a new problem, and over the past several decades supply chain disruptions have repeatedly plagued the U.S. health care system, costing health care systems millions of dollars per year, threatening the clinical research enterprise, and most importantly, imperiling the health and lives of patients. In 2020, a committee convened by the National Academies of Sciences, Engineering, and Medicine was charged to address this important issue by examining the root causes of medical product shortages and identifying ways to enhance the resilience and security of America's medical product supply chains—both in so-called normal times and during public health emergencies.

Because medical product supply chains are complex, multilevel, globally distributed systems that involve people, processes, technologies, and policies, they are vulnerable to many types of risk, as well as amenable to many types of remediation. To identify measures that will have the greatest impact on public health and safety, the committee focused on *supply chain critical* medical products, which are defined as those that are both medically essential and vulnerable to shortages. Market incentives play a key role in determining the vulnerability of medical product supplies. For example, high margins on patented drugs provide strong incentive for manufacturers to build in supply continuity protections, while low margins on generic drugs do not. Consequently, identifying supply chain critical medical products requires both an evaluation of medical need and an assessment of a mismatch between private and public incentives.

To prioritize the myriad ways the supply chains for these critical products can be made more resilient, the committee invoked basic concepts of system reliability and supply chain management to create a framework that categorizes measures into four layers of protection. These layers address the timeline from a disruptive event to impact on human health by considering awareness, mitigation, preparedness, and response (see Chapter 5).

Awareness measures identify, analyze, and share information essential to understanding and reducing medical product supply chain risks (see Chapter 6). As such, awareness is a prerequisite to mitigate, prepare for, or respond to supply chain disruptions. Mitigation measures reduce the likelihood or magnitude of disruptive events that could lead to medical product shortages (see Chapter 7). For example, a quality rating system that avoids a medical product recall is a mitigation measure that prevents a recall-induced shortage before it can happen. Preparedness measures are actions taken prior to a disruptive event that will reduce the negative impacts on health and safety if the event occurs (see Chapter 8). An example is inventory stockpiling, which does not stop a capacity disruption or demand surge event from occurring, but can prevent end users from experiencing a supply shortage. Response measures include steps taken after a shortage has occurred to prevent or reduce public harm (see Chapter 9). For example, crisis standards of care, which alter and prioritize use of scarce medical products, do not avoid or reduce a supply shortage, but when implemented, they can protect health by maximizing the effectiveness of the limited supply, and are therefore an important response measure. This medical product supply chain resilience framework can be used to identify a set of effective and complementary policies for enhancing supply resilience for a specific medical product.

The committee leveraged the framework to identify high-priority, high-impact recommendations within the four protective layers to build an integrated strategy to address the most significant gaps in medical product supply chain resilience.

- **Awareness:** To enhance awareness of medical product supply chain risks and remedies, the committee recommends the U.S. Food and Drug Administration (FDA) make sourcing, quality, volume, and capacity information publicly available for all medical products approved or cleared for sale in the United States (Recommendation 1) and establish a public database to share this information and to promote analyses of these data by interested parties (Recommendation 2). Novel approaches to mitigation, preparedness, and response will come from these analyses.

- **Mitigation:** To reduce the risk and magnitude of disruptive events that cause supply shortages, particularly under nonemergency conditions, the committee recommends that health systems deliberately incorporate quality and reliability, in addition to price, in contracting, purchasing, and inventory decisions (Recommendation 3).
- **Preparedness:** To prevent or reduce shortages from disruptive events that do occur, the committee recommends the Office of the Assistant Secretary for Preparedness and Response (ASPR) modernize and optimize inventory stockpiling management as protection against medical product shortages at the national and regional levels (Recommendation 4) and that ASPR and FDA complement stockpiling with capacity buffering policies to enhance cost efficiency and to improve protection in major emergencies (Recommendation 5).
- **Response:** To protect health against supply shortages that do reach end users, the committee recommends negotiating an international, plurilateral treaty with other major medical product exporters to make more effective use of limited global supplies by ruling out export bans on key medical products and components (Recommendation 6) and that ASPR and the Centers for Disease Control and Prevention establish a domestic working group to examine ways to improve effectiveness of the final delivery stage within the United States ("last mile") of medical product supply chains and to engage end users in planning for emergency response to medical product shortages (Recommendation 7).

Collectively, these seven recommendations will improve supply reliability for medical products during normal conditions and will protect public health and safety during emergencies.

Contents

ACRONYMS AND ABBREVIATIONS   xxv

SUMMARY   1

PART I: OVERVIEW OF GLOBAL MEDICAL PRODUCT
    SUPPLY CHAINS   23

1   INTRODUCTION   25
    Context for This Study, 29
    Study Approach, 32
    References, 43

2   UNDERSTANDING MEDICAL PRODUCT SUPPLY CHAINS   49
    Overview of the Medical Product Supply Chain System, 49
    Differences in Supply Chain Economics by Product Category, 53
    Policy Underpinnings of U.S. Medical Product Supply Chains, 55
    Concluding Remarks, 64
    References, 65

3   GLOBALIZATION OF U.S. MEDICAL PRODUCT
    SUPPLY CHAINS   69
    Global Landscape of Medical Product Supply Chains, 70
    Geographical Considerations for Medical Product
        Supply Chains, 74
    Impacts of Globalization, 83

Concluding Remarks, 87
References, 88

**4 CAUSES AND CONSEQUENCES OF
   MEDICAL PRODUCT SUPPLY CHAIN FAILURES** 95
   Mechanics of Medical Product Supply Chain Failures, 96
   Demand Surges, 100
   Capacity Reductions, 106
   Coordination Failure, 114
   Effects of Medical Product Shortages, 119
   Concluding Remarks, 124
   References, 125

**PART II: MEASURES FOR ENHANCING THE RESILIENCY
          OF MEDICAL PRODUCT SUPPLY CHAINS** 135

**5 A FRAMEWORK FOR RESILIENT MEDICAL
   PRODUCT SUPPLY CHAINS** 137
   Defining Resilience for Medical Product Supply Chains, 138
   Multilayered Protection, 142
   The Committee's Medical Product Supply Chains Resilience
      Framework, 144
   Concluding Remarks and Overview of Committee
      Recommendations, 159
   References, 161

**6 AWARENESS MEASURES FOR RESILIENT MEDICAL
   PRODUCT SUPPLY CHAINS** 163
   Transparency, 165
   Analytics, 170
   Communication, 171
   Current Efforts to Increase Awareness, 172
   Recommendations, 178
   References, 181

**7 MITIGATION MEASURES FOR RESILIENT MEDICAL
   PRODUCT SUPPLY CHAINS** 183
   Incentives for Quality and Reliability, 184
   Hardening Day-to-Day Medical Product Supply Chains, 185
   Diversification of Medical Product Supply Chains, 189
   Recommendation, 193
   References, 194

8	**PREPAREDNESS MEASURES FOR RESILIENT MEDICAL PRODUCT SUPPLY CHAINS**	197

Inventory Stockpiling, 200
Capacity Buffering, 204
But Buffer Flexibility, 209
Contingency Planning and Readiness, 212
Recommendations, 213
References, 216

9	**RESPONSE MEASURES FOR RESILIENT MEDICAL PRODUCT SUPPLY CHAINS**	221

Response Measures for Global Medical Product
    Supply Chains, 223
Response Measures for Last-Mile Delivery and End Users, 228
Recommendations, 233
References, 234

APPENDIXES

A	STUDY METHODS AND PUBLIC AGENDAS	239
B	SUMMARY OF RECOMMENDATIONS FROM CONTEMPORARY REPORTS	261
C	DETERMINING RISK VALUES WHEN EVALUATING MEDICAL PRODUCT SUPPLY CHAIN RESILIENCE	277
D	COMMISSIONED ECONOMIC ANALYSIS	285
E	COMMITTEE AND STAFF BIOSKETCHES	323
F	DISCLOSURE OF UNAVOIDABLE CONFLICT OF INTEREST	335

Boxes, Figures, and Tables

BOXES

S-1 Summary of Recommendations, 21

1-1 Statement of Task, 31
1-2 Key Terminology and Definitions, 34

2-1 Current Tools for FDA to Address Supply Chain Shortages, 56

3-1 Key Terminology and Definitions Regarding Geographic Location Based Production, 80
3-2 The Role of Global Collaboration in Developing Vaccines Against COVID-19, 85

4-1 Case Study on N95 Masks, 101
4-2 Case Study on Saline, 105
4-3 Case Study on Heparin, 108

5-1 Breakdown Example of a Multilayered Defense System, 143
5-2 Relative Economics of Inventory Stockpiling and Capacity Buffering, 151
5-3 Summary of Recommendations, 160

6-1 Benefits of Information Sharing in Supply Chain Management, 164
6-2 FDA's Site Selection Model: Risk Factors, 169

7-1 Resources for Addressing Medical Product Shortages and Quality Concerns, 186

8-1 Overview of Roadmap for Selecting Preparedness Measures, 199
8-2 3M's Use of Capacity Buffering, 205
8-3 Comparing the Economics of On-Shoring and Stockpiling, 206
8-4 Resources for Crisis Standards of Care, 213

9-1 Summary of Recommendations from *Regulating Medicines in a Globalized World*, 226

FIGURES

S-1 Simple schematic of medical product supply chains under normal conditions, 3
S-2 The three causes of shortages in medical product supply chains—demand surges, capacity reductions, and coordination failures—and examples of each, 7
S-3 Medical product supply chains resilience framework: potential trigger events and resilience measures, 9

1-1 Stakeholders in a medical product supply chain, 38

2-1 Simple schematic of a medical product supply chain under normal conditions, 51

3-1 U.S. imports of pharmaceuticals and medical equipment, products, and supplies in 2019, 71
3-2 Percentage of API and FDF manufacturing facilities for human drugs in the U.S. market by country or region, May 2020, 76

4-1 Simple schematic of a medical product supply chain under normal conditions, 96
4-2 Schematic of a typical shortage found in a medical product supply chain, 98
4-3 How shortages propagate through a medical product supply chain, 99
4-4 The three causes of shortages in medical product supply chains—demand surges, capacity reductions, and coordination failures—and examples of each, 100

5-1 Cumulative probability distribution of supply disruption time, 140
5-2 Swiss cheese model of system failure, 143
5-3 Swiss cheese model of medication error, 144
5-4 Medical product supply chains resilience framework: potential trigger events and resilience measures, 145
5-5 A layered protection strategy for matching resilience measures to medical products, 158

6-1 Medical product supply chain resilience framework: potential awareness measures, 163

7-1 Medical product supply chain resilience framework: potential mitigation measures, 184

8-1 Medical product supply chain resilience framework: potential preparedness measures, 198
8-2 Cost comparison of stockpiling and on-shoring, 207

9-1 Medical product supply chains resilience framework: potential response measures, 222

C-1 Cumulative probability distributions of shortage volume, 281
C-2 Conditional cumulative probability distributions of shortage duration for a reference scenario, 283

TABLES

1-1 Select Federal Agencies with Responsibilities in Medical Product Supply Chains, 40

3-1 Countries with the Largest Global Pharmaceutical Markets in the World, 87

Acronyms and Abbreviations

ADI	area deprivation index
AEP	Analytic Exchange Program
ANDA	Abbreviated New Drug Application
API	active pharmaceutical ingredient
ASHP	American Society of Health-System Pharmacists
ASIAS	Aviation Safety Information Analysis and Sharing
ASPE	Assistant Secretary for Planning and Evaluation
ASPR	Assistant Secretary for Preparedness and Response
BARDA	Biomedical Advanced Research and Development Authority
BSE	bovine spongiform encephalopathy
CARES Act	Coronavirus Aid, Relief, and Economic Security Act
CAGR	compound annual growth rate
CBRN	chemical, biological, radiological, and nuclear
CDC	Centers for Disease Control and Prevention
CDER	Center for Drug Evaluation and Research
CDRH	Center for Devices and Radiological Health
CI	consignment inventory
CIDRAP	Center for Infectious Disease Research and Policy
CGMP	current good manufacturing practice
CMS	Centers for Medicare & Medicaid Services
COI	conflict of interest
COVID-19	The disease caused by the virus SARS-CoV-2
CPU	central processing unit

CSC	crisis standards of care
CT	computerized tomography
DEA	Drug Enforcement Administration
DMAP	Data Modernization Action Plan
DoD	Department of Defense
DPA	Defense Production Act
DRG	diagnosis-related group
DSCSA	Drug Supply Chain Security Act
EU	European Union
FDA	U.S. Food and Drug Administration
FDAAA	Food and Drug Administration Amendments Act
FDASIA	Food and Drug Administration Safety and Innovation Act
FD&C Act	Federal Food, Drug and Cosmetic Act
FDI	foreign direct investment
FDF	finished dosage form
FEI	FDA Establishment Identifier
FEMA	Federal Emergency Management Agency
FIFO	first in, first out
GDUFA	Generic Drug User Fee Amendments
GM	General Motors
GPO	group purchasing organization
GUDID	Global Unique Device Identification Database
HCC	health care coalition
HHS	U.S. Department of Health and Human Services
HIDA	Health Industry Distributors Association
IAAE	International Academy of Automation Engineering
ICU	intensive care unit
ISPE	International Society for Pharmaceutical Engineering
IT	information technology
IV	intravenous
MCM	medical countermeasure
MDIC	The Medical Device Innovation Consortium
MRA	mutual recognition agreement
n.d.	no date
NDC	National Drug Code

NRCC	National Response Coordination Center
OPQ	Office of Pharmaceutical Quality
ORA	Office of Regulatory Affairs
OS	Office of Surveillance
OTE	The Bureau Industry and Security's Office of Technology Innovation
PDG	Partnership for DSCSA Governance
PPE	personal protective equipment
QALY	quality adjusted life year
QbD	quality by design
RFP	request for proposal
SCCT	Supply Chain Control Tower
SCRLC	Supply Chain Risk Leadership Council
SLEP	Shelf-Life Extension Program
SNS	Strategic National Stockpile
SOP	standard operating procedure
SSIL	Site Surveillance Inspection List
SVI	Social Vulnerability Index
TRIPS	Agreement on Trade-Related Aspects of Intellectual Property Rights
UDI	unique device identification
UK	United Kingdom
USP	United States Pharmacopeia
VA	U.S. Department of Veterans Affairs
VMI	vendor-managed inventory
WHO	World Health Organization
WTO	World Trade Organization
WWII	World War II

Summary[1]

Serious vulnerabilities have been present in global medical product supply chains for many years. Some of these have been highlighted by the ongoing COVID-19 pandemic—where shortages of masks and personal protective equipment for health care workers, medical products used to treat COVID-19, and medications to treat related conditions have put the lives of Americans at risk and compromised the U.S. health care system. In response, the U.S. government has urged a "whole-of-government approach to assessing the vulnerabilities in, and strengthening the resilience of, critical supply chains." Section 3101 of the Coronavirus Aid, Relief, and Economic Security (CARES) Act, signed into law on March 27, 2020, directed the secretary of the U.S. Department of Health and Human Services (HHS) to enter into an agreement with the National Academies of Sciences, Engineering, and Medicine (the National Academies) to establish an ad hoc committee to examine the security and resilience of U.S. medical product supply chains. The full charge to the committee is presented in Chapter 1 of this report.

In many ways, medical product supply chains resemble supply chains of other products. They consist of multiple stages, which are often carried out by different organizations in different parts of the world. However, because medical products are particularly important to human health, medical product supply chains have some unique characteristics, including higher levels of oversight and regulation. To date, the primary emphasis of regulatory oversight in the United States has been product quality, with

---

[1] This Summary does not include references. Citations for the discussion presented in the Summary appear in the subsequent report chapters.

a secondary focus on cost. But as the COVID-19 pandemic powerfully reminded the nation, supply reliability is also vital to human health. The investment, both financial and human capital, that government and private industry has made in the supply reliability of medical product supply chains has not been sufficient to meet the public health need. In keeping with the committee's charge, this report focuses specifically on the resilience of medical product supply chains, which is defined as the ability to prevent public health and safety from being compromised by disruptions to supplies of medical products.

Supply shortages of medical products can be the result of many types of events, including production process problems (at the final product level or at any prior level of the supply chain), inadequate or unacceptable quality, natural disasters, disease outbreaks, geopolitical events, and many more. To improve the resilience of medical product supply chains, the risks to such events need to be assessed and strategies identified to reduce those risks. However, because other social needs also demand resources, it is vital to consider cost.

DEFINING SUPPLY CHAIN CRITICAL MEDICAL PRODUCTS

To identify measures that will have the greatest effect on public health and safety per dollar invested, it is important to first determine which medical products warrant attention. The U.S. Food and Drug Administration (FDA) defines essential drugs and devices as those "that are medically necessary to have available at all times." However, a product that is medically essential under this definition, but already has a highly reliable supply chain, is a poor target for resilience investments. Therefore, the committee defines the term *supply chain critical* medical products as those that are both medically essential and vulnerable to shortages.

Chapter 5 describes a formal supply chain criticality score that represents risk as the expected patient harm attributable to the disruption of the supply of a given product. This score is given by the product of a measure of medical criticality and a measure of supply risk. By focusing attention on medical products that present the largest expected health risk to the public, this definition encourages cost-effectiveness through measures that protect large numbers of people. However, shortages of some products can present very grave risks to small groups of people. Other products present unlikely but extreme risks. In the interests of equity and national security, the committee advocates for including certain products on the list of supply chain critical medical products beyond those included for reasons of maximizing overall public health and safety. These considerations are discussed in more detail in Chapter 5.

UNDERSTANDING MEDICAL PRODUCT SUPPLY CHAINS

To increase the resilience of medical product supply chains, the causes of the supply disruption risks they face must first be understood. This in turn requires an understanding of the basic structure of medical product supply chains. Chapter 2 provides a high-level overview of medical product supply chains and how they differ depending on the product. These chains are complex, multistage, global systems that involve people, processes, technologies, and policies. Medical product supply chains facilitate the flow of drugs and devices from raw material or component suppliers (e.g., makers of ingredients or subassemblies) to producers (e.g., final assembly plants, fill-and-finish facilities) to distributors (e.g., wholesalers) to providers (e.g., health systems, pharmacies, retailers) and finally to patients (Figure S-1). A variety of stakeholders, including government agencies, raw material suppliers, manufacturers, distributors, group purchasing organizations, health systems, providers, and patients influence the behavior of medical product supply chains.

Medical product supply chains—which for the purpose of this report is an all-encompassing term that includes the supply chains for drugs, biologics, medical devices, and medical equipment—deliver a diverse array of drugs and devices, including the four main categories described in this

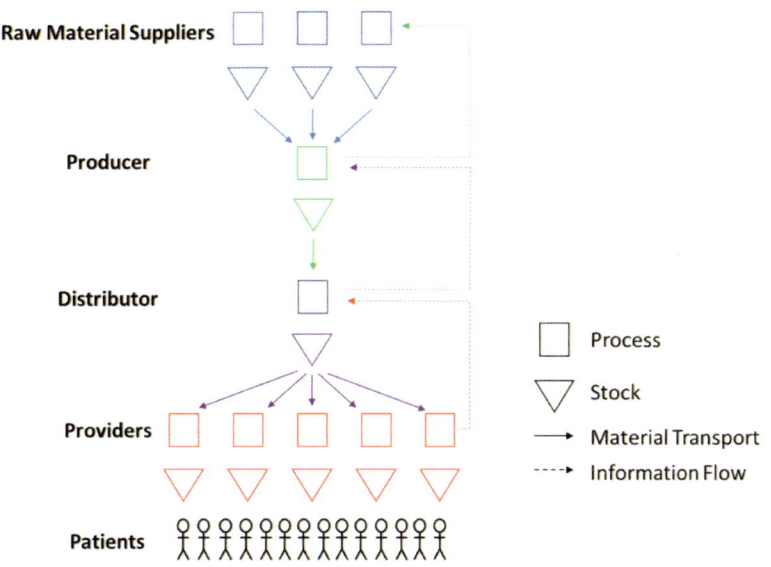

FIGURE S-1 Simple schematic of medical product supply chains under normal conditions.

report.[2] Product types have production processes and supply chains that vary considerably depending on product characteristics. When considering measures to increase supply chain resilience for a specific medical product, these characteristics can be important to consider. But when considering broader public policy measures, it is helpful to group products into classes.

Drugs can be divided into originator and generic products. A generic drug is a medication developed to be equivalent to an already marketed brand-name drug in dosage form, safety, strength, route of administration, quality, performance characteristics, and intended use so that the generic medicine works in the same way and provides the same clinical benefit as the brand-name medicine. In general, margins are much lower on generic drugs than on original drugs. Because this implies that generic drug producers have less financial incentive to protect supply continuity, generics are more prone to routine supply disruptions and quality deviations and are thereby more likely to warrant inclusion on the supply chain critical list. Within the supply chains of both generic and originator drugs, two basic steps occur: (1) the basic production of bulk-drug substances, commonly referred to as active pharmaceutical ingredients (APIs) and pharmaceutical excipients and (2) the pharmaceutical manufacturing of finished dosage form (FDF) drug products. This is important to supply chain risk assessment and remediation because API or incipient production may pose significant risks of shortages but is all but invisible to both buyers and regulators because the producer identity and location for inputs is not generally disclosed by drug manufacturers.

Medical devices are defined by FDA as any object or component used in the diagnosis, treatment, prevention, or cure of medical conditions or diseases, or that affects body structure or function through means other than chemical or metabolic reaction in humans or animals. For regulatory purposes, devices are divided into three classes. Class I medical devices present minimal potential for harm to the user and are often simpler in design than Classes II and III. Class II medical devices present moderate risk of harm to the patient or user. More than 50 percent of FDA-regulated medical devices are considered Class II. Class III medical devices are highly complex devices that also present a high safety risk to the patient and user. These classes

---

[2] This report does not focus in detail on supply chains for biologics or vaccines given the distinct features in their supply chains. However, as some biologics and vaccines are high-margin, patent-protected pharmaceuticals while others are not, the discussion of profit margins and incentives between originator and generic drugs is still applicable to these medical products. Furthermore, four new reports from the National Academy of Medicine focus on how to prepare for seasonal and pandemic influenza through lessons learned from COVID-19—with one report in particular focusing on globally resilient supply chains for pandemic and seasonal influenza vaccines. These reports can be accessed here: https://nam.edu/four-new-reports-from-the-national-academy-of-medicine-focus-on-how-to-prepare-for-seasonal-and-pandemic-influenza-through-lessons-learned-from-covid-19.

were established primarily to regulate product quality. However, the fact that Class III devices present the highest safety risks does not mean they present the highest supply disruption risk. Complex Class III devices, such as pacemakers, have high margins that motivate producers to protect their supply chains in order to protect their revenue streams. In contrast, less risky Class II devices, such as N95 respirators, have lower margins that lead producers to leave them vulnerable to shortages. As seen in the early months of the COVID-19 pandemic, shortages of relatively simple personal protective equipment (PPE) products can present serious public health risks.

There are two important insights from this overview of medical product supply chains. First, there is no one-size-fits-all strategy for increasing supply chain resilience for all medical products, which implies that a key challenge is to match resilience measures to products in a cost-effective manner. Second, current classification schemes for medical products are sometimes based solely on clinical importance, which implies the need to factor in shortage risks when making decisions about improving the resilience of medical product supply chains.

GLOBALIZATION OF U.S. MEDICAL PRODUCT SUPPLY CHAINS

As has been the case in other industries, the past several decades have been a time of rapid globalization for U.S. medical product supply chains. As described in Chapter 3, medical product companies have increasingly sourced production of products, components, and raw materials from locations around the globe that offer cost-effectiveness, skilled labor, and the necessary infrastructure to support manufacturing and distribution. This globalization has provided benefits to U.S. producers, consumers, investors, and health care providers, such as lower costs, expanded efficiency, and greater resources to invest in innovation in some cases, but also in the form of supply security because of diversification and innovation driven by competition.

However, globalization also has downsides. International production is more difficult to inspect and regulate than domestic production. This has contributed to a rash of quality problems in generic drugs that peaked in 2011 but remains an ongoing source of safety and supply problems. Long, global supply chains spread around the world are also less transparent than short, domestic ones. As a result, purchasers of medical products often do not know where they are produced and almost never know where the ingredients and components they contain are sourced from. Even FDA does not have detailed enough information about global medical product supply chains to enable assessment of vulnerabilities.

These issues have led to widespread calls for the on-shoring of medical product manufacturing. Unfortunately, many calls fail to specify what on-shoring actually means. Often it seems that the recommendations are to move final assembly to domestic sites without a recognition of the rest of the supply chain. By themselves, such moves will have a limited effect on supply reliability because they leave supplies vulnerable to disruptions in the supply of necessary inputs. Moving all stages of production to the United States would be highly daunting for supply chains with more than a few stages. Even if it were possible, it could significantly increase operating costs.

Consequently, on-shoring is not the panacea it is sometimes presented as. But this does mean that it cannot be part of a cost-effective strategy to improve the resilience of medical product supply chains. To properly determine if and when on-shoring is appropriate, on-shoring proposals need to be vetted financially against alternatives. To facilitate this, and more importantly to identify the components of a cost-effective strategy for medical product supply chains, a framework is needed for systematically enumerating alternatives.

CAUSES OF FAILURES OF MEDICAL PRODUCT SUPPLY CHAINS

A precursor to creating a framework for resilient medical product supply chains is to describe the mechanisms that lead to supply shortages. To do this, the committee examined how trigger events, including natural disasters, infectious disease outbreaks, or manufacturing process problems, can disrupt medical product supply chains in three primary ways:

1. Demand surge: An event drives demand for a medical product well above the normal level for an extended period of time. For example, a major natural disaster, such as a tornado or earthquake, can spike regional demand for certain medical products if these events result in a significant number of casualties requiring medical care. As seen during COVID-19, a pandemic can drive up global demand for many medical products.
2. Capacity reduction: One or more production or transport processes are impeded by lack of assets, power, or people. For example, a natural disaster could cause a factory to lose power and halt production or regulatory barriers or manufacturing quality problems could restrict the output of a supplier or producer, and could even eliminate inventory stock if a product is recalled. As seen during the COVID-19 pandemic, production of some products may have decreased because of lockdown measures or the need for workers to quarantine or be on sick leave.
3. Coordination failure: Events that prevent supply from being matched to demand can cause shortages of medical products even

when total supply is sufficient to meet total demand. For example, geopolitical issues or communication system failures during a hurricane or other natural disaster can reduce or obstruct the delivery of emergency supplies to the people that need them.

It is important to note that disruptions can overlap and interact—demand surges and capacity reductions may occur simultaneously, or capacity reductions may precipitate subsequent demand increases and vice versa. Additionally, disruptions do not cause medical product supply chains to shift instantly from the normal conditions to shortages. Because all supply chains contain at least some amount of inventory, and because decision makers will take steps to increase capacity or implement flexible strategies in response to an impending shortage, it will take time for a disruption to turn into a shortage experienced by patients. Chapter 4 describes the different causes of failures of medical product supply chains and provides examples of each (Figure S-2).

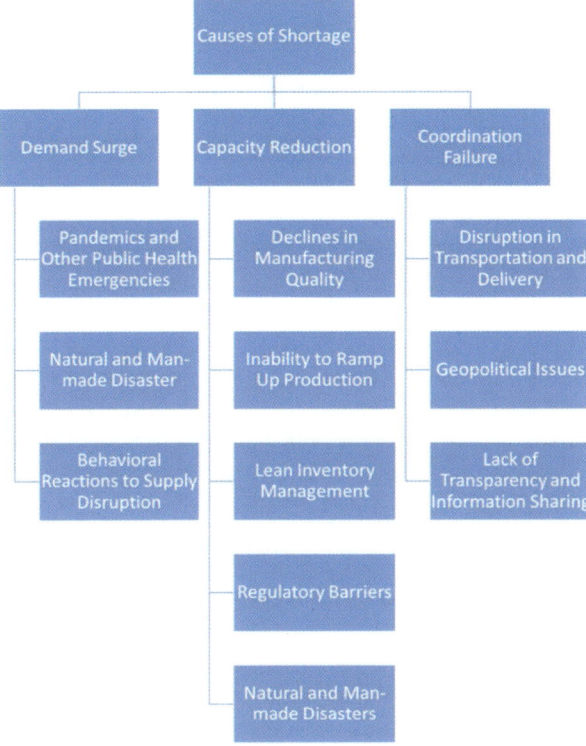

FIGURE S-2 The three causes of shortages in medical product supply chains—demand surges, capacity reductions, and coordination failures—and examples of each.

FRAMEWORK FOR IMPROVING THE RESILIENCE OF MEDICAL PRODUCT SUPPLY CHAINS

The key challenge of a medical product supply chains resilience framework is to identify the means for preventing trigger events from leading to human harm. As such, the resilience of medical product supply chains is an example of a reliability problem—albeit a complicated and difficult one because there are many resilience options available that fit together in intricate ways. Nevertheless, the basic concepts of system reliability and supply chain management can be invoked to create a framework that systematically categorizes means for providing a desired level of protection for a given medical product. Figure S-3 graphically illustrates such a framework by depicting the path from a potential trigger event (see Figure S-2) to public harm, with successive layers (or shields) of protection in between. In this figure, each shield represents a category of measures to prevent or reduce harm to the public's health and safety from shortages in medical product supply chains. The options within these categories comprise the building blocks of a resilience strategy for medical product supply chains.

Note that the shields in Figure S-3 are organized chronologically. The awareness category, shown as a foundation for the shields, is a precursor for the other three categories and includes measures that provide the information needed to implement them. The mitigation shield includes measures that reduce (possibly to zero) the extent to which a trigger event results in a supply shortage. The preparedness shield includes measures that reduce (possibly to zero) the extent to which a supply shortage reaches patients or providers. And finally, the response shield reduces (possibly to zero) the extent to which a supply shortage that reaches patients and providers causes harm to health and safety. The framework in Figure S-3 shows the shields deflecting the balls (threats caused by trigger events) to represent full prevention of harm, and also reducing the size of the balls to represent reduction in the magnitude of harm.

In addition to simply enumerating resilience options, overarching insights can be applied to help prioritize options for cost-effectiveness. In the framework of Figure S-3, a cost-effectiveness hierarchy is suggested among the protection shields in order of their timing. That is, in general, using awareness measures to give supply chain actors information to make better decisions is more efficient than using mitigation measures to avoid a shortage, which is more efficient than using preparedness measures to prevent shortages from reaching people, which is more efficient than using response measures to deal with shortage situations after the fact. This implies that a resilience strategy for medical product supply chains should carefully consider the awareness foundation and the early protection shields before thinking about the later shields.

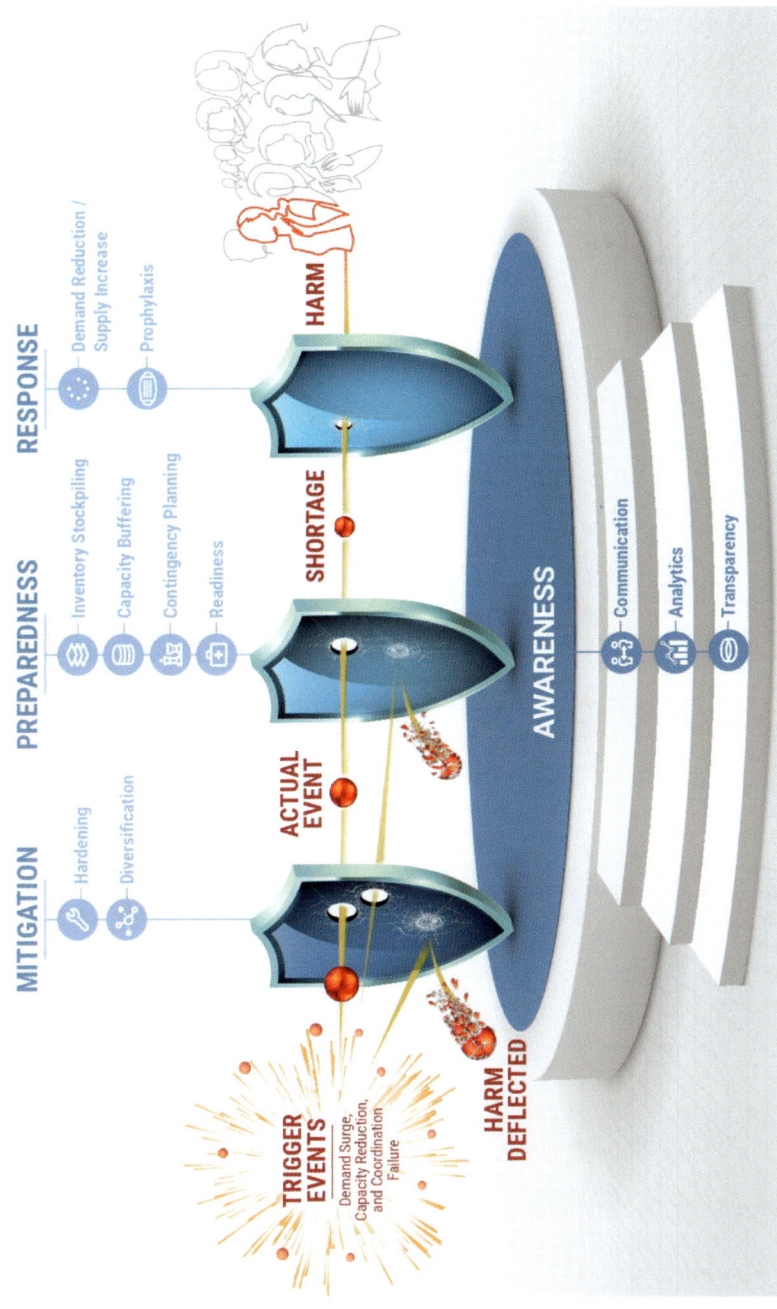

FIGURE S-3 Medical product supply chains resilience framework: potential trigger events and resilience measures.

However, the law of diminishing returns from economics implies that the cost-effectiveness of incremental investments in any single resilience measure will decrease as the amount of investment increases. For example, the cost of each additional unit of inventory in a stockpile is the same but the amount of protection provided decreases because the likelihood of needing the extra inventory declines. This suggests that a diversified strategy that uses a balance of different supply chain measures will be more cost-effective than one that relies on a single measure. Therefore, although while the protection shields should be considered in chronological order, it is also important to consider how far to go in each shield and how to fit measures from the different shields together. This process is discussed in Chapter 5 and is used to describe the connections between the committee's different recommendations in Chapters 6–9.

Finally, it must be acknowledged that shortages in medical product supply chains are in part the result of a market failure. Profit motives of manufacturers and vendors motivate a smaller investment in protection than is optimal from a public health perspective. Basically, firms have an incentive to protect supply continuity at a level that maximizes profits, while society has an incentive to protect supply continuity at a higher level that preserves public health. Consequently, the committee's recommendations include some necessary regulatory components. However, where possible, the committee's recommendations call for incentive-based solutions instead of behavior-forcing solutions that tap the power of the market to innovate and compete.

With the framework of Figure S-3 and the above observations, seven recommendations were identified as key to building resilient supply chains for medical products.

AWARENESS

Awareness across the entire medical product supply chain ecosystem requires transparency activities from regulators, suppliers, producers, distributors, and providers. The more transparency stakeholders bring into medical product supply chains, the better positioned they will be to identify vulnerabilities and proactively mitigate, prepare for, and respond to potential disruptions in medical product supply chains. As health system purchasing agents have long known, and the COVID-19 pandemic has made glaringly obvious, it is not always known where key components of the medical products are made or where in the supply chain medical products are. The current practice of keeping medical product supply chains confidential conflicts with public health needs and puts the public's health at risk. Improving the public's access to data that is important to their health and well-being is critical. Furthermore, lack of transparency and limited visibility into medical product supply chains have led to limited empirical evidence for identifying best strategies to address supply chain issues. These limitations also hamper the government's ability to work effectively with industry and other partners to increase the resilience of medical product supply chains.

Awareness measures can be broken into three categories: (1) transparency activities that make data available, (2) analytics activities that process data into useful information, and (3) communication activities that get the information into the hands of the people responsible for mitigation, preparedness, and response. Over the longer term, efforts should be established to collect, compile, and disseminate medical product supply chain data from these various stakeholders to increase end-to-end awareness to identify and mitigate risks. In the short, immediate term, the committee identifies upstream transparency efforts as a critical first step to increasing the resilience of medical product supply chains. The committee offers two recommendations pivotal to collecting, compiling, and disseminating the data on where and how medical products are made. Recommendation 1 (Public Transparency) addresses the significant gap in the data needed to assess and address risks in medical product supply chains by calling for both quality transparency (via risk-based site selection scores becoming public) and supply chain transparency (via all FDA Establishment Identifier [FEI] location data made public for where products are made).[3] These two dimensions of transparency (quality and supply chain) each have different sources. Quality data are currently kept by regulators, but they are not available to the public or manufacturers and distributors. Supply chain data are currently kept by manufacturers, but they are not available to the public or regulators. Recommendation 1 (Public Transparency) also calls for volume and capacity transparency to further assess risks directly related to medical product supply chains and to evaluate strategies for ameliorating these. Transparency is required both from manufacturers and from regulators so the public can be both informed about available medical products and empowered to act upon these data through data analysis and potentially put pressure on regulators and lawmakers. These data will enable the mapping of medical product supply chains, the identification of vulnerabilities such as supply concentrations, and the assessment of what

---

[3] Making certain data submitted to the FDA transparent to the public may also warrant certain legislative changes. For instance, it might necessitate a statutory amendment in the form of a change to section 301(j) of the FD&C Act (21 U.S.C. § 331(j)), which would be required only to the extent that the data that are proposed to be disclosed outside HHS are deemed as "concerning any method or process which as a trade secret is entitled to protection." In addition, 18 U.S.C. § 1905 (the Trade Secrets Act) would have to be amended to the extent the disclosed information "concerns or relates to ... trade secrets, processes, [or] operations ... or to the identity [or] confidential statistical data" of any company, unless disclosure of that information is otherwise "authorized by law."

medical products are most at risk. Specific data essential to transparency are discussed further in Chapter 6. Without this information, it is nearly impossible to make use of the supply chain resilience framework to identify measures for reducing risks to public health and safety.

Recommendation 1 (Public Transparency). The U.S. Food and Drug Administration (FDA) should take steps to make sourcing, quality, volume, and capacity information publicly available for all medical products approved or cleared for sale in the United States. These steps include the following:

    a. The manufacturer for a pharmaceutical drug should be required to publicly disclose the manufacturing location, in particular the FDA Establishment Identifier (FEI), the city, and the country, for the finished dosage form (FDF), active pharmaceutical ingredient (API), major excipients, and major packaging and delivery devices for all pharmaceutical drugs sold in the United States. API manufacturers shall be required to publicly disclose the sources of raw materials. This information should be made available on the labels for all pharmaceutical drugs and in a publicly accessible database. The National Drug Code should be associated with the primary FEI (where a majority of the volume is manufactured) in the database.

    b. FDA should make publicly available their risk-based Site Selection Model scores for all pharmaceutical drug manufacturing facilities that make drugs sold in the United States. FDA should also make public the Office of Pharmaceutical Quality (OPQ) scores. The risk-based Site Selection Model scores for the API and FDF plants (e.g., FEIs) should be made available on the labels for all pharmaceutical drugs and in a publicly accessible database, and the OPQ scores should also be included in this database.

    c. The manufacturer for a medical device should be required to publicly disclose the manufacturing location, in particular the FEI, the city, and the country, for the primary manufacturing and final assembly steps for all medical devices and major components sold in the United States. This information should be made available on the labels for all medical devices and in a publicly accessible database. The part number should be associated with the primary FEI (where a majority of the volume is manufactured) in the database.

    d. The risk-based Site Selection Model score for the primary manufacturing and final assembly plants (e.g., FEIs) should be made

available on the labels for all medical devices and in a publicly accessible database.
   e. Sourcing and quality information should be provided as part of the pharmaceutical drug or medical device approval or clearance processes and on an ongoing basis in order to retain a license or clearance to sell in the United States.
   f. Drug volume data reported to FDA, as mandated by the CARES Act, should be made available in a publicly accessible database. This requirement should be expanded to include reporting of capacity, in addition to volume, and should be required for medical devices, in addition to drugs.
   g. To the extent that amendments to the Trade Secrets Act at 18 U.S.C. § 1905 and to the Food, Drug, and Cosmetic Act at 21 U.S.C. § 331(j) are necessary to permit public disclosure of all the sourcing, quality, volume, and capacity information referenced in this recommendation, Congress should make such amendments.

However, data by themselves are not information. To enable stakeholders to make better decisions, data must be compiled into useful forms and disseminated to those who need it. Merely including supplier identity and location information on labels will not by itself enable health system purchasers to reduce their risk of supply disruptions or enable government officials to determine how and where to spend resources to protect the public health from such disruptions. Therefore, Recommendation 2 (Public Database) calls for the establishment of a publicly accessible database that summarizes supply chain information for medical products. Making the database public allows analyses and compilations to be done by both government actors and third parties. This will facilitate the use of sophisticated technologies, such as artificial intelligence, to process data and evaluate the type and degree of supply chain risks to medical product supplies.

Recommendation 2 (Public Database). The U.S. Food and Drug Administration (FDA), in cooperation with other U.S. government agencies, should establish a publicly accessible database containing the supply chain information acquired for medical products. FDA, in cooperation with other U.S. government agencies, should use the information on medical product supply chains it acquires to
   a. Understand better the vulnerabilities of medical product supply chains as a whole.
   b. Perform risk assessments regarding the risks to the total supply of particular medical products in both normal and emergency scenarios.

c. Coordinate, conduct, and compile research on the resilience of medical product supply chains, including by funding independent research that uses the established database.
d. Track the ways in which increased transparency, and the prediction of potential medical product shortages through data tracking, support improved supply chain resilience and functionality.
e. Incentivize the establishment of third-party rating system(s) for risk and quality.

Making this type of supply chain risk information publicly available will produce a host of predictable benefits. For example, a rating system that makes disruption risks visible will enable health system purchasers to factor supply reliability into their purchasing decisions. This in turn would provide an incentive for producers to improve supply chain reliability. Highlighting risks will also enable policy makers to prioritize programs for protecting public health by focusing on areas of greatest vulnerability. Finally, by placing more data into the hands of analysts, this public database creates the potential for new and useful insights. For instance, researchers may detect previously unknown risk predictors that could be used to design new and effective resilience measures for medical product supply chains.

MITIGATION

Mitigation includes actions taken prior to a disruptive event that helps prevent the event altogether or reduce its magnitude. Types of mitigation measures include hardening to reduce the likelihood or magnitude of disruptive events within stages of the system, and diversification to create parallel versions of stages to reduce the risk of catastrophic failure.

Because of a lack of transparency, medical product manufacturers currently have little incentive to harden their supply chains through updated techniques, processes, and controls that promote reliability and quality in medical products. The information that would be available in the public database proposed in Recommendation 2 would provide a key tool for improving the resilience of medical product supply chains. However, this information must be acted upon. A key place where this action is needed is in the purchasing decisions by health systems because a high percentage of medical product shortages, particularly in generic drugs, are encountered during normal times as a result of process disruptions caused by problems with quality. Hence, an important method to reduce the likelihood and magnitude of medical product supply shortages is by inducing health systems to incorporate reliability into their purchasing decisions.

The incentives that health systems have when managing their supply chains are misaligned with the incentives of the suppliers, distributors, and others participating in medical product supply chains. Health system contracts that focus on price alone can drive competitor products from the market in a "race to the bottom" pricing structure. This can lead to fewer suppliers, which in turn can weaken the resilience of the supply chain as no options are available to fill the void if a quality or manufacturing issue occurs. Health systems can address the "cost only" inertia by explicitly contracting for supply reliability in addition to price. Previous reports have issued recommendations that call for manufacturers to adopt updated manufacturing processes that would improve the quality and reliability of medical products (see Appendix B). Recommendation 3 (Resilience Contracting by Health Systems) builds on these by tasking health systems with actions that, when taken together with manufacturers and suppliers, will help build robust mitigation strategies into critical medical product supply chains.

> **Recommendation 3 (Resilience Contracting by Health Systems).** Health systems should promote a more resilient market for medical products by deliberately incorporating quality and reliability, in addition to price, in their contracting, purchasing, and inventory decisions. When quality ratings for medical products are available, accreditation organizations for health systems should use the ratings of the products sourced by health systems in their evaluations and ratings, as well as the frequency of shortages experienced at a health system that negatively affected patient care. Specifically,
>
> a. Health systems should fortify their contracts with medical product suppliers by including failure-to-supply penalties for contracts requiring a committed purchase or purchase volume, preferentially awarding contracts to suppliers that can demonstrate superior quality and reliability, awarding contracts to multiple suppliers of the same medical product, and requiring these same standards in contracts that are negotiated by group purchasing organizations on their behalf.
>
> b. Health systems should budget to adequately reward a select groups of products (e.g., low-cost, low-margin, off-patent, small molecule) if guarantees are met for higher quality and assured supply levels.
>
> c. Health systems and medical product wholesalers should routinely enter into emergency purchasing agreements for a specified list of emergency supplies or products that guarantees product delivery in the event of an unexpected supply demand or a substantial supply disruption. They should have a good understanding of the supplier's ability to meet demand, considering commitments to other buyers.

PREPAREDNESS

Preparedness includes actions taken prior to a disruptive event that will reduce the risks to health and safety if the event occurs. These actions can be grouped into four subcategories, two physical and two virtual. Physical preparedness measures include inventory buffering and capacity buffering, in which stock or productive capacity are held in readiness to fill a supply shortfall. Virtual preparedness measures include contingency planning, which establishes plans for dealing with specific scenarios, and readiness, which builds capabilities for dealing with scenarios without specific plans made in advance.

During the COVID-19 crisis, holding inventory in readiness was more complicated in practice than in theory. In the real world, problems with forecasting demand and monitoring stock levels, rotating stock to prevent expiration, and other practical details prevented inventory stockpiles from providing the intended level of protection in an emergency. Furthermore, capacity can be a cost-effective alternative or supplement to inventory as protection against shortages. The committee recommends action related to both stockpiling and capacity buffering. Stockpiling is already part of the national preparedness strategy, primarily in the form of the Strategic National Stockpile. Therefore, Recommendation 4 (Stockpiling) focuses primarily on refining and improving the ways inventory is held as protection against a medical product shortage.

Recommendation 4 (Stockpiling). The Office of the Assistant Secretary for Preparedness and Response should take steps to develop strategies to modernize and optimize inventory stockpiling management for the Strategic National Stockpile (SNS) and beyond to respond to medical product shortages at the national and regional levels. These steps include the following:
   a. Consider the recommendations provided in the National Academies report, *Ensuring the Effectiveness of the Public Health Emergency Medical Countermeasures Enterprise*, particularly those that focus on adopting a systems approach to managing the SNS.
   b. Analyze risk levels of supply chain critical medical products and the viability of other response strategies (e.g., capacity buffering).
   c. Examine key inventory stockpiling process considerations such as
      o Inventory system visibility.
      o Mechanisms and thresholds for the use, sharing, deployment, distribution, and allocation of stockpiled inventory in response to shortages (triggered by both emergencies and routine use) and to prevent product expiration.

- The risks and benefits of stockpiling ingredients or components as opposed to finished goods.
- The risks and benefits of just-in-time production or inventories in larger reserves.
- Funding levels to meet the required inventory levels and management tasks for the regional and national stockpiles as well as incentives for stakeholders for holding inventory.

d. Convene regional and local working groups composed of emergency health planners, clinicians, health care systems, and public health agencies, among others, to discuss and inform expectations for federal SNS support; national and regional stockpile content and pre-deployment positioning; regional supply capabilities and expectations; and roles and responsibilities for key stakeholders.

Recommendation 5 (Capacity Buffering) calls for measures to cultivate contingent capacity that can be brought online to supplement inventory buffers as needed. Such capacity buffering could be the result of direct contracts, such as advance arrangements to have specific manufacturers provide emergency capacity, as the auto manufacturers did during the pandemic by assembling ventilators. It could also be the result of a list of guaranteed "crisis prices" that the government would pay for certain products under specified conditions. This would provide an incentive for firms to find creative ways to deliver pop-up capacity during emergencies. Finally, the federal government should fund research on advanced manufacturing technologies that make it more economical to produce locally and easier to scale up capacity quickly. Both of these would make capacity buffering a more viable preparedness option, and hence would facilitate a partial shift away from expensive inventory and toward cheaper capacity.

As noted earlier, on-shoring is often espoused as a means for increasing the resilience of medical product supply chains via the argument that the more medical products a country produces domestically, the more control it has of supplies during an emergency. By reducing labor costs and promoting flexibility and scalability, the advanced manufacturing technologies advocated in Recommendation 5 (Capacity Buffering) may make on-shoring a good option for some products. Indeed, if technological capabilities permit efficient, small-scale production, then dispersed production in the country of consumption will be the natural market outcome. However, where this is not the case, on-shoring will impose a significant price penalty on an ongoing basis in return for a potentially small advantage during emergencies. If many developed countries pursue on-shoring strategies for many medical products, considerable resources will be spent that could be put to better use addressing other problems.

Therefore, on-shoring should be part of an integrated resilience strategy, rather than the option of choice.

Recommendation 5 (Capacity Buffering). The Office of the Assistant Secretary for Preparedness and Response (ASPR) and the U.S. Food and Drug Administration (FDA) should take steps to cultivate capacity buffering for supply chain critical medical products where such capacity is a cost-effective complement to stockpiling and as protection against long-lasting supply disruptions or demand surges. These steps include
   a. Government investments in capacity buffering should be aimed at all stages of the supply chain and at major public health emergencies.
   b. ASPR and FDA should develop and routinely maintain a crisis-prices list of supply chain critical medical products (i.e., medically essential and supply chain vulnerable) and identify which capacity measure is a practical supplement to the stockpiled inventory. Further, ASPR should develop and manage a database to coordinate inventory stockpiling and capacity buffering policies regarding crisis-prices list.
   c. ASPR and FDA should fund research and development for both advanced pharmaceutical and advanced medical technology manufacturing techniques to help make on-shoring more cost-competitive. By making capacity more easily scalable, these technologies would enable firms to respond to the need for capacity buffers more quickly and cost-effectively.
   d. ASPR and FDA should create public–private partnerships and support and fund capital and staff investments jointly, to implement these advanced manufacturing approaches to ensure production capacity. These partnerships will provide a great depth and breadth of expertise and can be leveraged for new economic incentives and regulatory clarity.
   e. ASPR should be responsible for anticipating and assessing public health emergency demand surge for supply chain critical medical products. They should clarify production capacity, identify vulnerabilities in supply chains, and engage producers in developing plans for surge response.

RESPONSE

Response includes actions taken after an event to minimize harm from the shortage and to resolve the shortage. These actions can be subdivided into prophylaxis measures, which protect human health while the shortage persists, and measures to close the supply gap through demand reduction and/or supply increase. Taken together, response activities seek to return the supply chain to normal (or to a "new normal") with as little harm as possible to end users and patients. The committee's recommendations about response include strategies at the global and end user levels to minimize harm from medical product shortages once they occur—both levels of response are needed to ensure the resilience of U.S. medical product supply chains. The key to both levels of response is effective communication and cooperation.

Because many medical product supply chains are global, some response actions must address production and supplies across international borders. The COVID-19 pandemic highlighted the vulnerability of global medical product supply chains to export bans and embargoes. By undermining trust that global medical product supply chains will function when they are needed most, these shortsighted measures promote both "tit-for-tat reciprocity" and "go-it-alone" behaviors that increase our collective vulnerability. The U.S. government must take on the task of better managing and reducing these risks, while maximizing the benefits of globalization. Recommendation 6 (International Treaty) calls for a plurilateral agreement by major exporters of medical products, including the United States, under the World Trade Organization that prohibits export bans on components of critical medical products. Although such an agreement cannot prevent a worldwide shortage from occurring, it can limit the risk to any individual country by "spreading the pain" across the global economy. Furthermore, if such an agreement increases the collective trust in global supply chains during an emergency, then it can be used in conjunction with Recommendation 5 (Capacity Buffering) to promote shared sources of contingent capacity. It is almost certainly more cost-efficient to build virtual capacity capabilities globally than locally. Hence, using the treaty as the basis for collaboration, major medical product exporting countries could further cooperate on providing capacity buffering for medical products likely to be in short supply during global emergencies.

Recommendation 6 (International Treaty). Major exporters of medical products, including the United States, should negotiate a plurilateral treaty under the World Trade Organization that prohibits export bans and restrictions on key components of global medical product supply chains. Any country that violates the terms of this agreement should be subject to sanctions by other signatories of the agreement. Specifically,
    a. **The treaty should provide incentives for countries to uphold commitments and cooperate in the event of a public health crisis.**
    b. **The treaty should provide disincentives or sanctions, such as reputational, economic, and legal sanctions, for violating the terms of the agreement.**

c. Treaty negotiators could consider adding provisions to this treaty that facilitate information sharing, particularly during medical emergencies.

While plurilateral cooperation will help ensure rational distribution of critical medical products among nations during emergencies, distribution of these supplies to end users, such as hospitals, clinicians, pharmacies, and patients, is also vital to protection of public health and safety. Consequently, these end users have important potential roles to play in addressing supply chain disruptions. Second, end users play critical roles in developing and using contingency plans when shortages arise that reduce the effect of shortages on patient and community health. Recommendation 7 (Last-Mile Management) advocates forming a working group of key stakeholders who represent the very end of medical product supply chains, to evaluate and improve the allocation and delivery of medical products during shortages. To protect public health it is vital to be ready to manage this final stage well in an emergency. One way this working group could improve the ability to manage the last mile of medical product supply chains in the next emergency is to collect, standardize, and disseminate best practices from past emergency events. Finally, this working group could lend its combined experience to the development of training and response readiness building programs for medical product shortages within health systems.

Recommendation 7 (Last-Mile Management). The Office of the Assistant Secretary for Preparedness and Response, in collaboration with the Centers for Disease Control and Prevention, should convene a working group of key stakeholders to examine and identify effective last-mile strategies to ensure end users are able to respond in the event of medical product shortages. The working group should
   a. Determine what information needs to be shared, with whom and in what form, in order for end users to be able to execute resource sharing, supply redistribution, substitution, adaptation, and other strategies for responding to medical product shortages at the local level.
   b. Develop a standard national ethical framework for allocating scarce medical products, building in previous crisis standards of care work, including attention to equity, efficiency, and additional ethical values.
   c. Develop and incorporate response plans and training for medical product shortages into public health and health care professional capabilities.

CONCLUDING REMARKS

Taken together, the committee's seven recommendations will increase the resilience of medical product supply chains by using all four protective shields of the resilience framework (see Box S-1). With proper coordination between them, these will substantially increase the nation's ability to maintain the supply of medical products and prevent harm during normal and emergency conditions.

BOX S-1
Summary of Recommendations

The following points collectively summarize the necessary actions recommended by the committee that are needed to increase the resilience of medical product supply chains:

Awareness
1. Public Transparency—Make sourcing, quality, volume, and capacity information publicly available for all medical products approved or cleared for sale in the United States.
2. Public Database—Establish a public database for the supply chain information acquired for medical products.

Mitigation
3. Resilience Contracting by Health Systems—Deliberately incorporate quality and reliability, in addition to price, in contracting, purchasing, and inventory decisions.

Preparedness
4. Stockpiling—Modernize and optimize inventory stockpiling management to respond to medical product shortages at the national and regional levels.
5. Capacity Buffering—Cultivate capacity buffering for supply chain critical medical products where such capacity is a cost-effective complement to stockpiling.

Response
6. International Treaty—Negotiate an international treaty with other major medical product exporters that rules out export bans on key components of global medical product supply chains.
7. Last-Mile Management—Establish a working group to examine last-mile and end user issues regarding medical product supply chains.

PART I: OVERVIEW OF GLOBAL MEDICAL PRODUCT SUPPLY CHAINS

1

Introduction

Medical product supply chains are essential for the national security and the health security of the United States, and ultimately, the continuity of society. The coronavirus disease 2019 (COVID-19) pandemic has exposed the fragility of U.S. medical product supply chains. Shortages of personal protective equipment for health care workers, medical devices, supplies, and drugs used to treat conditions associated with COVID-19 have put the lives of Americans at risk and have compromised the U.S. health care system. However, the vulnerabilities in U.S. medical product supply chains predate the current public health crisis. Over the past several decades, supply chain disruptions and drug shortages have repeatedly plagued the U.S. health care system, costing medical facilities millions of dollars per year (Vizient, 2019), threatening the clinical research enterprise (McBride et al., 2013), and most importantly, impacting the health and lives of patients (Phuong et al., 2019). These disruptions are the result of a lack of resilience and security of U.S. medical product supply chains and their inability to deliver essential medical products to patients who need them, both in so-called normal times and during disasters or public health emergencies (Accenture, 2021; Phuong et al., 2019).

Medical product supply chains share many characteristics with other modern supply chains. They involve multiple stages and steps, with different entities in different locations frequently being responsible for different portions of those stages rather than being performed within a single vertically integrated organization. These entities are subject to variation in supply and demand, and they are powerfully influenced by profit motives. At the same time, medical product supply chains are also integral to the health care system. Unlike supply chains for consumer goods, where profit motives and competition provide effective incentives to meet customer needs, medical product supply chains serve profit *and* public health objectives, which may be in conflict (Shah et al., 2021). Consequently, maintaining resilient medical product supply chains is not only about delivering products and generating profits, it is also about saving lives and protecting public safety. Failure in medical product supply chains can result in serious harm to patients or even death. As a result, *medical products*—which for the purpose of this report is an all-encompassing term that includes drugs, biologics, medical devices, and medical equipment—and manufacturing processes are subject to more government oversight and regulation than supply chains for many other consumer goods.

The U.S. Food and Drug Administration (FDA) plays critical roles in the regulation of development, manufacture, sale, and distribution of drugs, biologics, and medical devices. The manufacture of medical products is an increasingly complex process. For example, the share of newly approved devices that contain software increased from approximately 10 percent in 2002 to nearly 18 percent in 2016, and devices containing such software increasingly include cybersecurity content (Stern et al., 2019). Given these complexities, regulatory oversight plays a particularly important role in the medical product supply chain to ensure patient safety.

Medical product supply chains deliver a diverse array of products, including the four main categories described in this report[1]:

1. Originator drugs that are drug or biological products approved by FDA through an Abbreviated New Drug Application (ANDA) or a biologics license application (BLA) (FDA, 2017a, 2021a, 2022; WHO, 2008);
2. Generic drugs that are products approved by FDA through an ANDA or biosimilar products that are approved by FDA through a BLA (FDA, 2018a);
3. Simple medical devices (Class I) that pose the lowest risk to the patient and/or user according to FDA categories (FDA, 2017b); and

---

[1] This report does not focus in detail on supply chains for biologics or vaccines given the distinct features in their supply chains. However, as some biologics and vaccines are high-margin, patent-protected pharmaceuticals while others are not, the discussion of profit margins and incentives between originator and generic drugs is still applicable to these medical products. Furthermore, four new reports from the National Academy of Medicine focus on how to prepare for seasonal and pandemic influenza through lessons learned from COVID-19—with one report in particular focusing on globally resilient supply chains for pandemic and seasonal influenza vaccines. These reports can be accessed here: https://nam.edu/four-new-reports-from-the-national-academy-of-medicine-focus-on-how-to-prepare-for-seasonal-and-pandemic-influenza-through-lessons-learned-from-covid-19/.

INTRODUCTION 27

   4. Complex medical devices (Class II and III) that pose a progressively higher risk to the patient or user (FDA, 2017b).

These products vary widely with regard to the complexity of their supply chains as well as their vulnerability to disruption. Chapter 2 summarizes in more detail the ways in which medical product supply chains are structured.

Some of these vulnerabilities are the result of competition and modern cost control trends in supply chain management, including globalization. While the United States remains a world leader in drug discovery and development, the manufacturing of many medical products used in the United States has shifted overseas in recent decades.[2] For example, as of August 2019, only 28 percent of the manufacturing facilities producing active pharmaceutical ingredients (APIs)[3] to supply the U.S. market were domestic facilities,[4] which still does not provide insight into the domestic product volume. The COVID-19 pandemic exposed vulnerabilities in this global network. Facing worldwide shortages, producers of medical products, including the United States, European Union (EU), China, and India, limited exports to preserve access to medical products for their own citizens through export bans and other trade restrictions, which further crippled already overtaxed supply chains (CRS, 2021). As a result, countries that have underinvested in the resilience of their supply chains, like the United States and many other world countries, struggled to obtain the necessary medical products to combat COVID-19, a situation which placed all patients at risk, even those with unrelated conditions (Kaplan, 2020).

Insufficiently resilient medical product supply chains pose risks not only to public health but also to national security. Medical product supply chains are highly multinational and interdependent, with products commonly including inputs from multiple countries and manufacturing steps taking place in disparate locations. As a result, the United States depends upon other countries, including China, India, the EU, Mexico, and Canada, for medical products (CRS, 2020a, 2020b, 2020c). These other countries also often depend on the United States to play critical parts in complex and interdependent supply chains, but concerns have arisen that U.S. reliance on foreign governments for medical products, key components, manufacturing steps, or even transportation potentially could leave the United States vulnerable to the geopolitical and trade decisions of other nations (CRS, 2020b). Reducing reliance on international suppliers of critical drugs and

---

[2] Information given by testimony of Janet Woodcock (House Committee on Energy and Commerce, 2019).

[3] APIs are the drug substances formulated into tablets, capsules, and injections.

[4] Information given by testimony of Janet Woodcock (House Committee on Energy and Commerce, 2019).

devices by increasing domestic production (i.e., on-shoring), stockpiling, and diversifying the supply has been widely suggested as a way to increase supply chain resilience (Adler et al., 2020; Murphy, 2020).

While on-shoring may appear to be a simple fix to the supply chain disruptions experienced during COVID-19, the globalized and complex nature of medical product supply chains may limit the feasibility of an on-shoring strategy to improve their resilience. Relocating the final stage of production to the United States may provide limited protection against disruption if inputs are globally sourced (The White House, 2021). But on-shoring every step of a long, complex supply chain is likely to be difficult and expensive, especially when compared to other options for increasing supply chain resilience. Moreover, concentrating production inside the United States can make supplies more vulnerable to regional disasters, such as hurricanes (The White House, 2021). These issues cloud the picture of whether on-shoring for a given medical product might alleviate, have no effect on, or worsen supply chain disruptions.

Therefore, rather than looking for arguments for or against any specific remedy, the committee decided to approach the medical product supply chain vulnerability problem by starting with a clear goal and then considering a full range of alternatives in order to identify appropriate elements of an integrated strategy:

> The primary goal of resilient medical product supply chains is to prevent public health and safety from becoming compromised by disruptions to supplies of medical products.

Many trigger events, including production interruptions, natural disasters, disease outbreaks, and geopolitical events can produce supply shortages by either directly impacting medical product supplies or indirectly impacting supplies and components needed to manufacture medical products. Regardless, all trigger events lead to product shortages by decreasing supply, increasing demand, or impeding the ability to match supply with demand. This observation narrows the search for resilience options, as opposed to exploring every possible trigger event. Instead, successful resilience measures will be those that increase supply, decrease demand, or improve coordination of supply with demand. With this, the committee's task becomes one of finding a set of measures that increase the resilience of a medical product supply chain by making it capable of avoiding harm to the public under a wider range of disruptive events. Finally, because measures to improve resilience generally come with costs, the aim must be to select the most cost-effective measures that achieve a socially desirable level of protection.

CONTEXT FOR THIS STUDY

Section 3101 of the CARES Act, signed into law on March 27, 2020, directed the Secretary of the U.S. Department of Health and Human Services (HHS) to enter into an agreement with the National Academies of Sciences, Engineering, and Medicine (the National Academies) to establish an ad hoc committee to examine the security and resilience of U.S. medical product supply chains.[5] A number of other reports that examine medical product shortages and medical product supply chains were released prior to the COVID-19 pandemic and afterward in response to it. This study builds on and complements the recommendations from other contemporary reports (see Appendix B).

Trends in Medical Product Shortages

Data from the University of Utah Drug Information Service and the American Society of Health-System Pharmacists show that the number of new drug shortages reported in a year had been increasing until 2011, when the number peaked, and then it began to gradually decline (Fox and McLaughlin, 2018). Another study on drugs used for adult critical care found the same trend, with a moderate decline in new drug shortages through the middle of 2016 (Mazer-Amirshahi et al., 2017). Although the number of new drug shortages has been decreasing in recent years, the number of ongoing shortages remains high—mostly because of the long time it takes for drug shortages to be resolved. Mazer-Amirshahi and colleagues reported that the median duration of resolved drug shortages was 7.2 months, while those that were still ongoing at the end of their study had a median duration of 13.6 months.

Certain categories of drugs notably experience shortages more frequently than others. As discussed in Chapter 2, supplies of generic drugs are prone to shortages, particularly those drugs that are older or low priced (Dave et al., 2018; Ventola, 2011). Several factors may contribute to the higher frequency of shortages among older or low-price generics, including lack of incentives to maintain adequate supply of low-margin drugs, low reimbursement rates, and market consolidation. Clinical classes of drugs that are frequently in shortage include anesthesia medications, antibiotics, pain medications, nutrition and electrolyte products, and chemotherapy agents (Fox et al., 2014). Sterile injectable drugs are commonly in shortage, which may be explained by the manufacturing complexities and the high cost hurdle of entering the generic market (NASEM, 2018). FDA data show

---

[5] CARES Act, Public Law 116-136, § 301 (2020).

that anywhere between 20 and 80 percent of drug shortages are represented by sterile injectables (Fox et al., 2014; NASEM, 2018), though this wide range demonstrates the uncertainty of the data on drug shortages.

Data on the occurrence of medical device shortages are even more scarce than on drug shortages. Device manufacturers were not required to notify FDA of anticipated discontinuance or interruption in the production of medical devices until 2020 with the passage of the CARES Act.[6] Before the CARES Act, FDA mainly relied on manufacturers' voluntary notifications of devices shortages (FDA, 2011).

As has been put into high relief by the COVID-19 pandemic, emergencies such as natural disasters, geopolitical interventions, or pandemics can exacerbate existing medical product supply shortages and bring about new ones (Schondelmeyer et al., 2020). Over the course of the COVID-19 pandemic, the United States and the world witnessed both demand surges and supply constraints for medical products. Health care systems increased orders and began hoarding products in response to the pandemic, while the pandemic simultaneously prompted manufacturing facilities to close and slowed or halted trade. Drugs used to treat COVID-19 patients, mechanical ventilators, and personal protective equipment (PPE) are all examples of medical products that have experienced shortages during the COVID-19 pandemic (Branson et al., 2021; Kaplan, 2020). As of late 2021, 24 of the 40 (60 percent) critical drugs for the treatment of COVID-19 patients were under short supply (CIDRAP, 2022). While the extremely rapid development, production, and distribution of vaccines against COVID-19 has demonstrated the impressive capabilities of some global medical product supply chains, the pandemic has also laid bare the fragility of others, including supply chains that Americans depend on for their health and safety during emergencies and routine times.

Charge to the Committee

Congress charged this committee with the task of assessing and evaluating the effect of U.S. dependence on critical drugs and devices sourced or manufactured outside of the United States and to provide recommendations to address the vulnerabilities of medical product supply chains and increase their resilience (see Box 1-1).

To carry out this study, the National Academies convened the Committee on Security of America's Medical Product Supply Chain whose members have expertise in crisis standards of care, emergency and critical care medicine, drug and device development and manufacturing, drug short-

---

[6] 21 U.S.C. 356j. Discontinuance or interruption in the production of medical devices.

INTRODUCTION   31

BOX 1-1
Statement of Task

An ad hoc committee of the National Academies of Sciences, Engineering, and Medicine will conduct a study to examine the security of the United States medical product supply chain.

The committee will

1. Assess and evaluate the dependence of the United States, including the private commercial sector, states, and the federal government, on critical drugs and devices that are sourced or manufactured outside of the United States, which may include an analysis of
   - the supply chain of critical drugs and devices of greatest priority to providing health care;
   - any potential public health security or national security risks associated with reliance on critical drugs and devices sourced or manufactured outside of the United States, which may include responses to previous or existing shortages or public health emergencies, such as infectious disease outbreaks, bioterror attacks, and other public health threats;
   - any existing supply chain information gaps, as applicable; and
   - any potential economic impact and other considerations associated with increased domestic manufacturing.
2. Provide recommendations to improve the resilience of the supply chain for critical drugs and devices and to address any supply vulnerabilities or potential disruptions of such products that would significantly affect or pose a threat to public health security or national security, as appropriate, which may include strategies to
   - promote supply chain redundancy and contingency planning;
   - encourage domestic manufacturing, including consideration of economic impacts, if any;
   - improve supply chain information gaps;
   - improve planning considerations for medical product supply chain capacity during public health emergencies; and
   - promote the accessibility of such drugs and devices.

---

ages, regulatory policy, health economics, medical logistics, supply chain management, risk and emergency management, operations research, public health preparedness and response, and state and local public health (see Appendix E for biographical sketches of committee members). The project was supported by the Office of the Assistant Secretary for Preparedness and Response (ASPR) within HHS. This report presents the committee's conclusions and the evidence that supports them, as well as recommendations to a diverse set of stakeholders.

The Committee's Interpretation of the Charge

To identify effective and efficient ways to increase medical product supply chain security and resilience, the committee adopted a system-wide perspective that captures the fundamental dynamics of supply chain behavior. Sensible allocation of the finite resources available to improve supply chain resilience requires attention to costs. This in turn requires a framework to help systematically enumerate measures, to identify synergies between different policies, and to evaluate the relative cost-efficiency of alternatives to improve the resilience of medical product supply chains. An effective supply chain resilience strategy must be diversified and comprehensive to address the array of supply chain risks that threaten the public health and national security of the United States. This observation is the underlying motivation for the rest of this report that describes medical product supply chains, examines their vulnerabilities, and develops a systematic framework for building resilience in order to identify and motivate strategic, cost-effective recommendations.

STUDY APPROACH

In developing this report and the recommendations presented herein, the committee deliberated for over a year, holding five milestone committee meetings and monthly committee calls virtually. The committee held six meetings that included portions open to the public as well as one virtual, public workshop. These sessions provided the committee an opportunity to hear from the study sponsor (ASPR) and other medical product supply chain field experts and stakeholders on what they consider to be the most pressing issues within medical product supply chains, steps they are currently taking to alleviate these issues, and recommendations for building more resilient medical product supply chains. Public meeting agendas can be found in Appendix A. When researching and developing the report, the committee considered input from relevant government agencies.

The committee began by scoping the literature in the medical product supply chain field (see detailed study methods in Appendix A). The National Academies' Research Center staff and study staff conducted literature reviews to find relevant peer-reviewed and gray literature that fell under the statement of task. Additionally, committee members submitted peer-reviewed journal articles to study staff and the committee for consideration. A review of key terms in this study and their definitions is presented in Box 1-2.

The committee also commissioned an economic modeling analysis of policies and practices to improve the resilience of medical product supply chains as well as a series of case studies on critical drugs and devices to illustrate key issues related to improving the resilience of medical product supply chains. These case studies addressed COVID-19 vaccine, heparin, N95 masks (PPE), and saline. Throughout this report, the committee uses boxes to highlight insights from these case studies that illustrate gaps in resilience for specific supply chains. The economic modeling analysis is included in Appendix D.

Although the COVID-19 pandemic triggered this report, it does not solely focus on pandemic-specific medical product supply chain issues. This report discusses broader, systemic supply chain problems that existed prior to the COVID-19 pandemic, problems that led to drug and device shortages in noncrisis times and exacerbated them during the pandemic. To identify options for increasing resilience, the committee examined the full length of medical product supply chains—from raw materials to finished products, including all intermediate steps, plus transportation and the administration of the medical product to the end user and management of shortages by end users to mitigate their adverse effects.

Defining Key Terminology

The medical and supply chain fields on which this study is based do not always have consistent terms for the concepts discussed in this report. Therefore, to promote clarity, Box 1-2 presents the committee's definitions for core terms. In addition to these terms, the report defines other important terms throughout, alongside the relevant discussion.

Defining Supply Chain Critical Medical Products

Multiple groups, including FDA, the Center for Infectious Disease Research and Policy at the University of Minnesota, and the World Health Organization (WHO), have previously defined "critical acute drugs" and "essential medicines," and have created lists of such medical products (Schondelmeyer et al., 2020; WHO, 2019). In August 2020, Executive Order 13944 directed FDA to identify a list of "essential medicines, medical countermeasures, and critical inputs that are medically necessary to have available at all times, in an amount adequate to serve patient needs and in the appropriate dosage forms" (The White House, 2020). This Essential Medicines List established criteria for each of the categories in consultation with subject matter experts and multiple federal agencies and partners. While the list is currently being refined based on further consultations and public comments, the initial publishing in October 2020 focuses on products necessary to address immediately life-threatening medical conditions encountered in U.S. acute care facilities, rather than medicines to manage longer-term chronic conditions (FDA, 2020).

BOX 1-2
Key Terminology and Definitions

- **Active pharmaceutical ingredient (API):** "Any substance or mixture of substances intended to be used in the manufacture of a drug product and that, when used in the production of a drug, becomes an active ingredient in the drug product" (FDA, 2015a).
- **Anticompetitive behavior:** "Unfair business practices that are likely to reduce competition and lead to higher prices, reduced quality or levels of service, or less innovation. Anticompetitive practices include activities like price fixing, group boycotts, and exclusionary exclusive dealing contracts or trade association rules" (FTC, n.d.).
- **Awareness:** A supply chain resilience strategy that promotes an understanding of vulnerabilities in the supply chain that allows for a prioritization of resilience efforts.
- **Bottleneck:** The resource in a supply chain with the highest utilization as a percentage of capacity. The bottleneck defines an upper limit on the capacity of a supply chain (Mizgier et al., 2013).
- **Capacity buffering:** A preparedness strategy that requires that manufacturing facilities maintain the ability to expand production volume.
- **Capacity reduction:** A reduction in the quantity of product that can be produced or transported at a stage of a supply chain or through the supply chain as a whole.
- **Contingency planning:** A preparedness strategy in which procedures are developed to detail responses and responsible actors for specific, potential disruptive events, aiming to mitigate adverse effects of supply disruptions for specified resources.
- **Coordination failure:** A failure of the supply chain to meet demand despite sufficient supply.
- **Crisis standards of care:** "A substantial change in usual healthcare operations and the level of care it is possible to deliver, which is made necessary by a pervasive (e.g., pandemic influenza) or catastrophic (e.g., earthquake, hurricane) disaster" (Institute of Medicine, 2009).
- **Current good manufacturing practice:** "Provide for systems that assure proper design, monitoring, and control of manufacturing processes and facilities." These are based in law, regulation, and policy and are enforced by FDA (FDA, 2021b).
- **Demand reduction:** A response strategy to help alleviate shortages by reducing the need for a product via substitution, use of a therapeutic alternative, crisis standards of care, delaying treatments, or other means, which can also dampen hoarding by increasing trust in the system's ability to continue to supply products.
- **Demand surge:** A substantial increase in demand for a medical product or products triggered by an external event, such as a natural disaster or outbreak of disease.
- **Diversification:** A mitigation strategy that involves building reliability into the medical product supply chain by adding parallel capacity at some or all stages.

- **Drug:** "A substance recognized by an official pharmacopoeia or formulary; a substance intended for use in diagnosis, cure, mitigation, treatment, or prevention of disease; a substance (other than food) intended to affect the structure or any function of the body; a substance intended for use as a component of a medicine but not a device or a component, part, or accessory of a device; biological products are included within this definition" (FDA, 2017a).
- **Finished dosage form:** "A drug product in the form in which it will be administered to a patient, such as a tablet, capsule, or topical application; a drug product in a form in which reconstitution is necessary prior to administration to a patient, such as oral suspension or lyophilized powders; or any combination of an active pharmaceutical ingredient with another component of a drug product for purposes of production of such a drug product" (FDA, 2015b).
- **Hardening:** A mitigation strategy that involves building reliability into medical product supply chains through improved execution of existing stages.
- **Inventory stockpiling:** A preparedness strategy involving the acquisition and maintenance of surplus inventory.
- **Market concentration:** "The extent to which market shares are concentrated between a small number of firms. It is often taken as a proxy for the intensity of competition" (Organisation for Economic Co-operation and Development, n.d.).
- **Medical countermeasure (MCM):** "Medical countermeasures, or MCMs, are FDA-regulated products (biologics, drugs, devices) that may be used in the event of a potential public health emergency stemming from a terrorist attack with a biological, chemical, or radiological/ nuclear material, or a naturally occurring emerging disease. MCMs can be used to diagnose, prevent, protect from, or treat conditions associated with chemical, biological, radiological, or nuclear (CBRN) threats, or emerging infectious diseases" (FDA, 2021c).
- **Medical device:** "An instrument, apparatus, implement, machine, contrivance, implant, in vitro reagent, or other similar or related article, including part or accessory which is: recognized in the official National Formulary, or the United State Pharmacopoeia, or any supplement to them; intended for use in the diagnosis of disease or other conditions, or in the cure, mitigation, treatment, or prevention of disease, in man or other animals, or; intended to affect the structure or any function of the body of man or other animals, and which does not achieve its primary intended purpose through chemical action within or on the body of man or other animals and which is not dependent upon being metabolized for the achievement of any of its primary intended purposes" (FDA, 2018b).
- **Medical product shortage:** "a period of time when the demand or projected demand for the drug [or medical device] within the United States exceeds the supply of the drug" (FDA et al., 2014). A medical product shortage can also be characterized as "a supply issue that affects how the pharmacy prepares or dispenses a drug product or influences patient care when prescribers must use an alternative agent" (Fox and McLaughlin, 2018).
- **Mitigation:** A supply chain resilience strategy that involves actions taken prior to a disruptive event to prevent the event from occurring or reduce the likelihood of its occurrence.

continued

BOX 1 CONTINUED

- **On-shoring:** The act of either sourcing materials or producing materials and goods within a nation's borders. Sometimes called "reshoring" (Gray et al., 2013).
- **Preparedness:** A supply chain resilience strategy that involves actions taken prior to a disruptive event to reduce the negative effects on health and safety should the disruptive event occur.
- **Prophylaxis measures:** Improvised or inventive measures taken by health care professionals to protect human health while the shortage persists. These tend to be front-line, last-mile measures rather than upstream actions as they resolve the immediate issue but do not solve the supply shortage.
- **Raw materials:** The basic materials used for the production of intermediates, key starting materials, APIs, or device components (Altria, 1998).
- **Readiness:** A preparedness strategy that entails the establishment of capabilities to respond to various scenarios without specific plans in advance.
- **Resilience:** The ability to prepare and plan for, absorb, recover from, or more successfully adapt to actual or potential adverse events. In the context of this study, resilience is specifically the ability of medical product supply chains to match supply with demand under both normal and emergency conditions.
- **Response:** A supply chain resilience strategy that includes actions taken after the occurrence of a disruptive event in order to reduce the negative effects on health and safety.
- **Supply chain critical medical product:** A medical product that is both medically essential and vulnerable to supply chain disruptions.
- **Supply disruption:** "Unplanned and unanticipated events that disrupt the normal flow of goods and materials within a supply chain" (Craighead et al., 2007).
- **Supply increase:** A response strategy in which additional product supply is produced to meet demand.
- **Transparency:** Visibility and disclosure are the two components of transparency. Visibility refers to "accurately identifying and collecting data from all links in [the] supply chain" and disclosure involves "communicating that information, both internally and externally, at the level of detail required or desired" (Harbert, 2020).

All of the above definitions and lists focus exclusively on the clinical importance of medical products.[7] However, a product that is medically essential, but already has a highly reliable supply chain, is a poor target for resilience investments. Therefore, the committee defines "supply chain critical" medical products as those that are both medically essential and vulnerable to shortages.

---

[7] While this report briefly mentions WHO's Model List of Essential Medicines, more on this list and how it fits into the security of America's medical supply chains can be found in the proceedings of a workshop the committee held in the spring of 2021 (see NASEM, 2021).

INTRODUCTION   *37*

How to Use This Report

Owing to their complexity and interconnectedness, there are a variety of stakeholders involved in medical product supply chains. These stakeholders include government agencies, raw material suppliers, manufacturers, distributors, group purchasing organizations (GPOs), health systems, providers, and patients (see Figure 1-1).

The committee designed this report to help policy makers, manufacturers, government agencies, and other stakeholders understand and use the available evidence to inform their decision making. These different stakeholders play different roles and therefore can use the framework and results of this report in different ways.

Government Agencies

The U.S. government plays multiple roles in medical product supply chains: as a direct participant, as a policy maker, and as the regulator that dictates the ground rules by which supply chains must operate. A number of federal agencies have diverse responsibilities to oversee and regulate medical product supply chains (see Table 1-1); however, gaps in oversight of medical product supply chains remain. The roles and responsibilities of the various federal agencies for various aspects of medical product supply chains have been unclear causing confusion at the state and local levels—especially during COVID-19. Moving forward and as agencies form new supply chain-related offices and undertake relevant initiatives, it will be important that these roles are clarified and codified in guidance. Some government agencies also function as consumers, purchasing medical products for federally run health programs (e.g., U.S. Veterans Administration and the Centers for Medicare & Medicaid Services) and for stockpiling, such as the Strategic National Stockpile. Government agencies at the federal, state, territory, tribal, and local levels can use the report to identify and address gaps in medical product supply chains and plan for future public health emergencies. Policy makers may find the report useful in informing decisions regarding legislation and regulations aimed at promoting the security and resilience of the medical product supply chain during routine functioning and any potential emergency events that may occur.

Supplier/Manufacturers/Distributors

A medical product supply chain typically begins at the point of the raw materials supplier. While raw materials suppliers represent a wide variety of industries (e.g., latex, reagents, starting compounds, steel), these industries can be geographically concentrated making them vulnerable to disruptions from natural disasters (NASEM, 2018). Stakeholders can make use of the

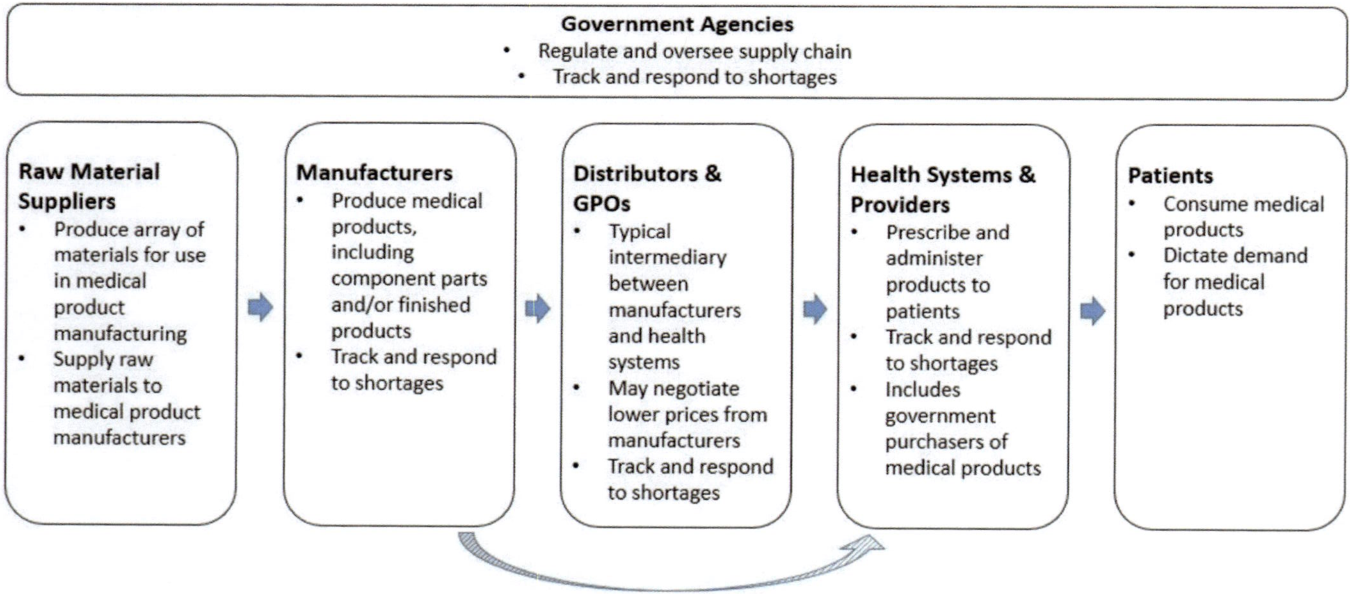

FIGURE 1-1 Stakeholders in a medical product supply chain.
NOTE: GPO = group purchasing organization.
SOURCE: Adapted from ASPR_TRACIE, 2019.

INTRODUCTION 39

framework of this report to identify ways to reduce risks of disruption as internal business continuity measures and as contributions to public health and safety initiatives.

Manufacturers of medical products are a diverse group of stakeholders, representing small and large firms, from manufacturers of APIs, excipients, and device components to finished dosage forms and medical devices. While some manufacturers actually make the individual components of the drug product that are used to make the finished drug product, other firms also referred to as "manufacturers" may work through one or more "contract manufacturing organizations" to coordinate and link together the various steps that lead to production of a drug as a finished dosage form. These stakeholders can make use of the framework of this report to assess vulnerabilities in their own supply chains and to increase their supply chain resilience for both business and compliance purposes.

Medical products may pass through a wholesale distributor, entities that purchase the product directly from the manufacturer before reselling it to a health system or a secondary distributor (Rockefeller et al., 2012). Similar to wholesale distributors, GPOs serve as an intermediary between health systems and the product manufacturers, though GPOs may also purchase from wholesale distributors (GAO, 2014). Health systems may choose to become a member of a GPO, which negotiates contracts for medical products on behalf of its members with the intent of sourcing from multiple suppliers in order to provide a more reliable supply to members at a lower cost. These stakeholders can use the report to identify areas within their supply chains that need to be secured, and improve the resilience of the supply chains they depend on to continue conducting business.

Health Systems, Public Health Agencies, and Providers

Ultimately, a medical product supply chain is designed to deliver products to consumers, which are composed of public health agencies, health systems, pharmacies, and nursing homes—in which physicians, nurses, pharmacists, and other care providers administer and deliver services to the patients that rely on them. Hospitals and medical facilities can use the report to develop and strengthen their business continuity plans and inform institutional guidelines and best practices.

Clinicians and Care Providers

Clinicians and care providers rely on medical product supply chains to be able to appropriately treat their patients. They may also play a role in the early detection and reporting of local shortages as well as in implementing contingency plans to mitigate the adverse effects of shortages. Practi-

TABLE 1-1 Select Federal Agencies with Responsibilities in Medical Product Supply Chains

Federal entity	Role	Medical Product Supply Chain Responsibilities
FDA	Awareness, Mitigation, Preparedness, Response	FDA has a number of authorities related to medical product supply chains, mainly in the pursuit of preventing shortages. During public health emergencies (i.e., COVID-19), FDA has the authority to track product shortages and mitigate shortages by developing strategic plans and exercising regulatory flexibility. FDA also has broad authority to prevent counterfeit or adulterated products from entering supply chains (FDA, 2021b).
ASPR	Awareness, Mitigation, Preparedness, Response	ASPR is responsible for the medical and public health preparedness for, response to, and recovery from disasters and public health emergencies. ASPR hosts the Supply Chain Control Tower Program to provide end-to-end visibility of the supply chain, aiming to improve monitoring, readiness, and response (ASPR, 2021b). Also under the authority of ASPR is the Supply Chain Logistics Operation Cell (SC-LOC) (ASPR, 2021a). SC-LOC works to monitor, analyze, and mitigate supply chain vulnerabilities in coordination with government partners, manufacturers, and distributors. Through the Industrial Base Expansion Program Office, ASPR is establishing integrated capabilities for a resilient domestic medical product supply chain and investing in the sustainability of domestic manufacturing of medical products.
VA	Awareness, Preparedness, Response	The Department of Veterans Affairs (VA) is a large purchaser of medical products in the United States. Because the Veterans Health Administration is a large and disperse health system, the VA maintains its own supply chains (Department of Veterans Affairs, 2020b). The Office of Logistics and Supply Chain Management within the VA oversees the logistics and policy development of the supply chain (Department of Veterans Affairs, 2020a). The VA is also standing up Regional Readiness Centers, to be able to quickly deploy medical products in the case of an emergency (GAO, 2021).
CDC	Awareness, Preparedness, Response	The Centers for Disease Control and Prevention (CDC) is responsible for developing standards for state, local, tribal, and territorial public health preparedness and response. These standards include content on the acquisition, distribution, and monitoring of medical products inventories during public health emergencies (CDC, 2019).

TABLE 1-1 Continued

Federal entity	Role	Medical Product Supply Chain Responsibilities
DoD	Awareness, Preparedness, Response	The Department of Defense (DoD) is responsible for monitoring and identifying potential disruptions to the medical product supply chain to mitigate the effects that a disruption might have on supply chain operations and the care beneficiaries receive (DoD, 2021). DoD also evaluates dependence on foreign manufacturers in the medical products supply chain as a potential disruption to operations. DoD manages the Warstoppers Program to mitigate shortages by negotiating priority contracts for certain critical medical products.
Commerce	Awareness, Mitigation	The Department of Commerce promotes domestic manufacturing of medical products in order to strengthen the competitiveness of U.S. manufacturing firms (Department of Commerce, 2016). The Department of Commerce also monitors the nation's dependence on foreign manufacturing for medical products to reduce the national security risk that dependence may confer (Department of Commerce, 2011).
DHS	Awareness, Response	The Department of Homeland Security (DHS) conducts research on the effects of disasters on medical product supply chains, and subsequently the nation's economy, infrastructure, and public health (Bryan, 2020). DHS also has a secondary role as a purchaser of medical products, often for emergency medical treatment (DHS, 2020).
BARDA	Mitigation, Response	Housed within ASPR, the Biomedical Advanced Research and Development Authority (BARDA) promotes the development of medical countermeasures to public health threats. BARDA's role in medical product supply chains has focused on making strategic investments to expand the infrastructure and capacity of domestic pharmaceutical manufacturing (BARDA, 2021).
SNS	Preparedness, Response	Within ASPR, the Strategic National Stockpile (SNS) procures and maintains a stockpile of medical products necessary to respond to certain public health threats (ASPR, 2021c). The SNS is also responsible for the distribution of supplies to communities in need of the additional resources that the SNS maintains.
FEMA	Response	The Federal Emergency Management Agency's (FEMA's) medical product supply chain responsibilities center on emergency and disaster response. FEMA helps to preserve and reroute supply chains during emergencies, assists with the distribution of supplies to affected communities, and works to expand manufacturing capabilities (FEMA, 2020). FEMA maintains a Logistics Supply Chain Management System designed to facilitate distribution of supplies during emergencies (DHS Office of Inspector General, 2014).

tioners may use the report to more fully understand the effects of medical product shortages and appreciate their role in contributing to supply chain resilience.

Patients

The final consumers in a medical product supply chain are patients. Patients require medical products for their health, and therefore drive demand for medical products. The general public can use this report to understand and recognize that medical product supply chains may have shortages, which can affect clinical outcomes for individual patients and broader communities. They can also use this report to inform their personal opinions on actions for security and resilience.

Organization of the Report

This report is organized into two parts and nine chapters. Part I provides an overview of global medical product supply chains and consists of Chapters 2 through 4. Chapter 2 provides an overview of medical products and the supply chains that deliver them. Chapter 3 examines medical product supply chain globalization and describes the implications for public health, supply chain resilience, and policy options. Chapter 4 enumerates the root causes of medical product shortages and discusses the effects of shortages.

Part II discusses measures for improving the resilience of medical product supply chains and consists of Chapters 5 through 9. Chapter 5 presents the committee's medical product supply chain resilience framework, which categorizes resilience policies into awareness, mitigation, preparedness, and response strategies. Chapter 6 addresses awareness measures for promoting supply chain resilience and discusses the importance of transparency in the medical product supply chains. It concludes with recommendations for improving transparency as a basis for many other medical product supply chain resilience measures. Chapter 7 addresses mitigation measures and focuses specifically on issues that plague medical product supply chains during nonemergency conditions, including quality concerns, infrastructure, and purchasing practices. This chapter concludes with a recommendation for how health systems, as consumers, can play an important role in improving the resilience of medical product supply chains. Chapter 8 addresses the full range of preparedness measures and concludes with two complementary recommendations for improving the ability of inventory stockpiling and capacity buffering measures (in conjunction with contingency planning and readiness) to protect people from harm caused by shortages of medical products. Finally, Chapter 9 addresses response measures for improving organizational capabilities to deal with major public health emergencies. It concludes with two recommendations focused on international cooperation and management of the "last mile" (i.e., delivery to patients) of medical product supply chains.

REFERENCES

Accenture. 2021. *Supply chain disruption.* https://www.accenture.com/us-en/insights/consulting/coronavirus-supply-chain-disruption (accessed December 16, 2021).

Adler, D., D. Breznitz, and S. Helper. 2020. *Policy options for building resilient U.S. medical supply networks.* https://equitablegrowth.org/policy-options-for-building-resilient-u-s-medical-supply-networks/ (accessed October 11, 2021).

Altria, K. D. 1998. Pharmaceutical raw materials and excipients analysis. In *Analysis of Pharmaceuticals by Capillary Electrophoresis*, Chromatographia CE Series, Vol. 2. Wiesbaden: Vieweg+Teubner Verlag. Pp. 133-152. https://doi.org/10.1007/978-3-322-85011-97.

ASPR (Assistant Secretary for Preparedness and Response). 2021a. *Division of logistics.* https://www.phe.gov/about/offices/program/office-of-operations-and-resources/Pages/Division-of-Logistics.aspx (accessed October 12, 2021).

ASPR. 2021b. *Information management division.* https://www.phe.gov/about/offices/program/icc/siim/Pages/Information-Management.aspx (accessed October 12, 2021).

ASPR. 2021c. *Strategic national stockpile.* https://www.phe.gov/about/sns/Pages/default.aspx (accessed October 12, 2021).

ASPR_TRACIE (Technical Resources, Assistance Center, and Information Exchange). 2019. *Partnering with the healthcare supply chain during disasters.* https://files.asprtracie.hhs.gov/documents/aspr-tracie-partnering-with-the-healthcare-supply-chain-during-disasters.pdf (accessed August 19, 2021).

BARDA (Biomedical Advanced Research and Development Authority). 2021. *Pharmaceutical manufacturing in America.* https://www.medicalcountermeasures.gov/barda/influenza-and-emerging-infectious-diseases/coronavirus/pharmaceutical-manufacturing-in-america/ (accessed October 12, 2021).

Branson, R., J. R. Dichter, H. Feldman, A. Devereaux, D. Dries, J. Benditt, T. Hossain, M. Ghazipura, M. King, M. Baldisseri, M. D. Christian, G. Dominigiuez-Cherit, K. Henry, A. M. O. Martland, M. Huffines, D. Ornoff, J. Persoff, D. Rodriquez, Jr., R. C. Maves, N. T. Kissoon, and L. Rubinson. 2021. The US Strategic National Stockpile ventilators in Coronavirus Disease 2019: A comparison of functionality and analysis regarding the emergency purchase of 200,000 devices. *Chest* 159(2):634-652.

Bryan, W. N. 2020. *Linking together the public and private sectors to strengthen global supply chains during COVID-19.* https://www.dhs.gov/science-and-technology/blog/2020/09/28/strengthen-global-supply-chains-during-covid-19 (accessed January 25, 2022).

CDC (Centers for Disease Control and Prevention). 2019. *Public health emergency preparedness and response capabilities: Capability 9: Medical materiel management and distribution.* https://www.cdc.gov/cpr/readiness/00_docs/CDC_PubHlthPrepCap_Oct2018_508_Cap9.pdf (accessed October 12, 2021).

CIDRAP (Center for Infectious Disease Research and Prevention). 2022. *Critical drug shortage dashboard.* https://www.cidrap.umn.edu/rds/critical-drug-shortages (accessed January 25, 2022).

Craighead, C. W., J. Blackhurst, M. J. Rungtusanatham, and R. B. Handfield. 2007. The severity of supply chain disruptions: Design characteristics and mitigation capabilities. *Decision Sciences* 38(1):131-156.

CRS (Congressional Research Service). 2020a. Appendix. U.S. imports of select medical products. In *COVID-19: China Medical Supply Chains and Broader Trade Issues*, edited by K. M. Sutter, A. B. Schwarzenberg, and M. D. Sutherland. CRS. https://crsreports.congress.gov/product/pdf/R/R46304?mod=article_inline (accessed December 16, 2021).

CRS. 2020b. *COVID-19: China medical supply chains and broader trade issues*. https://crsreports.congress.gov/product/pdf/R/R46304 (accessed December 16, 2021).

CRS. 2020c. *Medical supply chains and policy options: The data challenge*. https://www.everycrsreport.com/files/2020-09-16_IF11648_fadf375c447b7698544a1dac3dc999b5e8358617.pdf (accessed August 26, 2021).

CRS. 2021. *Export restrictions in response to the COVID-19 pandemic*, edited by C. A. Casey and C. D. Cimino-Isaacs. CRS. https://crsreports.congress.gov/product/pdf/IF/IF11551 (accessed September 29, 2021).

Dave, C. V., A. Pawar, E. R. Fox, G. Brill, and A. S. Kesselheim. 2018. Predictors of drug shortages and association with generic drug prices: A retrospective cohort study. *Value in Health* 21(11):1286-1290.

Department of Commerce. 2011. *Reliance on foreign sourcing in the healthcare and public health (HPH) sector: Pharmaceuticals, medical devices, and surgical equipment*. https://www.bis.doc.gov/index.php/documents/other-areas/642-department-of-homeland-security-dhs-assessment-impact-of-foreign-sourcing-on-health-related-infra/file (accessed December 20, 2021).

Department of Commerce. 2016. *2016 top markets report: Medical devices*. https://legacy.trade.gov/topmarkets/pdf/Medical_Devices_Top_Markets_Report.pdf (accessed January 25, 2022).

Department of Veterans Affairs. 2020a. *Office of Logistics and Supply Chain Management*. https://www.va.gov/oal/about/logistics.asp (accessed January 25, 2022).

Department of Veterans Affairs. 2020b. *Supply chain management operations*. https://www.navao.org/wp-content/uploads/2016/11/VHA-Directive-1761-Supply-Chain-Inventory-Mgmt-10-24-16.pdf (accessed January 25, 2022).

DHS (Department of Homeland Security). 2020. *Medical supplies*. https://www.dhs.gov/sites/default/files/publications/medical-supplies_dhsgov_webpage_12-31-2020.pdf (accessed January 25, 2022).

DHS Office of Inspector General. 2014. *FEMA's logistics supply chain management system may not be effective during a catastrophic disaster*. https://www.hsdl.org/?abstract&did=758407 (accessed October 12, 2021).

DoD (Department of Defense). 2021. *Evaluation of the Department of Defense's mitigation of foreign suppliers in the pharmaceutical supply chain*. https://media.defense.gov/2021/Sep/22/2002859154/-1/-1/1/DODIG-2021-126_REDACTED.PDF (accessed January 25, 2022).

FDA (U.S. Food and Drug Administration). 2011. *A review of FDA's approach to medical product shortages*. Silver Spring, MD: FDA. https://nyschp.memberclicks.net/assets/docs/Events Education/NYSCHP_NYACCP_drug%20shortages_efox.pdf (accessed December 20, 2021).

FDA. 2015a. Drug quality assurances: Active pharmacuetical ingredient (API) process inspection. In *FDA compliance program guidance manual*. FDA. P. 31. https://www.fda.gov/media/75201/download (accessed December 20, 2021).

FDA. 2015b. *GDUFA glossary*. https://www.fda.gov/industry/generic-drug-user-fee-amendments/gdufa-glossary (accessed October 12, 2021).

FDA. 2017a. *Drugs@FDA glossary of terms*. https://www.fda.gov/drugs/drug-approvals-and-databases/drugsfda-glossary-terms (accessed October 12, 2021).

FDA. 2017b. *Overview of medical device classification and reclassification*. https://www.fda.gov/about-fda/cdrh-transparency/overview-medical-device-classification-and-reclassification (accessed October 11, 2021).

FDA. 2018a. *Generic drug facts.* https://www.fda.gov/drugs/generic-drugs/generic-drug-facts (accessed September 14, 2021).
FDA. 2018b. *Medical device overview.* https://www.fda.gov/industry/regulated-products/medical-device-overview#What (accessed May 26, 2021).
FDA. 2020. *FDA publishes list of essential medicines, medical countermeasures, critical inputs required by executive order.* https://www.fda.gov/news-events/press-announcements/fda-publishes-list-essential-medicines-medical-countermeasures-critical-inputs-required-executive (accessed December 16, 2021).
FDA. 2021a. *Biologics license applications (BLA) process (CBER).* https://www.fda.gov/vaccines-blood-biologics/development-approval-process-cber/biologics-license-applications-bla-process-cber (accessed February 3, 2022).
FDA. 2021b. *Facts about the current good manufacturing practices (CGMPs).* https://www.fda.gov/drugs/pharmaceutical-quality-resources/facts-about-current-good-manufacturing-practices-cgmps (accessed June 10, 2021).
FDA. 2021c. *What are medical countermeasures?* https://www.fda.gov/emergency-preparedness-and-response/about-mcmi/what-are-medical-countermeasures (accessed June 8, 2021).
FDA. 2022. *First generic drug approvals.* https://www.fda.gov/drugs/drug-and-biologic-approval-and-ind-activity-reports/first-generic-drug-approvals (accessed February 3, 2022).
FDA, ASHP (American Society of Health-System Pharmacists), and University of Utah Drug Information Service. 2014. *FDA and ASHP shortage parameters.* https://www.ashp.org/Drug-Shortages/Current-Shortages/FDA-and-ASHP-Shortage-Parameters (accessed April 8, 2021).
FEMA (Federal Emergency Management Agency). 2020. *FEMA COVID-19 supply chain task force: Supply chain stabilization.* https://www.fema.gov/news-release/20200725/nhom-cong-tac-chuoi-cung-ung-trong-dai-dich-covid-19-cua-fema-dinh-chuoi-cung (accessed October 12, 2021).
Fox, E. R., and M. M. McLaughlin. 2018. ASHP guidelines on managing drug product shortages. *American Journal of Health-System Pharmacy* 75(21):1742-1750.
Fox, E. R., B. V. Sweet, and V. Jensen. 2014. Drug shortages: A complex health care crisis. *Mayo Clinic Proceedings* 89(3):361-373.
FTC (Federal Trade Commission). n.d. *Anticompetitive practices.* https://www.ftc.gov/enforcement/anticompetitive-practices (accessed August 31, 2021).
GAO (Government Accountability Office). 2014. *Group purchasing organizations: Funding structure has potential implications for Medicare costs.* https://www.gao.gov/assets/gao-15-13.pdf (accessed October 12, 2021).
GAO. 2021. *VA acquisition management: Comprehensive supply chain management strategy key to address existing challenges.* https://www.gao.gov/assets/gao-21-445t.pdf (accessed January 25, 2022).
Gray, J. V., K. Skowronski, G. Esenduran, and M. J. Rungtusanatham. 2013. The reshoring phenomenon: What supply chain academics ought to know and should do. *Journal of Supply Chain Management* 49:27-33.
Harbert, T. 2020. *Supply chain transparency, explained.* MIT Sloan School of Management. https://mitsloan.mit.edu/ideas-made-to-matter/supply-chain-transparency-explained (accessed December 10, 2021).
House Committee on Energy and Commerce. 2019. *Securing the US drug supply chain: Oversight of FDA's foreign inspection program: Congressional testimony of Janet Woodcock.* December 10. https://www.fda.gov/news-events/congressional-testimony/securing-us-drug-supply-chain-oversight-fdas-foreign-inspection-program-12102019 (accessed December 10, 2021).

Institute of Medicine. 2009. *Guidance for establishing crisis standards of care for use in disaster situations: A letter report.* Edited by B. M. Altevogt, C. Stroud, S. L. Hanson, D. Hanfling, and L. O. Gostin. Washington, DC: The National Academies Press.

Kaplan, D. A. 2020. How health systems are responding as COVID-19 squeezes the medical supply chain. *Supply Chain Dive.* https://www.supplychaindive.com/news/covid-19-health-medical-supply-chain/574787/ (accessed December 16, 2021).

Mazer-Amirshahi, M., M. Goyal, S. A. Umar, E. R. Fox, M. Zocchi, K. L. Hawley, and J. M. Pines. 2017. U.S. drug shortages for medications used in adult critical care (2001-2016). *Journal of Critical Care* 41:283-288.

McBride, A., L. M. Holle, C. Westendorf, M. Sidebottom, N. Griffith, R. J. Muller, and J. M. Hoffman. 2013. National survey on the effect of oncology drug shortages on cancer care. *American Journal of Health-System Pharmacy* 70(7):609-617.

Mizgier, K. J., M. P. Jüttner, and S. M. Wagner. 2013. Bottleneck identification in supply chain networks. *International Journal of Production Research* 51(5):1477-1490.

Murphy, J. 2020. *Learning the right lessons: Safeguarding the U.S. supply of medicines and medical products.* https://www.uschamber.com/issue-brief/learning-the-right-lessons-safeguarding-the-us-supply-of-medicines-and-medical-products (accessed October 11, 2021).

NASEM (National Academies of Sciences, Engineering, and Medicine). 2018. *Impact of the global medical supply chain on SNS operations and communications: Proceedings of a workshop.* Edited by A. Mack. Washington, DC: The National Academies Press.

NASEM. 2021. *The security of America's medical product supply chain considerations for critical drugs and devices: Proceedings of a workshop.* Washington, DC: The National Academies Press.

Organisation for Economic Co-operation and Development. n.d. *Market concentration.* https://www.oecd.org/daf/competition/market-concentration.htm (accessed August 31, 2021).

Phuong, J. M., J. Penm, B. Chaar, L. D. Oldfield, and R. Moles. 2019. The impacts of medication shortages on patient outcomes: A scoping review. *PLoS ONE* 14(5):e0215837.

Rockefeller, J. D., T. Harkin, and E. E. Cummings. 2012. *Shining light on the "gray market": An examination of why hospitals are forced to pay exorbitant prices for prescription drugs facing critical shortages.* https://www.commerce.senate.gov/services/files/AFA98935-2FF5-4004-88DC-BE70D1C22B5D (accessed December 16, 2021).

Schondelmeyer, S. W., J. Seifert, D. J. Margraf, M. Mueller, I. Williamson, C. Dickson, D. Dasararaju, C. Caschetta, N. Senne, and M. T. Osterholm 2020. Part 6: Ensuring a resilient us prescription drug supply. In *COVID-19: The CIDRAP viewpoint*, edited by J. Wappes. Minneapolis, MN: Regents of the University of Minnesota.

Shah, S., J. J. Qian, A. Navathe, and N. R. Shah. 2021. Public benefit corporations: A third option for health care delivery? *Health Affairs Blog.* Health Affairs. https://www.healthaffairs.org/do/10.1377/hblog20210317.310736/full/ (accessed December 16, 2021).

Stern, A. D., W. J. Gordon, A. B. Landman, and D. B. Kramer. 2019. Cybersecurity features of digital medical devices: An analysis of FDA product summaries. *British Medical Journal Open* 9(6):e025374.

Ventola, C. L. 2011. The drug shortage crisis in the United States: Causes, impact, and management strategies. *Pharmacy and Therapeutics* 36(11):740-757.

Vizient. 2019. Drug shortages and labor costs mesuring the hidden costs of drug shortages on U.S. hospitals. In *Vizient drug shortages impact report.* Irving, Texas: Vizient Inc.

The White House. 2020. *Executive order on ensuring essential medicines, medical countermeasures, and critical inputs are made in the United States.* https://trumpwhitehouse.archives.gov/presidential-actions/executive-order-ensuring-essential-medicines-medical-countermeasures-critical-inputs-made-united-states/ (accessed December 16, 2021).

The White House. 2021. *Building resilient supply chains, revitalizing american manufacturing, and fostering broad-based growth: 100-day reviews under Executive Order 14017.* Washington, DC: Department of Commerce, Department of Energy, Department of Defense, Department of Health and Human Services. https://www.whitehouse.gov/wp-content/uploads/2021/06/100-day-supply-chain-review-report.pdf (accessed October 20, 2021).

WHO (World Health Organization). 2008. Glossary. In *Measuring medicine prices, availability, affordability and price components*, 2nd edition, 234 pp. World Health Organization and Health Action International. https://apps.who.int/iris/handle/10665/70013 (accessed December 20, 2021).

WHO. 2019. Executive summary. The selection and use of essential medicines 2019. *Report of the 22nd WHO expert committee on the selection and use of essential medicines, 1-5 April 2019.* Geneva, Switzerland: WHO. https://apps.who.int/iris/bitstream/handle/10665/325773/WHO-MVP-EMP-IAU-2019.05-eng.pdf?ua=1 (accessed December 10, 2021).

2

Understanding Medical Product Supply Chains

Medical product supply chains are complex, global systems that involve people, processes, technologies, and policies. This chapter describes the ways different categories of medical product supply chains are structured and concludes with a brief overview of the various economic and policy spaces in which they operate. Medical product supply chains are designed for efficiency and cost, and do not always consider transparency or resilience. This can have negative consequences for public health and national security as evidenced by the ongoing COVID-19 pandemic as well as persistent medical product shortages that take place every year in the United States. To identify policies for making medical product supply chains more resilient, understanding their characteristics is essential. This background chapter is critical to understanding how to ensure a resilient supply chain as different products, different markets, and different risk profiles require different interventions. The key challenge will be to match interventions to products in a cost-effective manner.

OVERVIEW OF THE MEDICAL PRODUCT SUPPLY CHAIN SYSTEM

This section focuses primarily on the supply chains for (1) drugs, particularly active pharmaceutical ingredients (APIs) and finished dosage form

(FDF) drug products, and (2) medical devices.[1] While the general structure of these products' supply chains is similar (i.e., spanning the path from raw materials to manufacturers to distributor to end user), the details of each are as varied as the products themselves, warranting separate discussions for each. However, the framework presented in Chapter 5 is still flexible enough to be adapted to the assessment and remediation of individual supply chains. What follows will provide a background for how different types of medical product supply chains operate, the economic incentives that promote and support these structures, and finally, the current challenges each presents to building more resilient supply chains.

General Structure of Medical Product Supply Chains

As discussed in Chapter 1, owing to the complexity and interconnectedness of medical product supply chains, there are a variety of stakeholders involved in supply chain operations, including government agencies, raw material suppliers, manufacturers, distributors, group purchasing organizations, health systems, providers, and patients. These stakeholders make the decisions that enable medical product supply chains to facilitate the flow of medical products from raw material or component suppliers (e.g., makers of ingredients, subassemblies) to producers (e.g., final assembly plants, fill-and-finish facilities), to distributors (e.g., wholesalers), to providers (e.g., health systems, pharmacies, retailers), and finally, to patients. To coordinate these steps, the supply chain must transmit demand information upstream to use as guidance for production and transport decisions for the products downstream. An efficient supply chain matches supply with demand in a responsive and cost-efficient manner. As currently structured, medical product supply chains are typically inelastic, meaning that there is demand for products regardless of price (Haninger et al., 2011), leading to a financially imbalanced supply-and-demand setup. See Figure 2-1 for a graphical representation of a typical medical product supply chain under normal well-functioning conditions.

---

[1] As mentioned in Chapter 1, this report does not focus in detail on supply chains for biologics or vaccines given the distinct features in their supply chains. However, as some biologics and vaccines are high-margin, patent-protected pharmaceuticals while others are not, the discussion of profit margins and incentives between originator and generic drugs is still applicable to these medical products. Furthermore, four new reports from the National Academy of Medicine focus on how to prepare for seasonal and pandemic influenza through lessons learned from COVID-19—with one report in particular focusing on globally resilient supply chains for pandemic and seasonal influenza vaccines. These reports can be accessed here: https://nam.edu/four-new-reports-from-the-national-academy-of-medicine-focus-on-how-to-prepare-for-seasonal-and-pandemic-influenza-through-lessons-learned-from-covid-19.

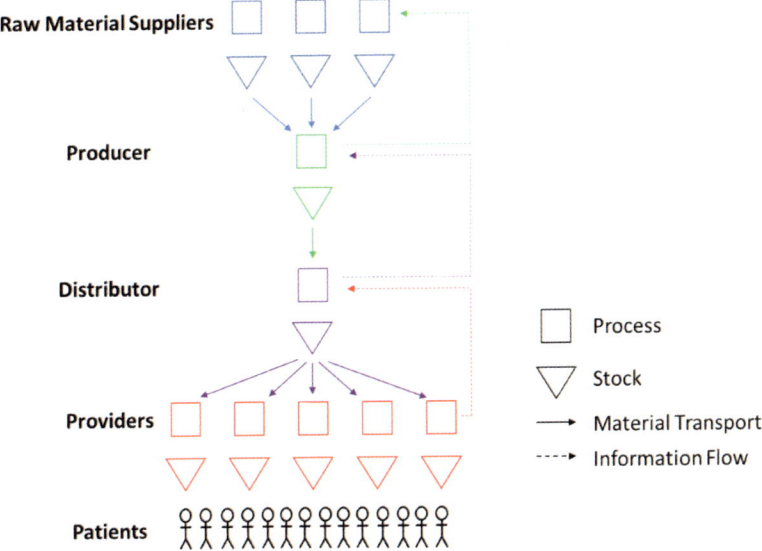

FIGURE 2-1 Simple schematic of a medical product supply chain under normal conditions.
SOURCE: Adapted from NASEM, 2020.

Pharmaceuticals (Originator and Generic)

Pharmaceutical manufacturing starts with the acquisition of raw materials, such as solvents, reagents, and other chemicals. These are combined by a series of reactions and then purified by a process designed to result in the desired APIs, or API intermediates (FDA, 2016). The APIs are then added to various excipients, shaped into a particular configuration, such as a tablet, capsule, or injectable, and apportioned into a particular dose to produce the drug product (FDA, 2012, 2016). Depending on the manufacturer, this process may occur in the same facility that manufactured the APIs or it may be outsourced to other drug manufacturing facilities. Regardless of where FDF production occurs, the timeframe for production, from raw materials to FDF, varies widely (from days to months) as many quality assurance and quality control tests are required before the drug products are deemed safe for distribution (FDA, 2016). To keep production efficiency high, produce less waste, and reduce inventory costs, raw materials are produced only as ordered and many drug manufacturers use just-in-time inventory management and receive the raw materials or APIs only as they need them (Dias et al., 2012; Stevens, 2020; The White House, 2021).

Pharmaceutical manufacturing can additionally be thought of as producing either originator or generic drugs. A generic drug is a medication developed to be the same as an already marketed brand-name drug in dosage form, safety, strength, route of administration, quality, performance characteristics, and intended use so the generic medicine works in the same way and provides the same clinical benefit as the brand-name medicine (FDA, 2021c). The manufacturing processes for originator and generic drugs are virtually identical, with the supply chains for each differing mainly by location, meaning the two kinds of drugs only differ *where* they are made or packaged, not *how* they are made. In the United States, off-patent, generic drugs are the most commonly used prescription pharmaceuticals and are the most frequently dispensed retail prescriptions (Berndt et al., 2017), accounting for 90 percent of all prescriptions filled and 20 percent of all prescription drug spending (AAM, 2021).

The last 3 decades have seen pharmaceutical manufacturing become a global enterprise (see Chapter 3 for further detail). In the United States, this shift toward relying on foreign manufacturing has been motivated mainly by the desire to control costs. This pressure to keep profits high deincentivizes generic drug manufacturers from using the highest-quality materials for production as these come at premium costs (Khan, 2020). Taken together, U.S. pharmaceutical companies were monetarily incentivized to either move their manufacturing offshore or rely on foreign manufacturers for their materials or both.

Medical Devices—Simple (Class I) and Complex (Class II/III)

Medical devices are defined by the U.S. Food and Drug Administration (FDA) as any object or component used in the diagnosis, treatment, prevention, or cure of medical conditions or diseases, or that affects body structure or function through means other than chemical or metabolic reaction in humans or animals (CDRH, 2018).[2] This broad definition includes a huge range of products, ranging from tongue depressors to computerized tomography scanners. Unlike pharmaceutical manufacturing, medical device manufacturing is highly varied depending on the product, and a one-process-flow description is not feasible. Furthermore, due to the large array of equipment classified as medical devices, FDA has no single standard to which a specific device must be manufactured. Instead, FDA created a standards guide that all manufacturers must follow, which includes requiring manufactures to develop comprehensive procedures within the FDA framework to produce devices that meet approved safety standards (CDRH, 2018). Approved medical devices are then categorized into one of three classes by these safety standards, according to the safety risks they pose.

---

[2] The statutory language from the Food, Drug, and Cosmetic Act (FD&C Act) 513(a) specifically distinguishes between the classes by defining medical devices as "as any instrument, apparatus, implement, machine, contrivance, implant, in vitro reagent, or other similar article (including a component of such article) intended for use in the diagnosis, cure, mitigation, treatment, or prevention or disease or other conditions, or intended to affect any structure or function of the body, that does not function primarily through chemical or metabolic reaction."

Class I medical devices present minimal potential for harm to the user and are often simpler in design than Classes II and III and are considered simple-design devices. Class II medical devices present moderate risk of harm to the patient or user. Most FDA-regulated medical devices are considered Class II (FDA, 2017). Class III medical devices are highly complex devices that also present a high safety risk to the patient or user. These devices usually sustain or support life, are implanted, or present potentially unreasonable risk of illness or injury. These represent 10 percent of medical devices regulated by FDA (FDA, 2017). As devices in Classes II and III are more complex in design than Class I devices, the medical devices that fall into Classes II and III are considered complex-design devices.

These product classifications are useful in protecting patient safety. But they are less helpful in assessing risks or building resilience in supply chains. One reason is that device complexity—simple (Class I) or complex (Class II or III)—does not always correlate with supply chain complexity. There is little similarity between where the devices are made/packaged and how they are made. Furthermore, the complexity of the supply chain for a medical device is not necessarily reflective of the complexity of the design of the device itself and few standards exist for interchangeable parts (e.g., ventilator tubing).[3] For instance, a simple, small adhesive bandage has a complex supply chain for production. Band-Aids, simple medical devices, have four components, each with its own raw materials sourcing and manufacturing processes (Lin et al., 2016). Production of the finished product requires the raw materials for each component (plastic strip, absorbent pad, adhesive, and release sheets), and therefore can be halted by the disruption of any of these supplies. Therefore, although supply chains are generally broader (more components) and deeper (more tiers) for complex products that contain more parts than for simple products with fewer parts, this is not always the case. Therefore, the simple/complex classifications will be used in the report as an approximation of supply chain complexity, recognizing that individual characteristics must be considered when assessing or remediating supply risks for specific products. All other things being equal, complex supply chains present greater risks of disruption.

DIFFERENCES IN SUPPLY CHAIN ECONOMICS BY PRODUCT CATEGORY

Supply chain complexity is not the only factor that affects the likelihood of a medical product supply disruption. Management decisions are also important. In low-margin products, which include many but not all generic drugs and simple devices, there is a heavy emphasis on cost control because of price pressures and profitability concerns. Consequently, many drug manufacturers rely on lean practices, such as just-in-time inventory

---

[3] 21 U.S.C. 807.81, when a premarket notification submission is required (amended December 28, 2007).

management, receiving raw materials or APIs only as they need them, to keep production efficiency high, produce less waste, and reduce inventory costs (Dias et al., 2012; Stevens, 2020). However, this makes supply chains more vulnerable to disruption because there is less protective inventory in the system. Although supply chain resilience and supply continuity may also be important considerations, there is variability in the extent to which the industry's concerns about continuity align with the concerns of customers or society at large. Moreover, the nature of the supply chain economics that shape decisions about investment in resilience and continuity differs by product category.

Producers of low-margin products, like generic drugs and simple medical devices, may have only a modest incentive to ensure supply continuity, even though patients and society may have high demand for and be dependent upon the availability of these products. For companies in the medical product industry—particularly those producing low-volume and low-margin products—lack of market insights about future demand can deter investment to expand manufacturing capacity to prepare for potential supply chain disruption (The PEW Charitable Trusts and ISPE, 2017). High costs can dissuade these same producers from upgrading facilities to comply with FDA current good manufacturing practice requirements, elevating the risk of quality issues that can precipitate shortages (The PEW Charitable Trusts and ISPE, 2017). Finally, cost pressures incentivize companies to shift the manufacturing of low-margin products to lower-cost countries, making quality oversight and assurance more difficult (The PEW Charitable Trusts and ISPE, 2017). This has led to shortages of low-margin products caused by issues at offshore manufacturing facilities. For all of these reasons, low-margin products—and generic drugs in particular—have been much more prone to supply disruptions than products with higher margins have been. It is possible to build just-in-case inventory or other business continuity protections into the supply chains for these products, but when margins are low, the returns on such investments do not justify the costs.

In contrast, for high-margin products—such as originator drugs and complex medical devices—producers are typically incentivized to ensure the continuity of their supply streams because this also protects their valuable revenue streams and market shares. For instance, when a disruption occurs, a company that already has market power will be more likely to maintain its leadership role if it is resilient enough to respond effectively and recover rapidly. Companies in this type of position can justify investment in strengthening their supply chain's resilience because their strong market role is linked to high-profit margins. Furthermore, companies that avoid disruptions may attract less attention from regulatory authorities (Sheffi and Rice, 2005). However, these incentives are most powerful when markets are competitive. If a producer has a monopoly on a product with few viable substitutes, it may still have an incentive to invest in business continuity measures to protect its revenue stream, but it will not have the added incentive to protect its market share.

The consequences of these differences in the supply chains of high- and low-margin products become particularly acute in emergencies, because they represent rare situations. From a financial perspective, it is difficult for companies to justify sufficient investment to ensure supply chain resilience and supply continuity in the event of a low-frequency but potentially high-consequence event, such as a large-scale natural or man-made disaster. This is a challenge for producers of products of all margins, but even more so for producers of low-margin products. As a result, rare events can pose serious risks to public health security if they disrupt the supply chains for products that are essential to health but are produced by industries that have limited financial incentives to ensure supply continuity.

Given these differences, an ideal starting point for identifying medical products at risk of shortages, due to capacity failures during normal times or lack of surge capacity to cope with demand surges during emergencies, is to focus on low-margin products. This generally means generic drugs and simple devices. But this is only an approximation, since some generic drugs and simple devices can have high margins. Also, some higher-margin products can have other risk factors, such as a high level of supply chain complexity or a low level of market diversification. Therefore, although the low-margin product categories will be used as partial predictors of supply risk, it also must be noted that there remains the need for more work to highlight medical products most vulnerable to shortages. The existing categories have been designed with quality and safety in mind. New categories can be developed to adapt or extend these to consider reliability. Alternatively, analytic techniques such as machine learning of past shortages can be used to identify product characteristics that predict shortages during normal conditions. Such analytic techniques will be less useful for predicting shortages in major disasters because the rarity of such events limits the data that are available. Therefore, to focus future medical product supply chain resilience efforts, new categories will likely be developed and analytics tools will be used for predicting risks.

POLICY UNDERPINNINGS OF U.S. MEDICAL PRODUCT SUPPLY CHAINS

The current U.S. policy landscape, and those specific to the ongoing COVID-19 pandemic, have significant implications for U.S. medical product supply chains. This section highlights the policies most relevant to medical product supply chains.[4]

---

[4] For a summary of existing U.S. legislation governing medical product supply chains and relevant legislation introduced in the 116th Congress see Appendixes A and B, respectively, at https://sgp.fas.org/crs/misc/R46507.pdf.

Federal Food, Drug, and Cosmetic Act

FDA is responsible for ensuring the safety and effectiveness of medical products marketed in the United States, and it plays a critical role in medical product supply chains. Box 2-1 details current tools at FDA's disposal to address supply chain shortages. The FD&C Act contains a number of statutory requirements relevant to the medical product supply chain. The

---

BOX 2-1
Current Tools for FDA to Address Supply Chain Shortages

Once a shortage or supply disruption is identified, FDA has several tools to respond:

- Working with the product manufacturer to identify actions it is willing and able to take to avoid or mitigate the shortage. Under certain conditions, FDA can exercise temporary regulatory flexibility and discretion as long as there is not a quality issue that could lead to an unacceptable clinical risk. Any temporary regulatory flexibility and/or discretion will involve thorough review by all relevant experts.
- Working with the approved manufacturer on any changes in specifications or additional lines, sites, or suppliers, and expediting review of these submissions to mitigate shortages.
- Determining whether there are any pending Abbreviated New Drug Applications that could be expedited and considering if there are discontinued applications or applications not currently being marketed that could relaunch or launch.
- For a product nearing expiry, working with the manufacturer on whether it has data to extend expiry on specific lots. FDA will post the lot numbers and new dating in the database on FDA's website.
- When a shortage involves a critical drug needed for patients and U.S. manufacturers are not able to resolve it immediately, FDA may consider allowing temporary importation of a product that is not approved for distribution in the United States. In these circumstances, FDA will consider a range of criteria to evaluate the product's safety and efficacy, including the formulation and other attributes of the drug, and the quality of the registered manufacturing establishment. FDA also encourages any firms temporarily importing a drug in these circumstances to apply to add an approved source to the market.
- In a public health emergency, issuing emergency use authorizations for therapeutics used to treat critically ill patients when the supply of the approved alternatives is insufficient to meet the emergency need.
- Outsourcing facilities under Section 503B of the FD&C Act, which may be an alternative source to help mitigate a shortage of an approved product.

SOURCE: The White House, 2021.

FD&C Act has been amended on several occasions to address medical product shortages and other issues related to the medical product supply chain.

For instance, in 2012, the Food and Drug Administration Safety and Innovation Act (FDASIA) amended the FD&C Act, giving FDA new authorities to address global supply chain challenges.[5] Among other things, FDASIA amended the FD&C Act to require that manufacturers notify FDA of discontinuance or interruption in the production of certain prescription drugs that are "life-saving, life-sustaining, or intended for use in the prevention or treatment of a debilitating disease or condition."[6] Additionally, FDASIA requires FDA to submit an annual report to Congress on drug shortages. The legislation called for the creation of a task force on drug shortages and set in motion a strategic plan to address drug shortages. FDASIA also introduced provisions aimed at improving the security of the drug supply chain, enumerating new requirements for facility registrations, risk-based facility inspections, and inspection reports. A 2021 study by Lee and colleagues empirically validated that this type of mandate-induced "operational transparency" was strongly associated with faster drug shortage recovery.

Below, some key aspects of this act are summarized in four categories—awareness, mitigation, preparedness, and response—in line with the committee's medical product supply chains resilience framework as detailed in Chapter 5.

Awareness of Medical Product Shortages

In response to the increasing frequency and threat of medical product shortages, the U.S. Congress passed legislation to improve the federal government's awareness of shortages. The FD&C Act requires that the secretary of the U.S. Department of Health and Human Services (HHS) publish a list of drugs and devices that are in shortage in the United States.[7,8] The FDA defines a drug and/or device shortage as a period of time when the demand or projected demand for the product within the United States exceeds the supply of the product (CDER, 2018). The shortage lists are to include the name of the drug or device, the name of the manufacturer, the reason for the shortage, and the estimated duration of the shortage. Furthermore,

---

[5] Food and Drug Administration Safety and Innovation Act, Public Law 112-144, 112th Congress (July 9, 2021).

[6] Food and Drug Administration Safety and Innovation Act, Public Law 112-144, 112th Congress (July 9, 2021).

[7] 21 U.S.C. 356e, Drug shortage list (amended March 27, 2020).

[8] 21 U.S.C. 356j, Discontinuance or interruption in the production of medical devices (amended March 27, 2020).

the HHS secretary is required to submit an annual report to Congress on the number of manufacturers reporting new drug shortages, the number of ongoing drug shortages, and the actions FDA has taken to prevent or alleviate shortages.[9]

Crucial to the government's ability to track product shortages is the requirement that manufacturers of drugs and devices that meet certain requirements,[10,11] such as being life supporting, life sustaining, or for use during a public health emergency, must notify the HHS secretary if the product will be permanently discontinued or is experiencing a meaningful disruption in its supply. This could be the result of a manufacturing disruption, a demand surge, and/or a mismatch in the location of available supply and demand need. Drug manufacturers are required to disclose reasons and risk factors for the discontinuation or interruption, as well as the sources of the API if that is a reason or risk factor for the interruption. These statutes also give the HHS secretary the authority to distribute nonproprietary information regarding the discontinuance or interruption to relevant groups, including patient organizations, health care providers, and prescribers. Of note, however, is that from 2014 to 2021, FDA has sent noncompliance letters to six different manufacturers who have failed to adequately notify of a discontinuance or interruption (FDA, 2021a), although manufacturers are not subject to fines or other disciplinary actions in cases of noncompliance.

During the COVID-19 pandemic, the FD&C Act was again amended under the Coronavirus Aid, Relief, and Economic Security (CARES) Act to provide more open communication and reporting between manufacturers and HHS. This is covered in more detail in the CARES Act section below.

Mitigation of Medical Product Shortages

In addition to measures to detect and track medical product shortages, the FD&C Act contains provisions to prevent shortages and blunt their effects. One such provision established a drug task force, which was charged with developing and implementing a strategic plan to prevent and mitigate shortages.[12] The legislation also calls for the strategic plan to include plans for

---

[9] 21 U.S.C. 356c-1, Annual reporting on drug shortages (amended December 13, 2016).

[10] 21 U.S.C. 356c, Discontinuance or interruption in the production of life-saving drugs (amended March 27, 2020).

[11] Food and Drug Administration Safety and Innovation Act, Public Law 112-144, 112th Congress (July 9, 2021).

[12] 21 U.S.C. 356d, Coordination; task force and strategic plan (amended July 9, 2012).

- interagency and intra-agency coordination,
- ensuring the consideration of drug shortages in regulatory actions,
- effective communication with external stakeholders,
- the effect of shortages on research and clinical trials, and
- examining the establishment of a qualified manufacturing partner program—a program that would use manufacturers with the capability and capacity to rapidly produce and supply drugs undergoing shortages.

In 2018, the FDA commissioner established the interagency Drug Shortages Task Force to focus more on drug shortages, to identify reasons why some shortages remain a persistent challenge, and to look for holistic solutions to addressing the underlying causes of the shortages (FDA, 2018). This task force produced a report on the root causes and potential solutions to drug shortages in 2019,[13] highlighting that on average, the number of ongoing drug shortages has been increasing and are lasting longer (FDA Drug Shortages Task Force, 2020). The task force also promoted several legislative proposals and FDA initiatives to help prevent and mitigate shortages, including improved data sharing and risk management plans.

Preparedness for Medical Product Shortages

The FD&C Act also gives the HHS secretary the authority to prioritize and expedite the review of drug or device applications,[14,15] or inspection of the facilities that produce them, when there is or is likely to be a shortage in which such an expedited review or inspection could mitigate or prevent the shortage. The relevant statutes create a system of accountability in requiring that FDA's annual report to Congress include information on the number of expedited reviews and inspections.[16] The annual reports also must contain the names of manufacturers that failed to notify the HHS secretary of interruptions or discontinuations, descriptions of the coordination between FDA and the Drug Enforcement Administration (DEA), and identify instances in which FDA exercised regulatory flexibility to prevent or alleviate shortages.

A provision of the FD&C Act also relegates responsibility to manufacturers of FDF drugs, APIs, or any associated medical device used for

---

[13] For more information and to read the full report, see https://www.fda.gov/media/131130/download (accessed August 19, 2021).

[14] Food and Drug Administration Safety and Innovation Act, Public Law 112-144, 112th Congress (July 9, 2021).

[15] For a summary of existing U.S. legislation governing the medical product supply chain and relevant legislation introduced in the 116th Congress see Appendixes A and B, respectively, at https://sgp.fas.org/crs/misc/R46507.pdf.

[16] 21 U.S.C. 356j, Discontinuance or interruption in the production of medical devices (amended March 27, 2020).

the preparation or administration of the drug to develop and maintain redundancy risk management plans and implement them as necessary.[17] The risk management plans are required to identify and evaluate the risks to the supply of the drug for each facility in which the FDF drug or API is manufactured. These plans are subject to inspection by the HHS secretary.

Various federal agencies, such as Departments of Commerce, Defense, Homeland Security, State, and Veterans Affairs, have developed and continue to develop regulations, guidance, standards, and other policy documents that complement the legal requirements regarding the medical product supply chain. These materials provide supply chain stakeholders with additional instruction for their role in the medical product supply chain.

Several gaps exist in the current legislation on medical product supply chains, leaving vulnerabilities unaddressed at the federal level. First, the reporting requirement for drug and device manufacturers focuses on disruptions to manufacturing, excluding downstream disruptions that could also lead to shortages, such as transportation disruptions, or disruptions that distributors detect. The President's Fiscal Year 2020 budget proposed levying financial penalties on manufacturers that failed to adequately notify FDA of a drug shortage (FDA Drug Shortages Task Force, 2020), but such penalties were not included in the CARES Act. Another notable gap is that, unlike drug manufacturers, device manufacturers are not required to develop risk management plans. Furthermore, the current statute only requires that risk mitigation management plans be available upon inspection. While companies are likely compelled to provide records to FDA to avoid official actions, the CARES Act does not require that manufacturers proactively submit their plans to FDA, which would allow the federal government to have a more comprehensive understanding of risks in the supply chain. FDA does however have the authority to initiate administrative, judicial, or other punitive actions when a firm refuses to provide access to records under the Federal Food, Drug, and Cosmetic Act (FDA, 2014).

Response for Medical Product Shortages

Finally, the FD&C Act provides authority for FDA and HHS to respond in the event of a medical product shortage. These provisions can be generally classified as ones for an expected shortage or those for active, ongoing shortages. The former are discussed in the preceding section.

Under the FDASIA-amended section 506C,[18] FDA and HHS can coordinate with the attorney general of DEA to increase production quotas for drugs should the nation experience a shortage of a controlled substance.

---

[17] Food and Drug Administration Safety and Innovation Act. Public Law 112-144, 112th Congress (July 9, 2021).

[18] 21 U.S.C. 356c-1, Annual reporting on drug shortages (amended December 13, 2016).

Furthermore, this section releases hospitals from registration requirements as "repackagers" of an FDF drug product, and saves them from some of the laborious nature of bureaucracy, if during response measures to a drug shortage, hospital pharmacies divide the volume of a drug into smaller amounts in order to extend its supply and safely transfer repackaged drugs to other hospitals within the same health system.[19] These policies enable medical supply chain resilience through flexibility in response measures.

Coronavirus Aid, Relief, and Economic Security Act

The shortages of medical products precipitated by the COVID-19 pandemic provided renewed urgency for addressing the resilience and transparency of medical product supply chains (Francis et al., 2021). Understanding this urgency, the U.S. government passed the CARES Act in March 2020, which called for the present study on the security of the medical product supply chain, and provided additional requirements for tracking and preventing medical product shortages.[20]

Due to a lack of transparency between manufacturers and HHS and incomplete reporting under existing regulations, the CARES Act amended the FD&C Act, adding certain API and device manufacturers to the categories of manufacturers that must notify the HHS secretary and Center for Devices and Radiological Health (CDRH) of device and drug shortages (FDA, 2020). It also added requirements for medical product manufacturers to develop risk management plans and annually report the amount of drug produced. The CARES Act also included provisions requiring (1) interagency notification of drug shortages, (2) facility inspection reports be sent to experts on drug shortages within FDA when drugs on the shortage list are produced at a specific facility, and (3) reporting the volume of each listed drug produced by each registered facility.

Defense Production Act

The Defense Production Act (DPA) enacted by Congress in 1950 was a post–World War II law, which gives the president emergency authority to manage U.S. industries and provide essential materials and goods to the government for national defense.[21] In response to the COVID-19 pandemic, President Trump used the DPA to address medical product supply shortages, by issuing several executive orders from March through August 2020, allowing numerous federal agencies (i.e., HHS, Homeland Security, Department

---

[19] 21 U.S.C. 356f, Hospital repackaging of drugs in shortage (amended July 9, 2012).
[20] Coronavirus Aid, Relief, and Economic Security Act of 2020, Public Law 116-136, 116th Congress (March 27, 2020).
[21] Defense Production Act of 1950, Public Law 81-774, 81st Congress (September 8, 1950).

of Commerce, etc.) to use DPA authorities to mitigate supply chain issues (GAO, 2020). These authorities included (1) identifying nationwide priorities and allocations of all health and medical resources needed to respond to COVID-19 within the United States; (2) preventing the hoarding and price gouging of resources such as personal protective equipment and disinfecting and sanitizing products; (3) expanding the production capacity of medical products such as ventilators; (4) providing loans to create, maintain, protect, expand, and restore the domestic industrial base capabilities; and (5) determining the priorities and allocations of essential medicines, medical countermeasures, and critical inputs, including APIs and raw materials (GAO, 2020).

Drug Supply Chain Security Act

The Drug Supply Chain Security Act (DSCSA), which was enacted by Congress in 2013, was intended to protect consumers from exposure to drug products that may be counterfeit, adulterated, or otherwise harmful to patients.[22] It lays out steps to create an electronic system to track and trace certain prescription drugs in the United States to help improve detection and removal of potentially dangerous drugs from the drug supply chain. The Partnership for DSCSA Governance, a nonprofit public–private partnership, was established to implement DSCSA traceability requirements over the coming years (FDA, 2021b). As of late 2021, the partnership had released a blueprint[23] with requirements and recommendations to meet the DSCSA's interoperability requirements that will take effect in 2023 (PDG, 2021).

Executive Orders

In addition to legislation on the medical product supply chain, several Presidential Executive Orders regarding the security of the supply chain have been released. These are discussed below.

Executive Order 13944 List of Essential Medicines, Medical Countermeasures, and Critical Inputs—August 6, 2020

The Trump administration released an executive order regarding the security of the medical product supply chain.[24] The order directed relevant

---

[22] Drug Quality and Security Act, Public Law 113-54, 113th Congress (November 27, 2013).

[23] For more information and to read the full blueprint, see https://dscsagovernance.org/wp-content/uploads/2021/07/PDG_Blueprint-v1.0-Final_071221.pdf (accessed October 11, 2021).

[24] Exec. Order No. 13944, 85 FR 49929 (August 6, 2020).

executive departments and agencies to identify and promote the procurement of essential medicines, medical countermeasures, and critical inputs from domestic sources, as well as to increase their production domestically. The administration also ordered the FDA commissioner and the director of the Office of Management and Budget to identify and mitigate vulnerabilities in the supply chain for essential medicines, medical countermeasures, and critical inputs. In October 2020, FDA published the list of essential medicines, medical countermeasures, and critical inputs required by the executive order.[25]

Executive Order 14001 A Sustainable Public Health Supply Chain—January 26, 2021

This executive order from the Biden administration focuses on the "strategy to design, build, and sustain a long-term capability in the United States to manufacture supplies for future pandemics and biological threats."[26] This order directs representatives from various departments and agencies to coordinate with the Assistant to the President for National Security Affairs and Assistant to the President for Domestic Policy to develop a strategy to ensure the functioning of the supply chain in the event of future pandemics or biological threats.

In July 2021, HHS and the Departments of Commerce, Defense, Homeland Security, State, and Veterans Affairs, as well as the White House Office of the COVID-19 Response, released a report in response to Executive Order (EO) 14011 addressing the resilience of the public health supply chain, outlining goals, objectives, and recommendations to improve resilience.[27] The recommendations are divided into three goals: (1) to build a diverse, agile public health supply chain and sustain long-term U.S. manufacturing capability for future pandemics; (2) to transform the U.S. government's ability to monitor and manage the public health supply chain through stockpiles, visibility, and engagement; and (3) to establish standards, systems, and governance to manage supply chains and ensure fair, equitable, and effective allocation of scarce resources. The committee of this National Academies of Sciences, Engineering, and Medicine (the National Academies) report provides recommendations that build upon the above three goals and additionally includes calls for international and global cooperation along with focusing resources at the last mile.

---

[25] See https://www.fda.gov/about-fda/reports/executive-order-13944-list-essential-medicines-medical-countermeasures-and-critical-inputs (accessed December 20, 2021).

[26] Exec. Order No. 14001, 86 FR 7219 (January 21, 2021).

[27] For the full report, see https://www.phe.gov/Preparedness/legal/Documents/National-Strategy-for-Resilient-Public-Health-Supply-Chain.pdf (accessed October 6, 2021).

Executive Order 14017 America's Supply Chains—February 24, 2021

Another executive order from the Biden administration took a broader approach, outlining the administration's vision for resilient, diverse, and secure supply chains.[28] The order calls for (1) the continuation of reporting to identify risks to the supply chain for drugs and the APIs that compose them, (2) policy recommendations to combat those risks, and (3) a report on the supply chains for the public health and biological preparedness industrial base. Ultimately, the goal of this executive order is to use the aforementioned reports to inform the Assistant to the President for National Security Affairs and the Assistant to the President for Economic Policy to be able to make recommendations regarding actions to make U.S. supply chains stronger and more resilient, such as regular supply chain reviews and international cooperation.

The report published in response to EO 14017 details some of the key risks and vulnerabilities to the pharmaceutical supply chain and offers potential solutions to address those vulnerabilities. The recommendations are divided into six categories: (1) rebuilding our production and innovation capabilities; (2) supporting the development of markets with high road production models, labor standards, and product quality; (3) leveraging the government's role as a market actor; (4) strengthening international trade rules, including trade enforcement mechanisms; (5) working with allies and partners to decrease vulnerabilities in the global supply chains; and (6) partnering with industry to take immediate action to address existing shortages.

CONCLUDING REMARKS

Medical product supply chains are vital to the nation's collective health and safety, in ordinary times as well as emergencies. But these supply chains are complex, varied, global, and constantly evolving. To an ever-greater degree, they are distributed enterprises managed by a network of organizations, rather than vertically integrated enterprises within a single entity. Particularly when profit margins are low, the private, profit-driven incentives to invest in supply resilience can differ widely from the public health and safety incentives to protect supplies of critical medical products. These factors all contribute to risks of supply disruptions, as evidenced by routine shortages and shortages during the COVID-19 pandemic.

Several acts of Congress and presidential executive orders have been enacted to address these risks. Although these instruments provide some authority, tools, and infrastructure for building medical product supply chain resilience, there is still much to do to better prepare for the next public health emergency. There have been continual policy fluctuations, and an

---

[28] Exec. Order No. 14017, 86 FR 11849 (March 1, 2021).

unclear role of the federal government (or federal assets) in a public health emergency—which serve a stunting role in investment in medical product supply chain resilience. Finally, as noted in this chapter, the product classifications used to monitor quality and safety are not ideal for assessing and remediating supply risks. This leads to a lack of clear sense of where resilience measures are needed most. There is also no systematic framework for enumerating, prioritizing, and combining measures into a medical product supply chain resilience strategy. The remainder of this report will focus on these questions in order to inform recommendations that will substantially increase the resilience of medical product supply chains.

REFERENCES

AAM (Association for Accessible Medicines). 2021. *2020 Generic drug & biosimilars access & savings in the U.S.* Washington, DC: Association for Accessible Medicines. https://accessiblemeds.org/sites/default/files/2020-09/AAM-2020-Generics-Biosimilars-Access-Savings-Report-US-Web.pdf (accessed October 20, 2021).

Berndt, E. R., R. M. Conti, and S. J. Murphy. 2017. The generic drug user fee amendments: An economic perspective. *Journal of Law and the Biosciences* 5(1):103-141.

CDER (Center for Drug Evaluation and Research). 2018. Drug shortage management. In *Manual of Policies and Procedures (MAPP 4190.1 Rev.3)*, edited by FDA (U.S. Food and Drug Adminstration). Silver Spring, MD. https://www.fda.gov/media/72447/download (accessed January 12, 2022).

CDRH (Center for Devices and Radiological Health). 2018. *Medical device overview*. https://www.fda.gov/industry/regulated-products/medical-device-overview#What%20is%20a%20medical%20device (accessed October 14, 2021).

Dias, V., J. D. Quick, and J. R. Rankin. 2012. Ch 23: Inventory management. In *MDS-3: Managing access to medicines and health technologies*, edited by M. Embrey. Arlington, VA: Management Sciences for Health. https://msh.org/resources/mds-3-managing-access-to-medicines-and-health-technologies/ (accessed December 21, 2021).

FDA (U.S. Food and Drug Adminstration). 2012. *Q11 development and manufacture of drug substances*, edited by Center for Drug Evaluation and Research. Silver Spring, MD: HHS. https://www.fda.gov/media/80909/download (accessed October 21, 2021).

FDA. 2014. *Guidance for industry FDA records access authority under sections 414 and 704 of the federal Food, Drug, and Cosmetic Act.* https://www.fda.gov/media/83083/download (accessed December 20, 2021).

FDA. 2016. *Q7 good manufacturing practice guidance for active pharmaceutical ingredients guidance for industry.* FDA-1995-D-0288 HHS. https://www.fda.gov/regulatory-information/search-fda-guidance-documents/q7-good-manufacturing-practice-guidance-active-pharmaceutical-ingredients-guidance-industry (accessed October 20, 2021).

FDA. 2017. *Learn if a medical device has been cleared by FDA for marketing.* https://www.fda.gov/medical-devices/consumers-medical-devices/learn-if-medical-device-has-been-cleared-fda-marketing (accessed December 9, 2021, 2021).

FDA. 2018. *Statement by FDA commissioner Scott Gottlieb, M.D., on formation of a new drug shortages task force and FDA's efforts to advance long-term solutions to prevent shortages.* HHS. https://www.fda.gov/news-events/press-announcements/statement-fda-commissioner-scott-gottlieb-md-formation-new-drug-shortages-task-force-and-fdas (accessed November 5, 2021).

FDA. 2020. *Medical device supply chain notifications during the COVID-19 pandemic.* https://www.fda.gov/medical-devices/coronavirus-covid-19-and-medical-devices/medical-device-supply-chain-notifications-during-covid-19-pandemic (accessed October 12, 2021).

FDA. 2021a. *Drug shortages: Non-compliance with notification requirement.* https://www.fda.gov/drugs/drug-shortages/drug-shortages-non-compliance-notification-requirement (accessed October 11, 2021).

FDA. 2021b. *Drug supply chain security act public-private partnership.* https://www.fda.gov/drugs/drug-supply-chain-security-act-dscsa/drug-supply-chain-security-act-public-private-partnership (accessed October 12, 2021).

FDA. 2021c. *Generic drugs: Questions & answers.* https://www.fda.gov/drugs/questions-answers/generic-drugs-questions-answers (accessed October 20, 2021).

FDA Drug Shortages Task Force. 2020. *Drug shortages: Root causes and potential solutions.* https://www.fda.gov/drugs/drug-shortages/report-drug-shortages-root-causes-and-potential-solutions (accessed December 16, 2021).

Francis, J. R., B. M. Mairose, and E. M. Tichy. 2021. 2020—the year the world was awakened to the importance of supply chain management. *Mayo Clinic Proceedings. Innovations, Quality & Outcomes* 5(1):187-192.

GAO (Government Accountability Office). 2020. *Defense Production Act: Opportunities exist to increase transparency and identify future actions to mitigate medical supply chain issues.* https://www.gao.gov/assets/gao-21-108.pdf (accessed October 12, 2021).

Haninger, K., A. Jessup, and K. Koehler. 2011. *Economic analysis of the causes of drug shortages*, edited by Office of Science and Data Policy and Office of the Assistant Secretary for Planning and Evaluation. Washington, DC: HHS. https://aspe.hhs.gov/reports/economic-analysis-causes-drug-shortages-0 (accessed October 20, 2021).

Khan, R. 2020. Unsustainable low prices causing generic drug market failure leading to supply chain disruptions and shortages. *Forbes*, July 6. https://www.forbes.com/sites/roomykhan/2020/07/06/unsustainable-low-prices-causing-generic-drug-market-failure-leading-to-supply-chain-disruptions-and-shortages/?sh=2f5c682a74d4 (accessed December 20, 2021).

Lee, J., H. S. H. Lee, H. Shin, V. Krishnan. 2021. Alleviating drug shortages: The role of mandated reporting induced operational transparency. *Management Science* 67(4):2326-2339. https://doi.org/10.1287/mnsc.2020.3857.

Lin, A., F. Ma, and M. Rees. 2016. *Life cycle of an adhesive bandage.* http://www.designlife-cycle.com/adhesive-bandage (accessed October 14, 2021).

NAM (National Academy of Medicine). 2021. *Four new reports from the National Academy of Medicine focus on how to prepare for seasonal and pandemic influenza through lessons learned from COVID-19.* NAM, November 17. https://nam.edu/four-new-reports-from-the-national-academy-of-medicine-focus-on-how-to-prepare-for-seasonal-and-pandemic-influenza-through-lessons-learned-from-covid-19/ (accessed January 11, 2022).

NASEM (National Academies of Sciences, Engineering, and Medicine). 2020. *Strengthening post-hurricane supply chain resilience: Observations from hurricanes Harvey, Irma, and Maria.* Washington, DC: The National Academies Press.

PDG (Partnership for Drug Supply Chain Security Act [DSCSA] Governance). 2021. *Partnership for DSCSA Governance (PDG) foundational blueprint for 2023 interoperability.* https://dscsagovernance.org/wp-content/uploads/2021/07/PDG_Blueprint-v1.0-Final_071221.pdf (accessed October 11, 2021).

The PEW Charitable Trust and ISPE. 2017. *Drug shortage: An exploration of the relationship between U.S. market forces and sterile injectable pharmaceutical products: Interviews with 10 pharmaceutical companies.* PEW and ISPE. https://www.pewtrusts.org/-/media/assets/2017/01/drug_shortages.pdf (accessed October 25, 2021). Sheffi, Y., and J. B. Rice, Jr. 2005. A supply chain view of the resilient enterprise. *MIT Sloan Management Review* 47(1):41.

Sheffi, Y., and J. B. Rice, Jr. 2005. A supply chain view of the resilient enterprise. *MIT Sloan Management Review* 47(1):41.

Stevens, C. 2020. *What is just-in-time (JIT) inventory management?* https://www.business.org/finance/inventory-management/what-is-just-in-time-inventory-management/ (accessed October 21, 2021).

The White House. 2021. *Building resilient supply chains, revitalizing American manufacturing, and fostering broad-based growth: 100-day reviews under Executive Order 14017.* Washington, DC: Department of Commerce, Department of Energy, Department of Defense, and Department of Health and Human Services. https://www.whitehouse.gov/wp-content/uploads/2021/06/100-day-supply-chain-review-report.pdf (accessed October 20, 2021).

3

Globalization of U.S. Medical Product Supply Chains

The past several decades have been a time of rapid globalization for U.S. medical product supply chains. The trend toward globalization has been driven by a range of factors, including incentives for individual firms and the market as a whole. The coronavirus disease 2019 (COVID-19) pandemic placed an unprecedented strain to cope with global demand for key goods as it far outpaced global supply, as well as highlighting long-standing supply chain resilience issues with medical product shortages (Ellis, 2021).[1] Challenges were exacerbated by export bans and countries, including the United States, favoring domestic use over foreign needs (Bown, 2021).

In response to the shortages of medical supplies that were spurred by the COVID-19 pandemic, Congress passed the Coronavirus Aid, Relief, and Economic Security (CARES) Act, addressing some of the gaps in medical product supply chains, as discussed in Chapter 2. COVID-19 also pushed several government actors to propose on-shoring of medical product supply chains—the domestic manufacture and production of medical products or critical components of those products—as a solution to make the supply chain more resilient.

The committee realized early in its deliberations that on-shoring entire medical product supply chains—from raw materials to finished production—would be logistically and economically challenging, while on-shoring only the final stage of production would not have a significant impact in reducing vulnerability to foreign shocks. Entirely domestic medical product supply chains, scaled to handle the expected demand in nonemergency times, would still be

---

[1] This chapter references a report commissioned by the Committee on Security of America's Medical Product Supply Chain titled *Where There's a Will: Economic Considerations in Reforming America's Medical Supply Chain*, by Phil Ellis (see Appendix D).

unable to immediately expand production sufficiently to meet the national needs in the case of a global health emergency (DoD et al., 2021). Proximity also does not necessarily imply resilience or scalability. Finally, if all nations responded to a U.S. on-shoring push by simultaneously trying to force the on-shoring of their own medical product supply chains, this could severely limit market opportunities for U.S. firms, fragment global production, cause severe shortages of manufacturing inputs, raise costs and reduce efficiency throughout the production system, and make an effective global response to the next pandemic even harder. This chapter provides context on the globalization of U.S. medical product supply chains and discusses the rationale for viewing on-shoring as one option among many, rather than as a panacea for improving global medical product supply chain resilience.

GLOBAL LANDSCAPE OF MEDICAL PRODUCT SUPPLY CHAINS

As mentioned in Chapter 1, the shift to overseas manufacturing of medical products is reflective of a broader trend on the part of the U.S. medical product industry. The shift to manufacturing outside of the contiguous United States began in the 1970s with production moving to Puerto Rico, then Europe, China, and India.[2] Since the 1990s, companies have moved to adopt lean manufacturing strategies and globalize sourcing and production in pursuit of cost reduction (Iakovou and White, 2020).

The medical product industry has grown to rely on multilateral relationships and international trade (Bhaskar et al., 2020; Gereffi, 2020). Although the United States is both an importer and exporter of medical products, the discussion that follows evaluates the dependence of the United States on medical products that are sourced or manufactured outside of the United States, per the statement of task. Further, the share of domestically produced and exported medical products or inputs versus those that are imported is difficult to accurately determine and varies greatly by product category (CRS, 2020b). Despite this lack of specific data, it is clear that the United States is heavily reliant on other countries for medical products, including China, India, the European Union (EU), Mexico, and Canada (CRS, 2020b). Whether a finished medical product is manufactured in the United States, Germany, or China, it is likely that the product is composed of component parts—active pharmaceutical ingredients (APIs), excipients, glass vials, device components—that were manufactured by different firms in various countries.

Regional Landscape

Estimates from 2019 indicate that the majority of the import revenue from pharmaceuticals, medical equipment and products, and related sup-

---

[2] Information given by testimony of Judith A. McMeekin (Senate Committee on Finance, 2020).

plies that the United States imports is from Europe (39.9 percent) and Asia (20 percent) (see Figure 3-1) (CRS, 2020a). Trends within these regions are discussed further in this section.

Europe

Medical research coming out of European institutions in the late 19th century led to groundbreaking discoveries, such as the X-ray and smallpox immunization, which helped pave the way for modern medicine (CDC, 2021; Karlsson, 2000; Peters, 1995; Tubiana, 1996). Given the region's long history of medical research, some of the world's largest medical product firms have European roots. For example, Philips & Co and Siemens Healthineers, two of the largest medical devices companies, were founded in Europe during the 1890s (Philips, 2022; Siemens, 2022). Several of the world's largest pharmaceutical firms, such as Roche, Merck KGaA, GlaxoSmithKline, and Bayer, have origins dating back to 17th–19th century Europe (Bayer, 2021; GlaxoSmithKline, 2022; Merck KGaA, 2022; Roche, 2022).

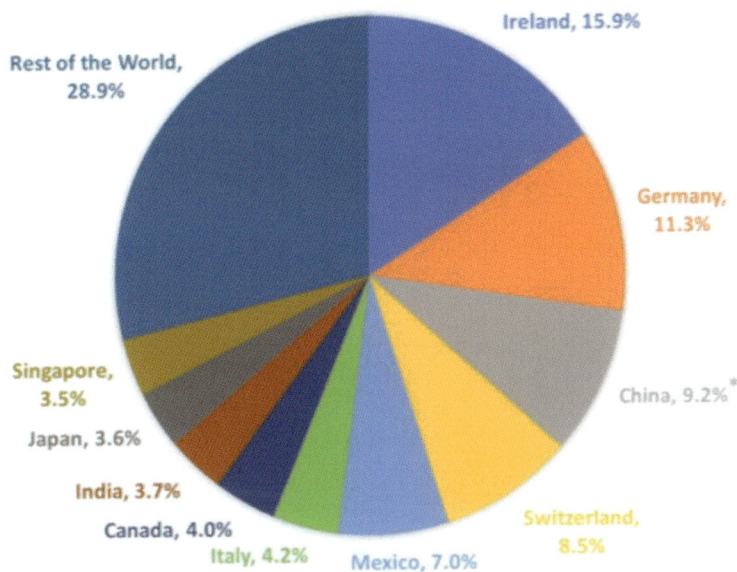

FIGURE 3-1 U.S. imports of pharmaceuticals and medical equipment, products, and supplies in 2019.
* China's 9.2% share of U.S. imports likely understates the extent to which the United States relies on China for pharmaceuticals and medical equipment, products, and supplies because of how these imports are classified.
SOURCE: CRS, 2020a.

Today, the United States relies on Europe for a significant portion of the medical products that it imports, particularly for more complex medical products, such as biologics and medical machinery (CRS, 2020a). Ireland in particular has been a prominent hub of medical device manufacturing (IDA Ireland, 2021). Since the late 1990s and early 2000s, Ireland was favored for medical device manufacturing due to its highly skilled, English-speaking workforce, and low tax rates. Ireland currently supplies €13 billion in exports annually and is the second largest exporter of medical technology products in Europe including diagnostic reagents, stents, artificial joints, and contact lenses (IDA Ireland, 2021).

Asia

In recent decades, Asian countries have come to represent a large portion of global medical product manufacturing because of a growing workforce that is both inexpensive and skilled, increased compliance with international standards, and local government incentives (NASEM, 2008). Multiple underlying factors are driving the shift toward globalization of drug manufacturing, particularly in China and India (Woo et al., 2008). A primary factor is that manufacturers are seeking to lower costs by sourcing finished dosage forms (FDFs), APIs, and other components from facilities in countries that can offer lower costs than U.S. facilities for labor, purchasing and shipping raw materials, and operations, including electricity, water, and coal (Marucheck et al., 2011).[3]

India

The emergence of India's pharmaceutical industry as a major global player in the global generic drug market provides an illustrative example of how globalization of supply chains can generate competition and drive down prices in the medical product market. Beginning in the 1970s, patent laws in India allowed the country's drug producers to engage in the practice of reverse engineering of drugs that were patent-protected by foreign companies, leading to rapid growth in its pharmaceutical sector. This practice was outlawed by changes to India's patent laws in 2005 that brought the country into compliance with the World Trade Organization Agreement on Trade-Related Aspects of Intellectual Property Rights (Greene, 2007). Other developing countries, to which India had traditionally exported its patent-infringing products, also adopted stronger pharmaceutical patent laws. To replace lost sales at home and abroad, many of India's leading drug

---

[3] Information also given by testimony of Janet Woodcock (House Committee on Energy and Commerce, 2019a,b).

producers turned to the production and export of generics to the United States and countries in Western Europe. As part of this transition, many of the producers in India engaged with foreign pharmaceutical companies through research and development agreements, mergers and acquisitions, and other types of alliances (Greene, 2007).

Today, India's pharmaceutical industry is one of the most price competitive in the world. With low labor costs, low barriers to entry, and small capital requirements, the number of pharmaceutical companies in the country burgeoned from 2,257 to more than 20,000 between 1970 and 2005. This pushed down prices and profit margins. By the late 2000s, reports suggested that compared to the United States and countries in Western Europe, pharmaceutical firms in India were offering 40 percent lower infrastructure costs and up to 20 percent lower fixed costs, enabling the production of bulk generic drugs at 60 percent lower costs. In the U.S. market, the price competitiveness in the Indian market and other lower-cost countries has parlayed into less expensive generic drugs and expanded choices for consumers (Greene, 2007).

A 2009 analysis of API manufacturing by the World Bank found that the wage index may be as little as 10 for Indian API manufacturers, compared to the average wage index of 8 for Chinese API manufacturers and 100 for API manufacturers in Western countries (Bumpas and Betsch, 2009). According to a 2011 U.S. Food and Drug Administration (FDA) report, U.S. manufacturers could reduce costs by 30 to 40 percent by sourcing APIs from manufacturers in India (FDA, 2011). Relentless cost pressures and the logistical challenges FDA faces in regulating India-based producers have led some Indian producers to sacrifice product quality in pursuit of low prices—an issue this report will consider later (Eban, 2019). Nevertheless, low-cost Indian producers have helped lower generic drug costs and boost access for millions of American consumers.

China

China's growing role in global medical product supply chains is particularly striking. The country has built up substantial industrial capacity in specific sectors through state-led industrial policies, such as a pharmaceutical "megaproject"—a large-scale goal-driven project led by China's Ministry of Health (Naughton, 2021). A strong Chinese pharmaceutical sector could make for a multipolar and more resilient global pharmaceutical supply chain. For example, safe and effective vaccines produced in China could bolster the world's insufficient supply by substantially expanding the number of vaccines on the market (Seligsohn et al., 2021).

Based on available data from China customs, China exported a total of $9.8 billion in medical supplies and $7.4 billion in organic chemicals to the United States in 2019 (CRS, 2020a). Of note, the classification "organic chemicals" includes both APIs and antibiotics. Additionally, the Congressional Research Service (CRS) has estimated that the United States imported around $20.7 billion in pharmaceuticals, medical devices, and other medical products from China in 2019, accounting for 9.2 percent of all U.S. imports in that year (see Figure 3-2) (CRS, 2020a). However, this probably underestimates the extent of the United States' reliance on China for medical products.

China produces almost all of the APIs used to manufacture such drugs as penicillin G, levodopa, and acetaminophen, and it produces two-thirds of the APIs used for other critical drugs such as antidiabetics, antihypertensives, and antiretrovirals (Ghangurde, 2020; Schondelmeyer et al., 2020). Other drugs that are highly reliant on Chinese manufacturers include heparin, chemotherapy drugs, antidepressants, and treatments for Alzheimer's disease and epilepsy (Thiessen, 2020). India, which is the largest provider of generic FDF products to the U.S. market, depends on China for more than 70 percent of its APIs (Schondelmeyer et al., 2020). As highlighted during the COVID-19 pandemic, the global supply chain also depends heavily on China for personal protective equipment such as respirators and surgical masks.

GEOGRAPHICAL CONSIDERATIONS FOR MEDICAL PRODUCT SUPPLY CHAINS

In response to rising wages abroad, transportation costs, and intellectual property concerns, the U.S. government and private-sector companies had been considering policies and initiatives to strengthen and "rebalance" medical supply chains through greater reliance on domestic medical product manufacturing well before the COVID-19 pandemic (Dolega, 2012).[4] However, the pandemic has sharpened the focus of these discussions as companies around the world have struggled to source APIs and other ingredients needed for medical product manufacturing, and global disruptions in medical product supply chains have threatened the U.S. health care system (Kajjumba et al., 2020; Lund et al., 2020). As a result, many policy makers have promoted on-shoring the production of medical product manufacturing, arguing that doing so would decrease America's dependence on foreign nations and give the United States more control in responding to shortages (Sardella and De Bona, 2021; The White House, 2020).

In 2020, former President Trump issued two executive orders addressing U.S. manufacturing of "essential medicines, medical counter measures, and critical inputs," and providing government agencies with additional flexibility to increase domestic procurement of certain medi-

---

[4] See Box 3-1 for definitions.

cal products to respond to the spread of COVID-19 (The White House, 2020). President Biden's 2021 Executive Order 14005, Ensuring the Future Is Made in All of America by All of America's Workers, launched a whole-of-government initiative to increase the use of federal procurement to support U.S.-based manufacturing. In addition to the United States, several other countries have implemented measures to encourage the on-shoring of manufacturing capacities (The White House, 2021). For example, in late 2020, the Japanese government allocated $2.4 billion to subsidize the process of strengthening domestic supply chains, including medical supplies (Takeo and Urabe, 2020). The Indian government also invested $6 billion in domestic manufacturing capacity to end dependence on China for bulk API materials (McRae, 2016). This effort to on-shore API production in India was re-endorsed in 2020 by the Indian government's "Production Linked Incentive Scheme" to promote domestic manufacturing of critical key starting materials, intermediaries, and active pharmaceutical ingredients by attracting large investments in the sector (McRae, 2016; Seth, 2020).

Dependence on Foreign Sourcing and Manufacturing

Foreign dependencies may manifest as dependence on a single nation for a particular source material, dependence on potential political adversaries, or dependence on foreign entities in a manner that exposes supply chains to geopolitical, economic, or climate shocks (The White House, 2021). In 2011, the Bureau of Industry and Security's Office of Technology Evaluation conducted an industrial base assessment of critical foreign sourcing in the Healthcare and Public Health Sector (Department of Commerce, 2011). The evaluation focused on the scope of foreign dependencies in the U.S. health care supply chain for 290 pharmaceuticals and 128 types of medical devices and surgical equipment considered critical in various emergency scenarios.[5] The study revealed a significant degree of foreign sourcing and dependency for critical components, materials, and finished products that are needed for U.S.-based manufacturing operations. Many of those components and products produced abroad had no alternative sources based in the United States. The breadth of these foreign dependencies was widely distributed. Pharmaceutical manufacturers reported suppliers in 47 countries, most commonly Italy, India, Germany, China, and France. Medical devices and surgical equipment manufacturers reported suppliers in 41 countries, most frequently China, Germany, Japan, Mexico, and the United Kingdom. About one-third of manufacturers reported mak-

---

[5] One hundred sixty-one companies that produced at least one of those commodities participated in the study (70 pharmaceutical manufacturers, 75 medical devices/surgical equipment manufacturers, and 16 manufacturers of both).

ing attempts to reduce their foreign dependency, but many said that it is challenging because the components they need are not available in the United States at all (Department of Commerce, 2011).

Historically, the United States has had a negative balance of trade for pharmaceuticals. In 2020, the United States imported nearly $94 billion, and exported almost $32 billion in human and animal drugs (FDA, 2020). The dependence on overseas production is particularly acute for APIs for generic drugs. According to FDA's Center for Drug Evaluation and Research (CDER) Site Catalog, only 46 percent of manufacturing facilities producing FDFs for U.S. consumption and 26 percent of facilities manufacturing APIs for U.S. consumption were located within the United States (CDER, 2021). The rest were located abroad (see Figure 3-2).[6]

Medical device manufacturing is also rapidly globalizing and increasingly reliant on complex, interconnected global networks of supply chains driven by specialization, global competition, and efficient capacity use. In 2020, the United States imported more than $68 billion and exported almost $59 billion in medical devices (FDA, 2020). The volume of imported products and components grew by an average of 25 percent annually between 2001 and 2007 (Seaborn, 2013). Likewise, the number of foreign Class I and II medical device manufacturing facilities nearly doubled during this same period, with an estimated 70 percent of medical device makers engaged in manufacturing arrangements with China (Rhea, 2007).

---

[6] Information given by testimony of Judith A. McMeekin (Senate Committee on Finance, 2020).

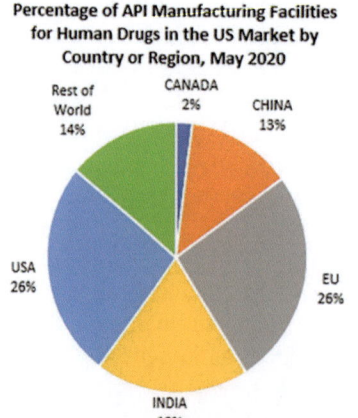
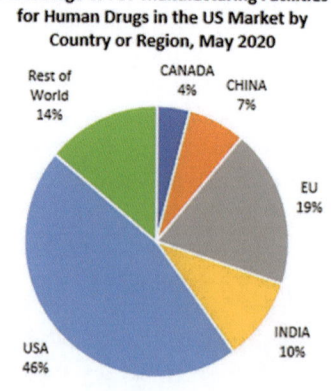

FIGURE 3-2 Percentage of API and FDF manufacturing facilities for human drugs in the U.S. market by country or region, May 2020.
NOTE: API = active pharmaceutical ingredient; FDF = finished dosage form.
SOURCE: Senate Committee on Finance, 2020a.

Geographical Concentration

Concentrating the production of individual products or components among a limited number of firms and sites can increase manufacturing efficiency through the realization of economies of scale for production (Gagnon and Volesky, 2017). However, across the links in supply chains for certain medical products, the increasing concentration of production in certain geographies, facilities, and suppliers also magnifies risks of disruption. Given the vast geography of such countries as India and China, the fact that a large share of medical products comes from these countries is not, in itself, a dangerous level of concentration. If, however, a large share of a product or material is concentrated in a single site or among few firms in the same location, a natural disaster, a localized health emergency, or political upheaval in that region could endanger the reliability of the entire global supply chain (Schondelmeyer et al., 2020). For example, Wuhan was a major center within China for PPE production and export. As the original epicenter of the global COVID-19 pandemic, its production shutdowns immediately disrupted global supply chains for these essential products (Bradsher and Alderman, 2020).

APIs and FDFs

As of August 2019, CDER's global geographic breakdown of the 1,788 API manufacturing facilities for all regulated drug products—including prescription, over-the-counter, and compounded drugs—indicated that 28 percent were located in the United States, 230 (13 percent) were in China, and 1,048 (59 percent) were in the rest of the world.[7] Since CDER does not measure or record the volume of production at any facility, a caveat to these figures is that the percentages of APIs actually produced at these facilities are indeterminate. The apparent global geographic dispersion of production sites could conceal high degrees of regional, national, or local concentration that could create bottlenecks inhibiting supply expansion and contribute to supply chain disruptions (NASEM, 2021). Furthermore, the markets can also be constrained and concentrated for certain products that require specific inert starting materials (e.g., talc for inhalers) or unique dosage forms (e.g., sterile injectables) (NASEM, 2021). The packaging and labeling needed to contain, transport, distribute, and administer products often relies on foreign sources for components such as resin-based bottles and films, paper cartons and labels, and stainless steel needles (Jung, 2020). The consistent availability of those components is necessary for uninterrupted supply of the finished product.

---

[7] Information given by testimony of Janet Woodcock (House Committee on Energy and Commerce, 2019a).

Generic Drugs

The generic drug manufacturing market has grown increasingly outside of the United States, with low-cost, off-patent generic drugs, likely to be outsourced to manufacturers in developing countries (Marucheck et al., 2011). In parallel, declines in manufacturing quality have led to an increased frequency of supply disruptions among some generic manufacturers in the global supply chain—particularly at the finished dosage level (Fox and McLaughlin, 2018).

Two recent studies have analyzed the geography of the foreign manufacture of generic drugs intended for the U.S. market. The first analyzed the locations of API and FDF facilities for generic drugs between 2013 and 2017 (Berndt et al., 2017). Data on the location of manufacturing provided under the Generic Drug User Fee Amendments of 2012[8] offered an "unprecedented window" into how generic drug manufacturing markets have evolved in recent years to become increasingly foreign. The proportions of both API and FDF facilities became increasingly foreign between 2013 and 2017. Almost 90 percent of API sites and around 60 percent of FDF sites for generics produced for use in the United States were located outside of the country. By 2017, the number of domestic FDF facilities was about 2.5-fold greater than the number of domestic API facilities. Moreover, there was a decrease in the total number of domestic and foreign registered API and FDF manufacturing facilities, with the greatest decline in the United States (Berndt et al., 2017). These data were confirmed to have remained unchanged by the White House's 100-Day Reviews under Executive Order 14017 (The White House, 2021).

The Berndt et al. study also explored the extent to which a small number of holding companies with huge portfolios own a disproportionate share of FDA-approved generic drug applications, called Abbreviated New Drug Applications (ANDAs) (Berndt et al., 2017). According to a list of ANDA sponsors publicly released by FDA in 2017, the 10 largest portfolio sponsors (of a total of 676) held more than 30 percent of the share of almost 10,000 approved ANDAs. Moreover, the number of API and FDF facilities declined by 10 to 11 percent between 2013 and 2017, further indicating growth in market concentration.

The second study used data made newly available by FDA to describe levels and trends in the manufacturing locations of the most commonly used prescription pharmaceuticals and off-patent generic drugs intended to be consumed by Americans (Kaygisiz et al., 2019). The analysis found that APIs for generics continued to be overwhelmingly manufactured outside the

---

[8] To implement fees under the Generic Drug User Fee Amendments of 2012, FDA required self-reported data to be submitted on generic manufacturing practices at API and FDF facilities (FDA, 2015).

United States. Between 2013 and 2019, foreign production of API intended for the U.S. market remained relatively stable at around 87 percent, largely concentrated in India (26 percent) and China (18 percent). During the same period, the number of U.S. sites producing API for generic drugs decreased by 10 percent. By 2019, the number of foreign FDF sites manufacturing drugs for consumption in the United States had increased by more than 5 percent—to about 60 percent of the overall share. The number of domestic FDF sites remained stable. FDF manufacturing was still dominated by the United States (41 percent), but India and China had growing shares of 21 and 8 percent, respectively. Again, the absence of production volume data means the true geographic distribution of production remains unknown to U.S. regulators (Kaygisiz et al., 2019).

Geographic Location Considerations for Manufacturing

In some instances, on-shoring and near-shoring (see Box 3-1 for definitions) may help to reduce supply chain risk and promote more efficient and robust markets. For example, geographical proximity can reduce transportation and shipping distances, which in turn may lower the risk of supply chain disruption. Shifting manufacturing capacity from overseas to U.S.-based locations may also enable more control and access to medical products for the U.S. government and health care systems and reduce the time to market. The impossibility, in the short term or the long term, of complete reconstruction of entire global medical product supply chains within the borders of any one country suggests that the United States will remain reliant on global supply chains for the foreseeable future.

Several of the inherent challenges related to globalization are broadly discussed further in Chapter 4. The committee concludes that *on-shoring, near-shoring, or friend-shoring may resolve some barriers, but these are not a one-size-fits-all solution to the problem of increasing the resilience of medical product supply chains. For example, transforming a diversified, global supply chain into a concentrated, domestic supply chain could reduce supply chain resilience.*

Furthermore, *on-shoring a supply chain in its entirety can be exceedingly expensive, both in terms of the fixed cost of moving facilities and infrastructure as well as the variable cost of production. These costs prevent the private sector from pursuing widespread on-shoring of its own accord and make it politically difficult for government to force on-shoring via regulatory or financial incentives.* Costs may include higher costs of production, which will be passed on to U.S. medical product consumers in some form, exacerbating the existing problem of high U.S. medical costs. If the higher costs of on-shored and near-shored production are offset by ongoing subsidies, this will divert public expenditure from other social

> **BOX 3-1**
> **Key Terminology and Definitions Regarding Geographic Location Based Production**
>
> There are strategies to promote medical product supply chain diversity based on the geographic location of manufacturing for source materials and/or final products. The following options can impact the cost-effectiveness, capacity, and sustainability of U.S. medical product supply chains (Austin and Dezenski, 2020; Gray et al., 2013; The White House, 2021).
>
> - *Far-shoring* is the act of sourcing materials or producing materials and goods in locations in geographically distant nations.
> - *Foreign direct investment* refers to a controlling equity investment made by a domestic company into a foreign company, allowing the domestic firm to control production (Trefler et al., 2005).
> - *Friend-shoring or ally-shoring* is the act of sourcing materials or producing materials and goods in nations that have existing economic partnerships and share values and strategic interests (Austin and Dezenski, 2020).
> - *Near-shoring* is the act of sourcing materials or producing materials and goods in locations in close proximity to a nation's borders, often sharing a border with a given nation.
> - *Offshoring* is the act of sourcing materials or producing materials or goods in locations outside of a nation's borders (Gray et al., 2013).
> - *Offshore outsourcing* refers to a transaction between a domestic company and a foreign company whereby the domestic firm essentially purchases the product from the foreign firm (Trefler et al., 2005).
> - *On-shoring* is the act of sourcing materials or producing materials and goods within domestic national borders to reduce the potential for supply chain disruption (Gray et al., 2013).
> - *Outsourcing* occurs when a firm obtains goods or services from another firm rather than from production internal to the company (Gray et al., 2013).
> - *Reshoring* is a reversal of offshoring; it is the act of relocating the sourcing of materials or the production of materials and goods to within a nation's borders (Gray et al., 2013).

priorities like education, infrastructure, and access to health care, and U.S trading partners could, under international trade rules, retaliate against the United States with tariffs or other sanctions for implementing trade-distorting subsidies. Other nations may also imitate American efforts to on-shore or near-shore, fragmenting global production in ways that lower efficiency and raise costs. Given the multiple stages of production involved in most medical products, and the geographic distribution of these stages across multiple countries, on-shoring or near-shoring only the final stage of production could still leave U.S. consumers as vulnerable to foreign supply disruptions as before the on-shoring or near-shoring because the production of final goods would be impossible without access to imports. Finally, the concentration of production within one region of the United States could expose U.S. consumers to disruption if that region suffers a natural disaster.

Multiple considerations are involved in choosing the appropriate relationship with a foreign service provider. For example, one approach holds that offshore outsourcing is the most suitable option if the project in question is routine and scoped (Trefler et al., 2005). However, foreign direct investment may be more appropriate if the project is too difficult or complex to fully describe and scope from the outset, as is more often the case with innovative projects with the potential to generate the greatest added value (Trefler et al., 2005).

The committee notes that *medical product supply chains consist of multiple stages. Even when on-shoring improves resilience, on-shoring a single stage of medical product supply chains, such as final assembly, can leave remaining aspects vulnerable to disruption.* The current push toward on-shoring is intended to assuage U.S. national security concerns, largely through "security-driven, China-focused policy and regulatory developments affecting private-sector businesses" (Gorelick and Preston, 2020). In the United States, increasing calls to support American manufacturing—coupled with a push to strengthen pandemic preparedness—may engender congressional support for initiatives, such as tax incentives or loans, for reshoring the manufacturing of medical products. Firms considering reshoring may perceive uncertainty and increasing risk in U.S. trade policy, which might work against on-shoring efforts for firms that serve global markets (Ellram et al., 2013). In some scenarios, reshoring could negatively affect employment for job seekers in the United States and other Western nations (Gray et al., 2013).

Economics of Geographical Location Considerations

On-shoring

Decisions about on-shoring require considering what can and cannot be on-shored at a reasonable cost. These decisions may be determined by the limits of the labor market, individual business considerations, national security policy, and federal on-shoring incentives. A nation's ability to implement on-shoring policies is limited by the availability of skilled labor on one end and prohibitive labor costs on the other. Developing countries may lack skilled labor that is available—but expensive—in developed countries (Kajjumba et al., 2020). For example, estimates suggest that in the United States domestically produced PPE and generic drugs may cost 20 to 50 percent greater than the price of these products produced abroad (Ellis, 2021). Thus, evaluating the economics of on-shoring, near-shoring, and offshoring decisions requires case-by-case business calculations that are context and company specific. On-shoring may optimize and streamline the supply chain and therefore add value for some companies with local, agile operations, but that is not always the case (Gyarmathy et al., 2020).

The economics of on-shoring can also be shaped by national security policy. COVID-19 has encouraged on-shoring by revealing supply chain insecurities to government and industry. The economics of on-shoring will likely be driven by national security and company-level supply chain risk assessments. Some have predicted that COVID-19 will give rise to a "rebirth of United States manufacturing in the form of the on-shoring of pharmaceutical and other critical manufacturing back to the United States as a national risk-reduction measure" (Zwiefel, 2020).

To protect national security, it is conceivable that the federal government could adjust national foreign policy to mandate that a proportion of the critical pharmaceutical manufacturing sector be on-shored (Zwiefel, 2020). Government action has deterred further outsourcing to China, but action could be taken to encourage the economics of on-shoring through tariffs and incentives. For instance, tariffs on Chinese exports have made manufacturing in China less profitable, leading many firms to explore other countries in the region with low-cost labor—but with similar potential for supply chain vulnerabilities—before considering on-shoring to the United States. Given that the pharmaceutical manufacturing base comprises private investment, the existing corporate tax incentives for on-shoring critical manufacturing will likely be insufficient (Zwiefel, 2020). Without substantial federal incentives, however, firms will not have the economic impetus to on-shore API production (Zwiefel, 2020). As the committee has already noted, however, efforts by the United States to induce on-shoring could (and likely would) be countered or copied by U.S. trading partners' policies in ways that could place additional stress on global supply chains.

Near-shoring and Friend-shoring

Definitions of "near-shoring" and "friend-shoring" involve a measure of ambiguity. For example, established proximity to qualify as "near-shoring" is not widely agreed upon. For European multinationals, "near-shoring" often moves activity to Eastern Europe or North Africa. For U.S. multinationals, "near-shoring" often moves activity to Latin America or the Caribbean. The committee also disagrees with the notion that a production site is necessarily more reliable or desirable simply because it is more geographically proximate to the United States mainland or its overseas territories. If a more proximate site is more prone to natural disasters or geopolitical upheaval or if it lacks the local skill base to meet requisite quality requirements or transportation infrastructure to receive components and export finished products, it could be strictly inferior to the more distant site it replaces in a supply chain, in terms of promoting resilience.

The same ambiguity applies to the notion of "friend-shoring." In discussions of "friend-shoring," it is uncertain as to what types of politically or economically motivated relationships qualifies a friend or ally. "Friendly" trade relationships are also not necessarily a proxy for "reliable" relationships. Notably, nations may change treaty relationships or impose restrictions in a time of crisis, as experienced during the COVID-19 pandemic. The reality of complex, multistage supply chains also makes the "near-shoring" or "friend-shoring" of the final stage of production of a drug or medical device of potentially little consequence if critical inputs remain concentrated in locations of questionable reliability.

To the extent that near-shoring actually improves the functioning of supply chains, firms are likely to pursue these opportunities on their own, without the need for government subsidy or coercion. This *laissez-faire* approach leaves the definition of "near" in the hands of the private-sector players whose capital investments create the supply chains in the first instance. Frequently cited benefits of near-shoring include shorter delivery times, faster product cycles, and easier communication largely due to reduced time zone differences and, in some cases, greater cultural similarity (Haar, 2021). Frequently, "near-shoring" involves reducing reliance on China, which can bring the added benefit of greater control over intellectual property. However, "near-shoring" generally results in increased costs (Haar, 2021). Given the capital at risk, firms managing supply chains have a strong incentive to balance potential benefits against costs in a cost-minimizing manner.

IMPACTS OF GLOBALIZATION

Decades of research in international economics have established multiple impacts of globalization that can benefit consumers and society at large. Firstly, moving from a national economy to a global economy enlarges the potential set of competitors. More competition means lower prices and greater variety, both of which benefit consumers (Krugman, 1980). Greater competition among input suppliers can also benefit firms that use these products as inputs. Greater quality and variety of inputs (and lower costs of inputs) can—and generally does—lead to firm productivity gains (De Loecker et al., 2016; Goldberg et al., 2010). Because global markets are larger than national ones, a shift from national markets to global ones also leads to an expansion of production by the most productive firms, the exit of the least productive firms, and the displacement in a national market of less productive domestic firms by the products of more productive foreign ones. This leads to increases in industry productivity within countries and across countries, also providing consumers with better products at better price levels (Melitz, 2003).

There is also strong evidence that increasing globalization has spurred the invention and production of new medical devices and new drugs far beyond what access to only a national market would have induced (Bertrand and Mol, 2013; Department of Commerce, 2016; Nieto and Rodríguez, 2011; Vrontis and Christofi, 2021). The prospect of exporting to a bigger market can induce firms to invest more in raising their quality or lowering their price than they would in the absence of export opportunities (Lileeva and Trefler, 2010). If these forces lead to increased incentives for research and development and an increased flow of better ideas, then globalization could induce a faster growth rate for an industry or even an entire national economy (Grossman and Helpman, 1993; Sampson, 2016). There is also growing evidence that exporting firms can obtain useful ideas from foreign customers and partners that make them more productive (Atkin et al., 2017).

Incentives for Innovation

Global markets create greater rewards for successful producers. Operating at a global level, producers can achieve greater economies of scale and producers of specialized inputs have a greater incentive to compete. Increasing globalization has laid the groundwork for the United States to take a leading role as an innovator in the biomedical field. When the United States is engaged in open trade with other countries by, for instance, purchasing less expensive medical products abroad, it also allows the United States to focus its medical device manufacturing industry on the export of innovative products around the globe. In 2015, the U.S. medical device market was valued at more than $140 billion, accounting for nearly 45 percent of the global market (Department of Commerce, 2016). U.S. and European firms, biotech startups, universities, and the U.S. National Institutes of Health also play a growing role in the development of new drugs for the global market—a phenomenon illustrated by the role of American companies in collaborating with other firms, as well as U.S. government investment to bring new, effective vaccines to market in the immediate aftermath of the COVID-19 crisis (see Box 3-2 for example).

Continued investment to spur innovation by U.S. firms is critical for maintaining the domestic industry's competitive advantage in the global market (Trefler et al., 2005). In some cases, research into advanced manufacturing technologies that enable efficient and scalable small-scale production would promote diversified foreign and domestic production without limiting incentives for innovation, primarily because of reasons of efficiency rather than as a result of trade restrictions. However, a large push for U.S. on-shoring through regulatory requirements, if followed suit by other countries, would fragment markets for medical products, resulting in higher prices, poorer health care, and greater vulnerability to shortages during regional disasters.

> **BOX 3-2**
> **The Role of Global Collaboration in Developing Vaccines Against COVID-19**
>
> The technology of the Comirnaty vaccine, which has been marketed in the United States by Pfizer, was discovered and initially developed by BioNTech—a German biotechnology company (Browne, 2020). Pfizer collaborated with BioNTech to provide support with clinical trials, logistics, manufacturing, and marketing (Thomas et al., 2021). Another vaccine available to the American public comes from Moderna, a U.S. company that developed an mRNA therapeutics platform in 2013 through partnership with AstraZeneca, a UK pharmaceutical. AstraZeneca provided technology and funding to discover, develop, and commercialize mRNA for various types of treatments (AstraZeneca, 2018). In addition to this support from AstraZeneca, Moderna was heavily funded by the U.S. National Institute of Allergy and Infectious Diseases and the Biomedical Advanced Research and Development Authority (Garde, 2016; Pollack, 2013; Weisman, 2013). Moderna then partnered with Swiss contract manufacturer Lonza Group to produce as many as 1 billion doses in 2021 (Garde, 2016; Miller, 2021; Pollack, 2013; Weisman, 2013).

Competition and Resilience

The degree of competition in a global market is greater than what would exist in just one national market, even one as large as the United States. This greater competition reduces medical product costs, lowers health care costs for American consumers, and creates more choices in terms of specialized drugs and medical products. Foreign drug manufacturers have the potential to help expand and sustain affordable access to essential off-patent drugs of appropriate quality in the United States even more than they currently do (Gupta et al., 2018). In 2015, Medicaid spent almost $700 million on generic drugs that did not have sufficient competition from other domestic manufacturers. However, there were foreign manufacturers approved by peer regulatory agencies abroad that could have brought generics to the U.S. market to bolster competition and bring down prices (Gupta et al., 2018).

A global market, whose production assets are distributed across multiple countries, may also be more resilient in the face of certain kinds of shocks. Natural disasters can disrupt supply chains where they occur—but if other sources of supply exist in countries far from the site of a national disaster confined to one country, the world can substitute foreign sources of supply while the domestic production facilities are rebuilt after the disaster (see case studies in Chapter 4). A similar logic can apply in the case of certain human-engineered disasters, such as acts of terrorism, war, or political instability.

Economic Growth

Global trade in medical products has grown over the past few decades as a result of increasing trade across all industries. Imports of finished pharmaceutical products grew by nearly 14 percent in the two decades following adoption of the 1994 Agreement on Trade in Pharmaceutical Products (WTO, 1994). In 2017, the global pharmaceutical drug market was valued at $934.8 billion, which is expected to triple by 2060 (Ledger and Opler, 2017). As of 2020, imports and exports of medical goods were valued at $2,343 billion (WTO, 2020).

Worldwide demand for medical devices, attributed to increasing health care spending in lower-income countries and aging populations in middle- and upper-income countries, has also contributed to a doubling of the global market (Bamber et al., 2020; Fortune Business Insights, 2021). Since 2015, this market has expanded at an annual rate of more than 4 percent compound annual growth rate (CAGR) (Jiang and Hassoun, 2021). Market research estimates suggest that in 2019, the global market for medical devices achieved $457 billion in sales (Jiang and Hassoun, 2021). This growth in the global medical device market has also helped to create further investment opportunities for U.S. device manufacturers. According to data from the Pharmaceutical Research and Manufacturers of America's annual membership survey, biopharmaceutical companies invested $500 billion in research and development between 2010 and 2020 (PhRMA, 2020).

Certain countries have benefited from global markets. Exports of PPE and medical devices from countries such as Belgium, France, Germany, Italy, Japan, the Netherlands, the United Kingdom, and the United States increased by 45 percent between 2008 and 2018. At the same time, exports from large, newly industrialized manufacturing hubs, such as China and Mexico, as well as smaller specialized manufacturing locations, such as Costa Rica, Malaysia, New Zealand, and Singapore, grew twice as fast (Bamber et al., 2020). As of 2020, the United States, Japan, China, Switzerland, and the United Kingdom had the largest pharmaceutical markets globally (see Table 3-1) (Wee, 2017).

Between 2017 and 2022, growth in the global market for pharmaceuticals has been catalyzed by the continued growth in developing markets such as the Indian subcontinent—which is expected to have a CAGR of 10 percent—as well as the Commonwealth of Independent States (8 percent CAGR), Latin America (7.8 percent CAGR), and Africa (7.3 percent CAGR). Significant growth is also predicted in existing markets such as North America (estimated 6.4 percent CAGR) (Ledger and Opler, 2017).

The committee concludes that *market forces create powerful incentives for medical product supply chains to remain globalized. These global supply chains provide efficiency, innovation, and, in some cases, diversification benefits. However, such global supply chains also pose transparency and*

TABLE 3-1 Countries with the Largest Global Pharmaceutical Markets in the World

Rank	Country	Value of Pharmaceutical Market (in millions of $)
1	USA	339,694
2	Japan	94,025
3	China	86,774
4	Germany	45,828
5	France	37,156
6	Brazil	30,670
7	Italy	27,930
8	UK	24,513
9	Canada	21,353
10	Spain	20,741

SOURCE: Wee, 2017.

coordination challenges. International cooperation can help address these challenges, strengthen medical product supply chain resilience, and minimize the effect of shortages. To achieve this, nations and manufacturers must be better equipped to understand and manage the challenges of global medical product supply chains, including issues related to transparency, regulatory authorities, and national security. In Part II of this report, the committee discusses ways that benefits of globalization can be harnessed while contending with the transparency challenges that globalized markets bring. The committee recommends steps the federal government can take, within its own jurisdiction, to increase transparency within medical product supply chains (see Chapter 6). The committee also recommends the exploration of possibilities for international information sharing between governments, especially during global public health emergencies (see Chapter 9).

CONCLUDING REMARKS

The globalization of U.S. medical product supply chains has brought supply chain efficiencies, expanded market access, and greater affordability. Increasing the resilience of medical product supply chains will require multiple solutions and cooperation across sectors and borders. Policy makers and other key decision makers should reconsider the trade-offs between offshoring and on-shoring medical product supply chains. An effective supply chain resilience strategy must be more nuanced, diversified, and comprehensive than simply incentivizing or mandating more domestic production. This observation motivates the remainder of the report, which develops a systematic framework for building increased resilience into medical product supply chains in order to identify and motivate strategic, cost-effective recommendations.

REFERENCES

AstraZeneca. 2018. *What science can do: Astrazeneca annual report.* https://www.astrazeneca.com/content/dam/az/Investor_Relations/annual-report-2018/PDF/AstraZeneca_AR_2018.pdf (accessed December 20, 2021).

Atkin, D., A. K. Khandelwal, and A. Osman. 2017. Exporting and firm performance: Evidence from a randomized trial. *The Quarterly Journal of Economics* 132(2):551-615. https://doi.org/10.1093/qje/qjx002.

Austin, J., and E. Dezenski. 2020. Re-forge strategic alliances and check China abroad, rebuild economy at home. *Newsweek*, July 12.

Bamber, P., K. Fernandez-Stark, and D. Taglioni. 2020. *Four reasons why globalized production helps meet demand spikes: The case of medical devices and personal and protective equipment.* https://blogs.worldbank.org/developmenttalk/four-reasons-why-globalized-production-helps-meet-demand-spikes-case-medical (accessed December 20, 2021).

Bayer. 2021. *History of Bayer.* https://www.bayer.com/en/history (accessed January 24, 2022).

Berndt, E. R., R. M. Conti, and S. J. Murphy. 2017. The generic drug user fee amendments: An economic perspective. *Journal of Law and the Biosciences* 5(1):103-141.

Bertrand, O., and M. J. Mol. 2013. The antecedents and innovation effects of domestic and offshore R&D outsourcing: The contingent impact of cognitive distance and absorptive capacity. *Strategic Management Journal* 34(6):751-760.

Bhaskar, S., J. Tan, M. L. A. M. Bogers, T. Minssen, H. Badaruddin, S. Israeli-Korn, and H. Chesbrough. 2020. At the epicenter of COVID-19—The tragic failure of the global supply chain for medical supplies. *Frontiers in Public Health* 8(821).

Bown, C. P. 2021. How COVID 19 medical supply shortages led to extraordinary trade and industrial policy. *Asian Economic Policy Review* 9999:1-22.

Bradsher, K., and L. Alderman. 2020. The world needs masks. China makes them, but has been hoarding them. *The New York Times*, March 14, B05.

Browne, R. 2020. What you need to know about Biontech—The European company behind Pfizer's COVID-19 vaccine. In *Health and Science*. CNBC.

Bumpas, J., and E. Betsch. 2009. Exploratory study on active pharmaceutical ingredient manufacturing for essential medicines. In *The World Bank's Human Development Network*. The World Bank. https://documents.worldbank.org/en/publication/documents-reports/documentdetail/848191468149087035/exploratory-study-on-active-pharmaceutical-ingredient-manufacturing-for-essential-medicines (accessed December 20, 2021).

CDC (Centers for Disease Control and Prevention). 2021. *History of smallpox.* https://www.cdc.gov/smallpox/history/history.html (accessed January 25, 2022).

CDER (Center for Drug Evaluation and Research). 2021. *Report on the state of pharmaceutical quality: Fiscal year 2020*, edited by CDER's Office of Pharmaceutical Quality. Silver Spring, MD: FDA. https://www.fda.gov/media/151561/download (accessed December 20, 2021).

CRS (Congressional Research Service). 2020a. *COVID-19: China medical supply chains and broader trade issues.* https://crsreports.congress.gov/product/pdf/R/R46304 (accessed December 16, 2021).

CRS. 2020b. *Medical supply chains and policy options: The data challenge.* https://www.everycrsreport.com/files/2020-09-16_IF11648_fadf375c447b7698544a1dac3dc999b5e8358617.pdf (accessed August 26, 2021).

De Loecker, J., P. K. Goldberg, A. K. Khandelwal, and N. Pavcnik. 2016. Prices, markups, and trade reform. *Econometrica* 84(2):445-510.

Department of Commerce. 2011. *Reliance on foreign sourcing in the healthcare and public health (HPH) sector: Pharmaceuticals, medical devices, and surgical equipment.* https://www.bis.doc.gov/index.php/documents/other-areas/642-department-of-homeland-security-dhs-assessment-impact-of-foreign-sourcing-on-health-related-infra/file (accessed December 20, 2021).

Department of Commerce. 2016. *2016 top markets report: Medical devices.* https://legacy.trade.gov/topmarkets/pdf/Medical_Devices_Top_Markets_Report.pdf (accessed December 20, 2021).

DoD (U.S. Department of Defense), HHS (U.S. Department of Health and Human Services), DHS (U.S. Department of Homeland Security), and VA (U.S. Department of Veterans Affairs). 2021. *National strategy for a resilient public health supply chain*, edited by Department of Health and Human Services, Department of Defense, Department of Homeland Security, Department of Commerce, Department of State, Department of Veterans Affairs, and The White House Office of the COVID-19 Response. Washington, DC. https://www.phe.gov/Preparedness/legal/Documents/National-Strategy-for-Resilient-Public-Health-Supply-Chain.pdf (accessed October 29, 2021).

Dolega, M. 2012. *Offshoring, onshoring, and the rebirth of American manufacturing.* Council of Development Finance Agencies, TD Economics. https://www.cdfa.net/cdfa/cdfaweb.nsf/pages/13816/$file/md1012_onshoring.pdf (accessed December 20, 2021).

Eban, K. 2019. *Bottle of lies: The inside story of the generic drug boom.* New York City, NY: HarperCollins.

Ellis, P. 2021. *Where there's a will: Economic considerations in reforming America's medical supply chain.* Commissioned by the Committee on Security of America's Medical Product Supply Chain.

Ellram, L. M., W. L. Tate, and K. J. Petersen. 2013. Offshoring and reshoring: An update on the manufacturing location decision. *Journal of Supply Chain Management* 49(2):14-22.

FDA (U.S. Food and Drug Administration). 2011. *Pathway to global product safety and quality.* https://www.hsdl.org/?view&did=4123 (accessed December 20, 2021).

FDA. 2015. *GDUFA glossary.* https://www.fda.gov/industry/generic-drug-user-fee-amendments/gdufa-glossary (accessed October 12, 2021).

FDA. 2020. *FDA at a glance: Regulated products and facilities.* https://www.fda.gov/media/143704/download (accessed December 20, 2021).

Fortune Business Insights. 2021. *Medical devices market size, share & COVID-19 impact analysis.* https://www.fortunebusinessinsights.com/industry-reports/medical-devices-market-100085 (accessed December 20, 2021).

Fox, E. R., and M. M. McLaughlin. 2018. ASHP guidelines on managing drug product shortages. *American Journal of Health-System Pharmacy* 75(21):1742-1750.

Gagnon, M.-A., and K. D. Volesky. 2017. Merger mania: Mergers and acquisitions in the generic drug sector from 1995 to 2016. *Globalization and Health* 13(1):62.

Garde, D. 2016. Ego, ambition, and turmoil: Inside one of biotech's most secretive startups. *STAT News*, September 13.

Gereffi, G. 2020. What does the COVID-19 pandemic teach us about global value chains? The case of medical supplies. *Journal of International Business Policy* 1-15.

Ghangurde, A. 2020. *How India API manufacturing stacks vs China, addressing challenges.* https://scrip.pharmaintelligence.informa.com/SC142101/How-India-API-Manufacturing-Stacks-Vs-China-Addressing-Challenges (accessed December 20, 2021).

GlaxoSmithKline. 2022. *Our history.* https://www.gsk.com/en-gb/about-us/our-history/ (accessed January 24, 2022).

Goldberg, P. K., A. K. Khandelwal, N. Pavcnik, and P. Topalova. 2010. Imported intermediate inputs and domestic product growth: Evidence from India. *The Quarterly Journal of Economics* 125(4):1727-1767.

Gorelick, J., and S. Preston. 2020. *US decoupling from China and the onshoring of critical supply chains: Implications for private sector businesses.* https://www.mondaq.com/unitedstates/inward-foreign-investment/988594/us-decoupling-from-china-and-the-onshoring-of-critical-supply-chains-implications-for-private-sector-businesses#:~:text=The%20effects%20of%20this%20decoupling%20from%20China%20and,to%20microprocessors%2C%20rare%20earth%20minerals%20and%20permanent%20magnets (accessed December 20, 2021).

Gray, J. V., K. Skowronski, G. Esenduran, and M. J. Rungtusanatham. 2013. The reshoring phenomenon: What supply chain academics ought to know and should do. *Journal of Supply Chain Management* 49(2):27-33.

Greene, W. 2007. *The emergence of India's pharmaceutical industry and implications for the US generic drug market.* Washington, DC: US International Trade Commission, Office of Economics Washington, DC. https://www.usitc.gov/publications/332/EC200705A.pdf (accessed December 20, 2021).

Grossman, G. M., and E. Helpman. 1993. *Innovation and growth in the global economy.* Cambridge, MA: MIT Press.

Gupta, R., T. J. Bollyky, M. Cohen, J. S. Ross, and A. S. Kesselheim. 2018. Affordability and availability of off-patent drugs in the United States—the case for importing from abroad: Observational study. *BMJ (Clinical Research Ed.)* 360:k831.

Gyarmathy, A., K. Peszynski, and L. Young. 2020. Theoretical framework for a local, agile supply chain to create innovative product closer to end-user: Onshore-offshore debate. *Operations and Supply Chain Management: An International Journal* 13(2):108-122.

Haar, J. 2021. Nearshoring: Panacea, quick fix or something in between? *The Hill*, November 22.

House Committee on Energy and Commerce and Subcommittee on Health. 2019a. *Safeguarding pharmaceutical supply chains in a global economy. Testimony of Janet Woodcock, MD, Director of the Center for Drug Evaluation and Research.* October 30. https://www.fda.gov/news-events/congressional-testimony/safeguarding-pharmaceutical-supply-chains-global-economy-10302019 (accessed December 20, 2021).

House Committee on Energy and Commerce. 2019b. *Securing the US drug supply chain: Oversight of FDA's foreign inspection program: Congressional testimony of Janet Woodcock.* December 10. https://www.fda.gov/news-events/congressional-testimony/securing-us-drug-supply-chain-oversight-fdas-foreign-inspection-program-12102019 (accessed December 10, 2021).

Iakovou, E., and C. C. White. 2020. *How to build more secure, resilient, next-gen U.S. supply chains.* Brookings. https://www.brookings.edu/techstream/how-to-build-more-secure-resilient-next-gen-u-s-supply-chains/ (accessed December 20, 2021).

IDA Ireland. 2021. *Medical technology sector in Ireland.* https://www.idaireland.com/doing-business-here/industry-sectors/medical-technology (accessed December 20, 2021).

Jiang, K., and H. Hassoun. 2021. The globalization of medical devices and the role of US academic medical centers. *MedTech Outlook* January–March:8-9.

Jung, A. 2020. *COVID-19: Risks and resiliency in the drug supply chain.* https://www.ey.com/en_us/strategy-transactions/covid-19-risks-and-resiliency-in-the-drug-supply-chain (accessed January 5, 2021).

Kajjumba, G. W., O. P. Nagitta, F. A. Osra, and M. Mkansi. 2020. Offshoring-outsourcing and onshoring tradeoffs: The impact of coronavirus on global supply chain. *IntechOpen.* doi:10.5772/intechopen.95281.

Karlsson, E. 2000. *The Nobel Prize in physics 1901–2000.* https://www.nobelprize.org/prizes/themes/the-nobel-prize-in-physics-1901-2000 (accessed January 23, 2022).

Kaygisiz, N. B., Y. Shivdasani, R. M. Conti, E. Bernt, and National Bureau of Economic Research. 2019. *The geography of prescription pharmaceuticals supplied to the U.S: Levels, trends and implications.* National Bureau of Economic Research.

Krugman, P. 1980. Scale economies, product differentiation, and the pattern of trade. *The American Economic Review* 70(5):950-959.

Ledger, M., and T. Opler. 2017. *The future of the global pharmaceutical industry.* New York, NY: Torreya. https://torreya.com/publications/torreya_global_pharma_industry_study_october2017.pdf (accessed December 20, 2021).

Lileeva, A., and D. Trefler. 2010. Improved access to foreign markets raises plant-level productivity… for some plants. *The Quarterly Journal of Economics* 125(3):1051-1099.

Lund, S., J. Manyika, J. Woetzel, E. Barriball, M. Krishnan, K. Alicke, M. Birshan, K. George, S. Smit, and D. Swan. 2020. *Risk, resilience, and rebalancing in global value chains.* McKinsey Global Institute. https://www.mckinsey.com/business-functions/operations/our-insights/risk-resilience-and-rebalancing-in-global-value-chains (accessed December 20, 2021).

Marucheck, A., N. Greis, C. Mena, and L. Cai. 2011. Product safety and security in the global supply chain: Issues, challenges and research opportunities. *Journal of Operations Management* 29(7-8):707-720.

McRae, N. 2016. *India plans to end dependence on China bulk imports by 2020.* https://scrip.pharmaintelligence.informa.com/SC089232/India-Plans-To-End-Dependence-On-China-Bulk-Imports-By-2020 (accessed January 18, 2022).

Melitz, M. J. 2003. The impact of trade on intra industry reallocations and aggregate industry productivity. *Econometrica* 71(6):1695-1725.

Merck KGaA. 2022. *History.* https://www.emdgroup.com/en/company/history.html (accessed January 24, 2022).

Miller, J. 2021. Moderna plans mix of COVID-19 vaccine doses with new Lonza deal. *Reuters,* June 2.

NASEM (National Academies of Sciences, Engineering, and Medicine). 2008. *The offshoring of engineering: Facts, unknowns, and potential implications.* Washington, DC: The National Academies Press.

NASEM. 2021. *The security of America's medical product supply chain: Considerations for critical drugs and devices: Proceedings of a workshop—In brief,* edited by A. Nicholson, E. Randall, L. Brown, C. Shore, and B. Kahn. Washington, DC: The National Academies Press.

Naughton, B. 2021. *The rise of China's industrial policy (1978-2020).* Ciudad de México: Universidad Nacional Autónoma de México. https://dusselpeters.com/CECHIMEX/Naughton2021_Industrial_Policy_in_China_CECHIMEX.pdf (accessed December 20, 2021).

Nieto, M. J., and A. Rodríguez. 2011. Offshoring of R&D: Looking abroad to improve innovation performance. *Journal of International Business Studies* 42(3):345-361.

Peters, P. 1995. W.C. Roentgen and the discovery of x-rays. In *Textbook of radiology.* New York: GE Healthcare. https://archive.is/20080511205052/http:/www.medcyclopaedia.com/library/radiology/chapter01.aspx (accessed January 24, 2022).

Philips. 2022. *Our history.* https://www.philips.com/a-w/about/our-history.html (accessed January 24, 2022).

PhRMA. 2020. *2020 Biopharmaceutical research industry profile.* https://phrma.org/-/media/Project/PhRMA/PhRMA-Org/PhRMA-Org/PDF/G-I/Industry-Profile-2020.pdf (accessed December 20, 2021).

Pollack, A. 2013. Astrazeneca makes a bet on an untested technique. *The New York Times,* March 21.

Rhea, S. 2007. US-Sino safety pact called 'modest start'. Experts say more must be done to ensure safe drug, medical device imports. *Modern Healthcare* 37(50):12-13.

Roche. 2022. *Roche milestones.* https://www.roche.com/about/history.htm (accessed January 24, 2022).

Sampson, T. 2016. Dynamic selection: An idea flows theory of entry, trade, and growth. *The Quarterly Journal of Economics* 131(1):315-380.

Sardella, A., and P. De Bona. 2021. *Safeguarding the United States pharmaceutical supply chain and policy considerations to mitigate shortages of essential medicines.* St. Louis: Washington University in St. Louis. https://wustl.app.box.com/s/wpqr6704f02eywivqsz7h1vfn8seb848 (accessed August 26, 2021).

Schondelmeyer, S. W., J. Seifert, D. J. Margraf, M. Mueller, I. Williamson, C. Dickson, D. Dasararaju, C. Caschetta, N. Senne, and M. T. Osterholm. 2020. Part 6: Ensuring a resilient us prescription drug supply. In *COVID-19: The CIDRAP viewpoint*, edited by J. Wappes. Minneapolis, MN: Regents of the University of Minnesota. https://www.cidrap.umn.edu/sites/default/files/public/downloads/cidrap-covid19-viewpoint-part1_0.pdf (accessed December 16, 2021).

Seaborn, A. 2013. *FDA imports overview—APO import forum.* FDA—Division of Import Operations. https://www.fda.gov/media/86269/download (accessed October 15, 2021).

Seligsohn, D., J. L. Ravelo, D. Russel, E. Uretsky, and E. Noor. 2021. *Will China be a global vaccine leader?* https://www.chinafile.com/conversation/will-china-be-global-vaccine-leader (accessed December 20, 2021).

Senate Committee on Finance. 2020. COVID-19 and beyond: Oversight of the FDA's foreign drug manufacturing inspection process: Congressional testimony of Judith A. McMeekin. June 2, 2020. https://www.fda.gov/news-events/congressional-testimony/covid-19-and-beyond-oversight-fdas-foreign-drug-manufacturing-inspection-process-06022020 (accessed January 25, 2022).

Seth, A. 2020. *India promotes domestic manufacturing of APIs to become 'self-reliant'.* https://generics.pharmaintelligence.informa.com/GB150106/India-Promotes-Domestic-Manufacturing-Of-APIs-To-Become-Self-Reliant (accessed January 18, 2022).

Siemens. 2022. *Our innovation legacy.* https://www.siemens-healthineers.com/company#innovation-legacy (accessed January 24, 2022).

Takeo, Y., and E. Urabe. 2020. Japan allocates $2.4 billion to beef up supply chains. *Bloomberg Law*, November 20.

Thiessen, M. 2020. It's time to practice social and economic distancing from China. *The Washington Post*, March 19.

Thomas, K., D. Gelles, and C. Zimmer. 2021. Pfizer's early data shows vaccine is more than 90% effective. *The New York Times.* https://www.nytimes.com/2020/11/09/health/covid-vaccine-pfizer.html (accessed February 15, 2022).

Trefler, D., D. Rodrik, and P. Antràs. 2005. Service offshoring: Threats and opportunities [with comments and discussion]. Paper read at Brookings trade forum.

Tubiana, M. 1996. Wilhelm Conrad Röntgen et la découverte des rayons X [Wilhelm Conrad Röntgen and the discovery of X-rays]. *Bulletin de L'Académie Nationale de Médecine* 180(1):97-108. French.

Vrontis, D., and M. Christofi. 2021. R&D internationalization and innovation: A systematic review, integrative framework and future research directions. *Journal of Business Research* 128:812-823.

Wee, R. Y. 2017. *Biggest pharmaceutical markets in the world by country.* https://www.worldatlas.com/articles/countries-with-the-biggest-global-pharmaceutical-markets-in-the-world.html (accessed January 23, 2022).

Weisman, R. 2013. Moderna in line for $240M licensing deal. *Boston Globe.*

The White House. 2020. *Combating public health emergencies and strengthening national security by ensuring essential medicines, medical countermeasures, and critical inputs are made in the United States.* https://www.federalregister.gov/documents/2020/08/14/2020-18012/combating-public-health-emergencies-and-strengthening-national-security-by-ensuring-essential (accessed December 20, 2021).

The White House. 2021. *Building resilient supply chains, revitalizing American manufacturing, and fostering broad-based growth: 100-day reviews under Executive Order 14017.* Washington, DC: Department of Commerce, Department of Energy, Department of Defense, and Department of Health and Human Services. https://www.whitehouse.gov/wp-content/uploads/2021/06/100-day-supply-chain-review-report.pdf (accessed October 20, 2021).

Woo, J., S. Wolfgang, and H. Batista. 2008. The effect of globalization of drug manufacturing, production, and sourcing and challenges for American drug safety. *Clinical Pharmacology and Therapeutics* 83(3):494-497.

WTO (The World Trade Organization). 1994. The WTO's pharma agreement. In *Trade topics.* The World Trade Organization. https://www.wto.org/english/tratop_e/pharma_ag_e/pharma_agreement_e.htm (accessed October 20, 2021).

WTO. 2020. *Trade in medical goods in the context of tackling COVID-19: Developments in the first half of 2020.* https://www.wto.org/english/tratop_e/covid19_e/medical_goods_update_e.pdf (accessed September 17, 2021).

Zwiefel, J. 2020. *Anticipated new phase in U.S. manufacturing.* https://info.burnsmcd.com/white-paper/pharma-onshoring (accessed December 20, 2021).

4

Causes and Consequences of Medical Product Supply Chain Failures

In preceding chapters, this report articulated an overarching goal of increasing the resilience of medical product supply chains and it described key characteristics of these supply chains. This chapter turns to the first step in identifying a strategy for achieving this goal, which is to understand why medical product supply chains fail. Medical product shortages can represent a significant threat across the landscape of public health and health care delivery by undermining the ability to provide timely and high-quality care to patients. This has been brutally clear in the context of the COVID-19 pandemic. However, long before COVID-19, medical product supply chains contended with a series of product shortages. The persistence of shortages in the United States and worldwide—caused by a confluence of complex factors—underscores the need to better understand the root causes and effects of shortages to inform more effective strategies to mitigate and protect against shortages, and respond to them when they do arise.

This chapter begins by outlining the mechanics of shortages in medical product supply chains and then explores the three main causes of shortages: demand surges, capacity reductions, and coordination failures. Finally, the chapter examines the effects of these shortages from the perspectives of patients, health care facilities and providers, and medical product manufacturers and suppliers. These discussions will provide the foundation for the development of the medical product supply chains resilience framework described in Chapter 5.

MECHANICS OF MEDICAL PRODUCT SUPPLY CHAIN FAILURES

As noted in Chapter 2, medical product supply chains facilitate the flow of medical products from raw material or component suppliers to producers to distributors to providers and finally to patients. See Figure 4-1 for a graphical representation of a typical supply chain under normal, nondisrupted conditions.

The field of supply chain management views a network like the one shown in Figure 4-1 as an end-to-end system, with the overarching goal of managing the flow of goods from the supplier to the end consumer through cooperation of the supply chain as a unified entity (Mentzer et al., 2001). However, it is rare to find supply chains for almost any product type that are contained entirely within a single vertically integrated organization. For medical products, the levels in Figure 4-1 are usually operated by separate entities—often with multiple entities at some levels. This means that supply chains are not centrally controlled systems but are instead distributed networks with multiple decision makers that have different objectives. This can lead to mismatches in supply and demand, even under normal conditions. The challenges presented by decentralization during

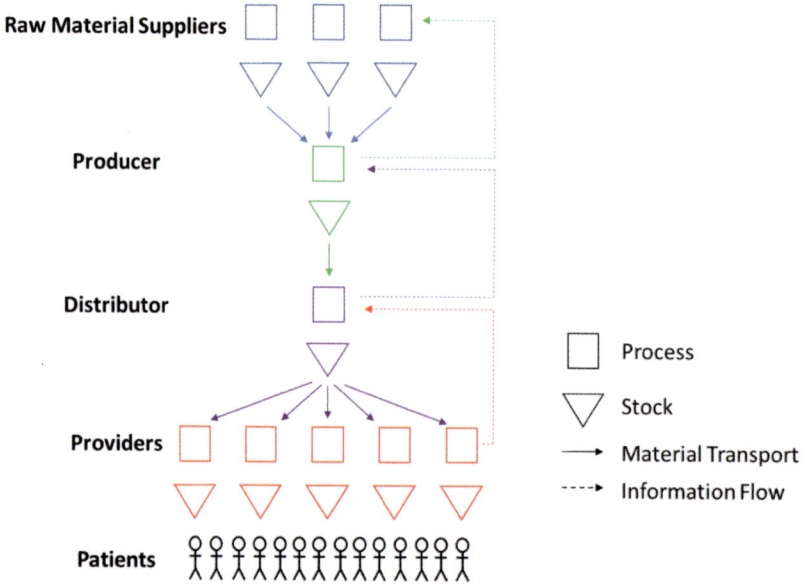

FIGURE 4-1 Simple schematic of a medical product supply chain under normal conditions.
SOURCE: Adapted from NASEM, 2020.

normal times become even greater when the supply chain is disrupted by a natural disaster, infectious disease outbreak, manufacturing process problem, or other event. At a high level, a disruptive event can cause a mismatch between supply and demand—a shortage—in medical product supply chains in three ways:

1. Demand surge: An event drives demand for a medical product well above the normal level for an extended period of time. For example, a major natural disaster, such as a tornado or earthquake, can spike regional demand for certain medical products if these events result in a significant number of casualties requiring medical care. As seen during COVID-19, a pandemic can drive up global demand for many medical products.
2. Capacity reduction: One or more production or transport processes are impeded by lack of assets, power, or people. For example, a natural disaster could cause a factory to lose power and halt production or regulatory barriers or manufacturing quality problems could restrict the output of a supplier or producer, and could even eliminate inventory stock if a product is recalled. As seen during the COVID-19 pandemic, production of some products may have decreased because of lockdown measures or the need for workers to quarantine or be on sick leave.
3. Coordination failure: Events that prevent supply from being matched to demand can cause shortages of medical products even when total supply is sufficient to meet total demand. For example, geopolitical issues or communication system failures during a hurricane or other natural disaster can reduce or obstruct the delivery of emergency supplies to the people that need them.

A central concept for describing the capacity of flow in a supply chain is a bottleneck. In general, bottleneck is the stage in a supply chain with the highest utilization (demand as a percentage of capacity) (Hopp, 2008). Under normal conditions, the bottlenecks in medical product supply chains can be the supply of raw materials, a production process of a supplier, a final assembly plant, or a distribution process. Under normal conditions, all stages of a supply chain, including the bottleneck, remain safely below 100 percent of capacity. However, an event that causes a demand surge or capacity reduction can push the use of one or more production or transport resources above 100 percent. A resource with use above 100 percent capacity is said to be *overloaded* (NASEM, 2020). When this happens, supply will not be able to keep up with demand. At first, this will cause stock levels at various points in the supply chain to decline. When this eventually depletes stock at the health care provider level, patients experience shortages (NASEM, 2020).[1]

Figure 4-2 illustrates a snapshot of a supply chain that is experiencing a shortage. In this scenario one of the raw material suppliers has become overloaded. This could be the result of a capacity reduction affecting that supplier, such as an earthquake damaging a facility or a manufacturing quality problem that has restricted shipments. It could also be the result of a demand surge that caused the supplier, which was already the bottleneck, to become overloaded. In either case, the bottleneck resource will define the overall capacity of the supply chain. If that capacity is insufficient to keep up with demand, patients will experience a shortage once any inventories in the supply chain are exhausted. Finally, note that Figure 4-2 indicates that some providers are experiencing shortages, while others are not. This could be the result of some nodes holding more buffer inventory or some receiving higher priority in the distribution of limited supplies.

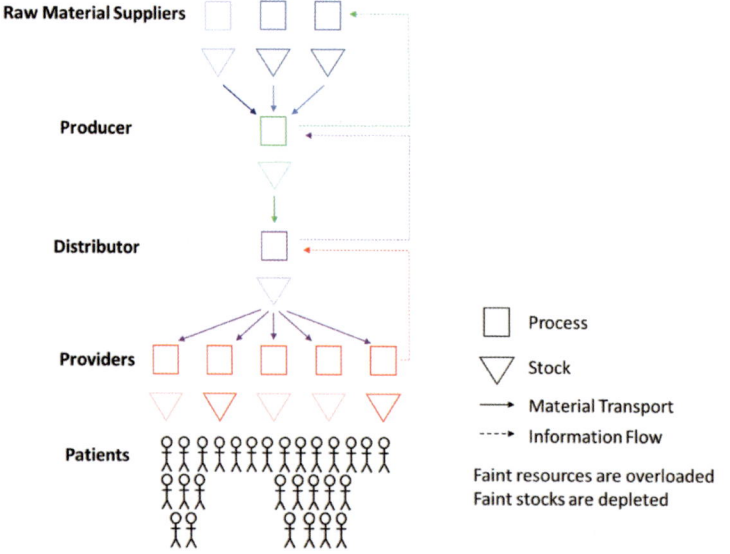

FIGURE 4-2 Schematic of a typical shortage found in a medical product supply chain.
SOURCE: Adapted from NASEM, 2020.

---

[1] Note that a disruptive event can cause the bottleneck to move. For example, under normal conditions, the bottleneck of a supply chain might be the final manufacturing step, which limits the amount of product that can be produced. However, if a fire damages a component plant, vastly reducing its output, this plant may become the bottleneck. Worse, it could become an overloaded bottleneck that prevents the entire supply chain from keeping up with demand.

It is important to note that disruptions can overlap and interact—demand surges and capacity reductions may occur simultaneously, or capacity reductions may precipitate subsequent demand increases and vice versa. Additionally, disruptions do not cause medical product supply chains to shift instantly from the normal conditions of Figure 4-1 to the shortages of Figure 4-2. Because all supply chains contain at least some amount of inventory, and because decision makers will take steps to increase capacity, such as run overtime shifts, in response to an impending shortage, it will take time for a disruption to turn into a shortage experienced by patients. Figure 4-3 gives a graphic illustration of how a capacity overload of a raw material supplier might propagate through the supply chain to affect patients as a shortage.

The time-phased nature of failures in medical product supply chains has important implications for building supply chain resilience. First, steps that increase the time from a disruption to a product shortage may help avoid shortages altogether; for example, if the length of the disruption is shorter than the timeframe covered by the inventory held in the supply chain, then inventory provides a buffer against a shortage. Second, even if a shortage does occur, inventory buffers delay the shortage from reaching patients and thereby provide time to execute contingency plans and response measures to protect patients. Chapter 5 will build on these insights to create a medical product supply chains resilience framework. This chapter will first explore types of demand surges, capacity reductions, and coordination failures, along with examples of each (see Figure 4-4).

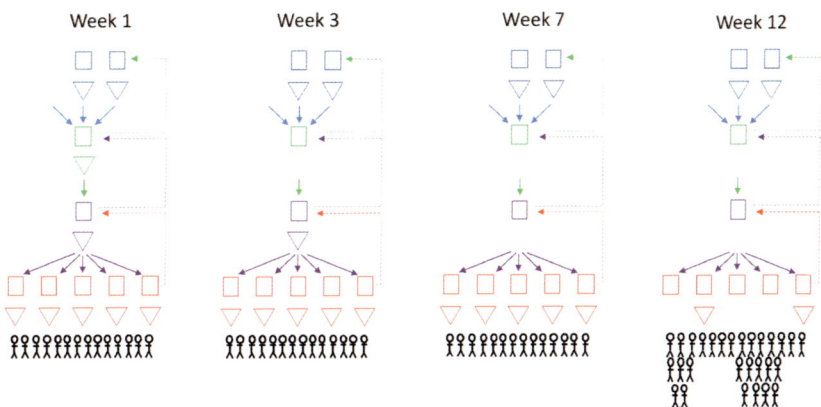

FIGURE 4-3 How shortages propagate through a medical product supply chain.
SOURCE: Adapted from NASEM, 2020.

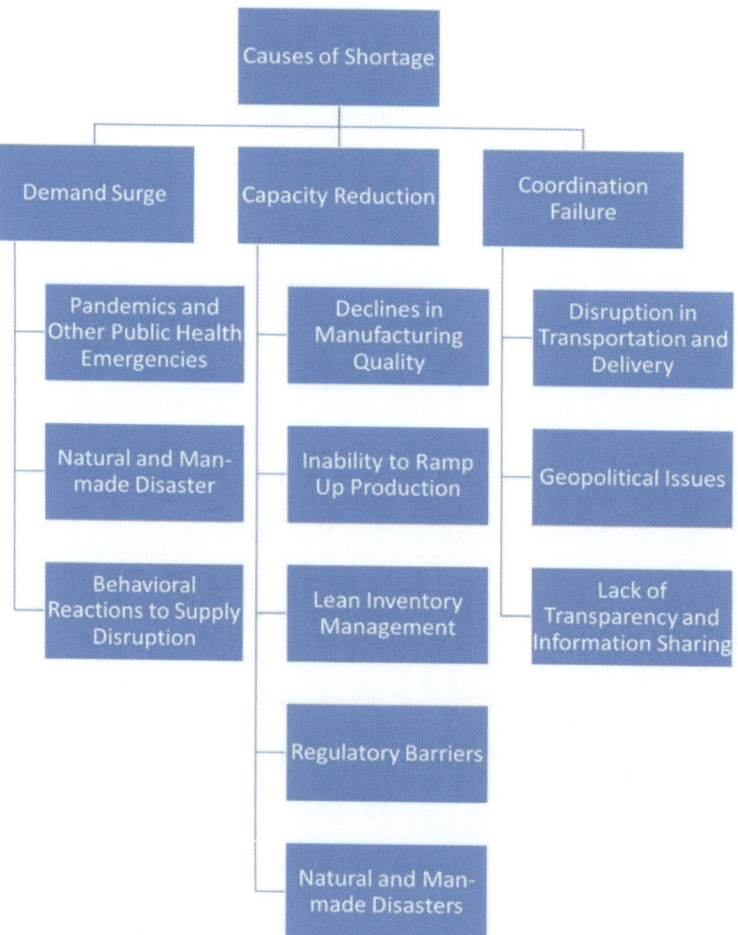

FIGURE 4-4 The three causes of shortages in medical product supply chains—demand surges, capacity reductions, and coordination failures—and examples of each.

DEMAND SURGES

When an event drives demand for a medical product well above the normal level for an extended period of time, a demand surge occurs. Whether a demand surge results in shortages or not depends on whether the various actors in the medical product supply chains have enacted mitigation and preparedness measures, such as hardening of the supply chain, building sufficient inventory or capacity buffers, and planning for contingencies (as will be discussed in detail in Chapter 5). Three types of events can cause demand surges: pandemics and other public health emergencies, natural and man-made disasters, and behavioral reactions to supply chain disruptions (FDA Drug Shortages Task Force, 2020; Socal et al., 2020).

Pandemics and Other Public Health Emergencies

As seen during the COVID-19 pandemic and previous infectious disease outbreaks, a pandemic or other public health emergency can severely strain medical resources at different levels—locally, regionally, nationally, and internationally—when the demand for health care services increases dramatically (IOM, 2009). The COVID-19 pandemic directly led to a demand surge for personal protection equipment (PPE), ventilators, and medications required for critical care (Ammar et al., 2021; Farrell et al., 2021; Ranney et al., 2020). Subsequent shortages led to intense competition for products in short supply, which in turn caused price increases and in some cases price gouging (Butler et al., 2020; Linskey et al., 2020). See Box 4-1 for a case study on the surge in demand for N95 masks. These shortages highlighted the effect of demand surges in the context of a major public health emergency (Schondelmeyer et al., 2020), the risks of having a single source for an item, the need to better manage supply risk, and the importance of end-to-end transparency across the supply chain (NASEM, 2021).

BOX 4-1
Case Study on N95 Masks

N95 respirators (N95) are face masks used in health care and construction settings, and in early 2020 they became one of the most important and in-demand tools in preventing the spread of COVID-19. An N95 forms a tight seal around the face and filters 95 percent of airborne particles larger than 0.3 microns (CDC, 2021a). The filters in N95 masks are made from nonwoven polypropylene, which is made by melting plastic pellets to create a liquid that is blown through perforated metal; this creates filaments that form a dense mat of fibers known as meltblown (Clark, 2021). An electrostatic charge is then added to help capture particles, and the filter is sealed between two protective layers (Clark, 2021). N95s are a generic product, and specifications and regulations differ between manufacturers and industries. The performance of N95s used in health care settings must meet criteria set by both the U.S. Food and Drug Administration (FDA) and the National Institute for Occupational Safety and Health (NIOSH).

Prior to the COVID-19 pandemic, about 50 percent of the world's supply of N95s came from China and the average cost of an N95 was $1 or less (Bradsher and Alderman, 2020; Clark, 2021; Hufford, 2020a). Within the United States, 10 companies made N95 masks domestically, accounting for 10 percent of the American supply (Evstatieva 2021).

continued

BOX 4-1 Continued

Inventory and Stockpiling

At the start of the pandemic, there were reported to be 12 million medical grade N95s in the Strategic National Stockpile, compared to an estimated need of 3.5 billion for a year-long pandemic (Goodnough, 2020). One reason for this gap was because 85 million N95s were used in 2009 during the H1N1 outbreak and were not replaced (Khazan, 2020). States, local jurisdictions, and hospitals sometimes maintain their own stockpiles of N95s. Although hospitals typically keep some level of surge inventories, these are typically small owing to just-in-time inventory control practices (Khazan, 2020). California created a state stockpile in 2006 that included 51 million N95s (Brunell, 2020). However, that stockpile was dismantled in 2011 because of a budget deficit, and the supplies were sold or donated to hospitals and local health departments (Brunell, 2020).

Demand Surge During the COVID-19 Pandemic

When COVID-19 initially spread in China in February 2020, China began importing and receiving donations of millions of N95s (Bradsher and Alderman, 2020) and PPE exports to the United States fell by 20 percent (Evans, 2020). Manufacturers with facilities in China, including 3M and the Medicom Group, were temporarily banned from sending N95s outside of China and instead were forced to sell to local governments (Evstatieva, 2021; Hufford and Evans, 2020). While China was able to ramp up production quickly, it did not immediately return to exporting PPE at prepandemic levels (Bradsher and Alderman, 2020). As COVID-19 spread throughout the United States, demand for N95s surged. Health systems were unable to purchase enough masks and other PPE, resulting in a severe and enduring shortage (Parshley, 2020).

Efforts to Reduce Demand

Faced with a huge shortage, health systems across the country quickly pivoted from single use to reuse with sterilization between uses. Ad hoc sterilization procedures, ranging from storage in a paper bag for 3–4 days to steaming or boiling and air-drying emerged. In July 2020, FDA issued multiple Emergency Use Authorizations (EUAs) for decontamination systems, such as vaporized hydrogen peroxide, ethylene oxide, and ultraviolet light (Chaudhuri, 2020) that facilitated N95 reuse (Hufford, 2020b), and also permitted their use beyond the expiration date (FDA, 2021b). By enabling reuse for up to 20 to 30 cycles of open-room processing, these policies reduced demand to far below what it would have been without them.

Efforts to Increase Supply

In addition to moderating demand, the government and private firms made efforts to increase supply. NIOSH allowed nonmedical N95 masks to be used in health care settings (Goodnough, 2020), with the federal government assuming liability on behalf of the companies (AMA, 2020). NIOSH also began issuing EUAs in March 2020 to allow the use of certain non-NIOSH approved respirators from countries with similar standards to those in the United States (FDA, 2021b).

Some American manufacturers, such as 3M, Honeywell, and Prestige America, were able to increase production in the United States (Evstatieva, 2021; Hufford and Evans, 2020). The federal government placed an order for 500 million N95s in March, to be delivered over 18 months, as a means to spur domestic production (Goodnough, 2020). In his first use of the Domestic Production Act, in April 2020 President Trump directed 3M to produce N95s for the Federal Emergency Management Agency (FEMA), to stop exporting them to Canada and Latin America, and to import more from foreign factories. 3M did not cease exporting N95s under existing contracts (Jacobsen, 2020).

Some manufacturers, however, were initially reluctant to ramp up N95 production in the early weeks of the pandemic. Manufacturer Prestige Ameritech ramped up production during the 2009 H1N1 influenza pandemic, and was left with excess product when that demand suddenly disappeared. The company did eventually ramp up their production in response to demand during the COVID-19 pandemic, but initial delays slowed efforts to increase the available supply of masks after they secured multiyear contracts (Noguchi, 2021).

The lack of a national online PPE clearinghouse meant that the federal government, states, hospitals, and individuals were all competing with one another for supplies. Among the many problems this created, small clinics and nursing homes could not compete with hospitals for PPE (Weber and Kaiser Health News, 2020). There were unclear criteria for federal shipments to states or reasons for intermittent interventions into shipments procured by state and local governments were absent (Linskey et al., 2020). There were numerous reports of FEMA rerouting shipments (Butler et al., 2020). As a result of the confusion, price gouging occurred (Butler et al., 2020).

As new companies entered the market, some had difficulty matching their supply to meet demand. Restrictions on sales and advertising on sites including Facebook and Google, and restrictions on Amazon, prevented companies from reaching consumers (Jacobs, 2021; Sathya, 2021).

Ad hoc efforts were made to improve transparency in the N95 market. For example, a group of emergency physicians created a website, GetUsPPE, in March 2020 to track and attempt to fill PPE needs of health care workers (Sathya, 2021). States such as California developed their own clearinghouses for PPE (California ACEP, 2021), and the Strategic National Stockpile has its own information technology system (King, 2020).

By spring 2021, the available supply of N95s increased sufficiently that the Centers for Disease Control and Prevention stopped recommending crisis capacity strategies including reuse of masks (CDC, 2021b).

Natural and Man-Made Disasters

Natural disasters—such as fires, floods, earthquakes, and hurricanes—and man-made disasters—such as war and bioterrorism—have the potential to cause demand surges for health care services that overwhelm local and regional medical and public health systems as well as the capacity of medical product supply chains (IOM, 2009). Even prior to the COVID-19 pandemic, there were shortages of N95 masks and air filters in areas where wildfire smoke caused poor air quality (CBS News, 2018). In 2011, a tsunami triggered by an earthquake off the coast of Japan led to a surge in demand for basic food items, blankets, sanitary pads, diapers, and toilet paper (Cavallo et al., 2014). Disasters are major disruptions to the supply chain, so without adequate preparedness and planning measures in place, demand surges can quickly turn into shortages.

Behavioral Reactions to Supply Disruption

Behaviors such as hoarding and panic buying can create demand surges and exacerbate existing supply disruptions. Hoarding can be both a result of a shortage and increase the likelihood that a disruption will become a shortage (Childs, 2019; Fox and McLaughlin, 2018). During a shortage, hoarding by institutions or individuals may be driven by concerns about maintaining or acquiring an adequate supply of products, particularly if there is a lack of awareness and transparency about the severity of the shortage, its expected duration, and any ongoing mitigation strategies. A national survey of more than 700 hospital pharmacy managers looked at rationing practices during shortages at U.S. hospitals. Eighty one percent of respondents reported using hoarding of the available supply of a drug in shortage as a mitigation strategy (Hantel et al., 2019). In turn, hoarding exacerbates a shortage by making the product unavailable for others, which can result in black and gray markets that can be counterproductive and potentially dangerous. Furthermore, frequent updates to clinical guidance and touting of potential treatments during a public health emergency can make demand difficult to predict (Callaway Kim et al., 2021). For example, the 2001 anthrax attacks led to a demand surge attributable to panic buying of ciprofloxacin (Weschsler, 2001). The ciprofloxacin shortage was not caused by widespread medical use of the drug to treat anthrax victims, it was the result of panic buying and limits on expanded production owing to intellectual property rights (Herper, 2001). See Box 4-2 for an additional example of health care providers hoarding saline solutions as a response to, and an exacerbation of, an existing shortage.

BOX 4-2
Case Study on Saline

Saline solutions are intravenous (IV) solutions made from low molecular weight salts or sugars used to maintain or replace fluids and electrolytes, and to carry medications into the bloodstream (Ward, 2019). IV solutions come in a variety of sizes, and a large hospital can use hundreds to thousands of IV bags each day (Armour and Burton, 2018; Mazer-Amirshahi and Fox, 2018). Though their components are simple, IV solutions are complex to manufacture, because they need to be both sterile and free from particulate matter (Mazer-Amirshahi and Fox, 2018). Manufacturing each batch of saline requires carrying out 29 steps over 10 days and includes 350 regulatory checks (Fry, 2015). In addition, the weight and size of saline bags makes them expensive to ship via air (Mazer-Amirshahi and Fox, 2018) and difficult to stockpile (Lee, 2014; Weber, 2018).

Market Concentration

Approximately 43 to 44 percent of the IV solutions in the United States are manufactured in Puerto Rico by Baxter, which holds the largest share of the U.S. market (AEP, 2018; Armour and Burton, 2018; CBS News, 2017; Wendelbo and Blackburn, 2018). Two other manufacturers, Hospira Inc (now ICU Medical) and B. Braun Medical, are the second and third largest suppliers in the United States, and both have manufacturing plants in the mainland United States (Armour and Burton, 2018; Palmer, 2019).

In early 2017, the U.S. Department of Justice launched an investigation into possible collusion among IV solution manufacturers and whether this affected pricing and shortages (Armour and Burton, 2018). This investigation has been closed with an unknown outcome (Raymond, 2019). As of 2019, Baxter and Hospira still faced a class-action lawsuit related to accusations of price fixing (Langreth and Koons, 2017; Raymond, 2019).

Capacity Reductions

Beginning in the 2013-2014 flu season, an increased demand for IV saline and several product recalls caused by poor manufacturing quality led to shortages (Fry, 2015; Lee, 2014; Wendelbo and Blackburn, 2018). The contaminations were severe, sickening and even causing patient deaths (Caspi, 2015; Sacks et al., 2018). Three months prior to Hurricane Maria, B. Braun Medical announced a supply disruption (Armour and Burton, 2018). It had been previously warned by FDA because of quality problems in its bags, such as leaky and moldy IV bags, and violations of good manufacturing practices (Armour and Burton, 2018; Langreth and Koons, 2017).

In September 2017, Puerto Rico was hit by Hurricane Maria, shutting down the electrical grid and damaging roads, the fuel supply, and airports (AEP, 2018). Baxter's plants lost power and were shut down (CBS News, 2017); power was not fully restored until January 2018 (NASEM, 2020). In the immediate aftermath, FDA helped manufacturers secure generators and fuel for plants and coordinated with the local government to help clear roads and secure transportation for raw ingredients (Paavola, 2017). To help address the shortage, FDA allowed Baxter to import products from other countries like Mexico, Ireland, and Australia (Paavola,

continued

> BOX 4-2 Continued
>
> 2017). FDA also approved saline products from two additional manufacturers (Mazer-Amirshahi and Fox, 2018) and considered extending expiration dates for available supply (Sacks et al., 2018; Scutti, 2018). However, there was not enough extra capacity in the industry to make up for the disruption in supply caused by the hurricane (Armour and Burton, 2018).
>   At the time, Baxter supplied 50 percent of U.S. hospitals with small volume saline bags (250 ml or less) (Langreth and Koons, 2017; Mazer-Amirshahi and Fox, 2018), and the shortage primarily affected the 0.9 percent saline injection bags, as their larger volume bags (0.5 and 1 liter) were not made in Puerto Rico (Scutti, 2018). The delivery delays caused by the hurricane were compounded by a bad 2017-2018 flu season (Wendelbo and Blackburn, 2018), and the planned shutdown of the three main manufacturers for maintenance before the end of the year (CBS News, 2017; Lee, 2014). The shortage was then worsened when some providers began hoarding IV bags, and hospitals were forced to delay elective procedures (Armour and Burton, 2018). After Hurricane Maria, Baxter invested $1 billion in its manufacturing network and now ships finished product to the U.S. mainland for storage, instead of storing it in Puerto Rico (Edney, 2020).

CAPACITY REDUCTIONS

A capacity reduction occurs when one or more production or transport processes are impeded by lack of assets, power, or people. Capacity reductions can arise at any part of the supply chain, including raw material production, component production, final assembly, and transportation (FDA Drug Shortages Task Force, 2020). Each of these steps can be disrupted by factors such as declines in manufacturing quality, inability to ramp up production, lean inventory management practices, regulatory barriers, and natural and man-made disasters.

Declines in Manufacturing Quality

The single biggest cause of drug product supply chain disruptions under routine conditions is a failure to maintain manufacturing quality, according to an analysis by FDA (FDA Drug Shortages Task Force, 2020). The 2020 update of the FDA Drug Shortages Report found that quality problems are responsible for 62 percent of the drugs that went into shortage between 2013 and 2017. Declines in quality are often attributable to factors such as the use of older facilities, the introduction of new products that require companies to share production facilities, contracting practices that lead to poor oversight, and increased price competition (Woodcock and Wosinska, 2013). In a market with a small number of manufacturers, a capacity reduction or market exit by a single manufacturer due to quality problems places pressure on the other manufacturers to fill the gap in supply, which they may not be able to do (Childs, 2019). Furthermore, the market currently does not recognize or incentivize robust quality management systems. The entry of low-cost competitors can cause a ripple effect that affects established manufacturers and ultimately forces some of them to exit the market because of price decreases (Childs, 2019).

Declines in manufacturing quality and consequent supply disruptions occur frequently among generic manufacturers—particularly disruptions at the finished dosage level. Generic drugs administered by injection are the most common products in shortages, largely because there are fewer manufacturers of these drugs and because the manufacturers that do produce them typically operate at full capacity, making it difficult to respond to and recover from disruptions (Fox and McLaughlin, 2018). Box 4-3 provides a case study of the anticoagulant heparin, which illustrates how quality issues led to both direct and indirect health effects owing to a supply shortage. This case also highlights difficulties in monitoring and regulating quality in global supply chains and some challenges and successes in both diversifying and on-shoring supplies.

All manufacturers must adhere to FDA's current good manufacturing practice regulations, which include "minimum requirements for methods, facilities, and controls used in manufacturing, processing, and packing of a drug product" (FDA, 2020a). Buyers, therefore, assume the product is safe for use and contains the ingredients at the strength it claims to have and do not distinguish between the quality of any given generic drug. As a result, the market does not reward for production quality. Without a price premium for quality, and with low margins that minimize the value of protecting continuity of supply, generic manufacturers typically do not invest enough in quality systems or equipment modernization to prevent quality failures.

The expansion of multiple foreign manufacturing sites presents new challenges in FDA's work to ensure the quality and safety of imported products entering the domestic market (Woo et al., 2008). To address these challenges, FDA relies on a number of measures to ensure quality and safety of medical products in facilities around the world including preapproval inspections, surveillance inspections, and for-case inspections.[2] FDA also relies on automated systems to screen import shipments of drugs, biologics, and medical devices at the U.S. port of entry for compliance with regulatory requirements. These electronic systems review import entries and flag products that may require additional information, a physical exam, or sample analysis (FDA, 2017).

The lack of visibility into the quality of the manufacturing processes used for medical products, and therefore the quality of the products them-

---

[2] Information given by testimony of Judith A. McMeekin (Senate Committee on Finance, 2020).

BOX 4-3
Case Study on Heparin

Heparin is the most widely used nonoral anticoagulant in the United States (McCarthy et al., 2020). Unfractionated heparin is given intravenously, often during surgery or hemodialysis, to treat blood clots. Heparin can also be given subcutaneously to prevent blood clots in hospitalized patients and is also used to coat certain medical devices, including stents (Fareed et al., 2019; McCarthy et al., 2020; The PEW Health Group, 2011).

Originally approved in 1959, heparin was manufactured from bovine lung tissue for 50 years until bovine spongiform encephalopathy (BSE) appeared in cows in the United Kingdom in the late 1980s (Szajek et al., 2015). Fears of transmitting prion diseases to patients led heparin manufacturers to withdraw bovine heparin from the market in the late 1990s. Currently, only porcine heparin is approved for use in the United States (Szajek et al., 2015).

Heparin Shortages

China produces 80 percent of the worldwide supply of heparin (McCarthy et al., 2020) and 60 percent of the U.S. supply (Szajek et al., 2015). In 2007, an outbreak of porcine reproductive and respiratory syndrome or "blue-ear pig disease" in Asia caused widespread loss of herds (Cha, 2007; McCarthy et al., 2020), severely reducing the capacity of the heparin supply chain and causing a shortage (McCarthy et al., 2020). The price of heparin doubled between May and November 2007 (The PEW Health Group, 2011).

In late 2007 and into early 2008, CDC and FDA received reports of allergic reactions in dialysis patients correlated with heparin use (Kishimoto et al., 2008; McCarthy et al., 2020). It was revealed that heparin contaminated with oversulfated chondroitin sulfate (OSCS) had entered the United States from China. OSCS also acts as an anticoagulant and is 100 times cheaper to produce than crude heparin, and was likely added in an attempt to capitalize on high prices and meet demand during the shortage (Usdin, 2009; Vilanova et al., 2019). The contamination resulted in over 80 deaths and an additional 800 serious adverse events in the United States (Kishimoto et al., 2008; Le et al., 2018; McCarthy et al., 2020; Vilanova et al., 2019). Fifteen companies worldwide recalled 11 drug products and 72 medical devices (The PEW Health Group, 2011). Elective surgeries were canceled to conserve heparin supply as regulators determined the extent of the contamination, in an attempt to reduce demand for the product (Zhu et al., 2019).

OSCS was initially not detected by standard testing assays, as it mimics some of heparin's chemical properties, highlighting gaps in testing protocols at the time. OSCS was likely introduced during crude heparin consolidation, as it was eventually identified in the crude material supplied to the producer, but the source of the adulteration was never confirmed. Standard heparin testing now includes screening for OSCS (The PEW Health Group, 2011).

Swine flu outbreaks continue to cause heparin shortages. An outbreak of the African swine flu in Europe and Asia in 2018 caused the loss of about half of China's swine breeding herds and led to shortages (Fareed et al., 2019; Patton, 2021), and another outbreak in the first quarter of 2021 resulted in shortages over the summer (Patton, 2021).

Barriers to FDA Oversight

In addition to the effect of widespread illnesses in Chinese swine herds, the current heparin supply chain is also challenged by its complexity and the difficulty of inspecting manufacturing facilities abroad. At the time of the OSCS crisis, it was very difficult (if not impossible) to trace a given batch of heparin to a specific pig farm, although some Chinese suppliers claimed to be able to do so (Fairclough and Burton, 2008).

Consolidators collect crude heparin lots, combine them, and sell them to manufacturers (or to brokers to sell to manufacturers) to produce active pharmaceutical ingredients (APIs) (Fareed et al., 2019; GAO, 2010). In China, not all heparin makers are overseen by drug regulators, because some are registered as chemical makers, as was the case for the site implicated in the 2008 crisis (Fairclough and Burton, 2008; The PEW Health Group, 2011).

The API in the tainted heparin, sold by Baxter Healthcare, was both manufactured in the United States by Scientific Protein Laboratories and sourced from a Chinese company (Usdin, 2009; Zhu et al., 2019). Although approved to produce APIs for the U.S. market, the Chinese manufacturer had not been inspected by FDA because of a clerical error, although an inspection would not have prevented subsequent OSCS contamination (The PEW Health Group, 2011; Usdin, 2009). During its investigation of the contaminated heparin, FDA was denied access to some facilities in China (The PEW Health Group, 2011). The inspection eventually uncovered multiple violations of current good manufacturing practices (Usdin, 2009).

Attempts to Diversify and Increase the Supply of Heparin

The global pig supply is geographically limited, and there do not appear to be viable options to expand porcine heparin manufacturing to other locations (Szajek et al., 2015). One way to diversify the heparin supply chain is to reintroduce bovine heparin to the market. FDA is encouraging applications from bovine heparin manufacturers, though there are challenges that come with this approach (FDA, 2019a; Szajek et al., 2015).

Bovine heparin was used in Brazil until 2013, and 70 percent of Argentina's heparin comes from cows (Szajek et al., 2015). No known cases of BSE have ever been linked to heparin, as this risk is tightly managed through measures related to tissue harvesting and chemical processing (Szajek et al., 2015). Having both porcine- and bovine-derived heparin on the market may carry safety risks, however. Bovine heparin is less potent by weight, so a larger dose must be given to achieve the same effect as a lower dose of porcine heparin (Szajek et al., 2015). Accidental misdosing may be responsible for the increase in adverse events seen in Brazil when bovine heparin was introduced on short notice in Brazil in 2008, leading to its removal from the market in Brazil in 2013 (Szajek et al., 2015). Heparin can also be extracted from other animals including sheep, camels, chickens, turkeys, and salmon though the efficiency in production and efficacy of the product varies widely across species (van der Meer et al., 2017). There have been efforts to bioengineer heparin, but it has been challenging to scale up manufacturing while keeping costs down (Westly, 2011; Zhu et al., 2019).

Some efforts have also been made to on-shore the heparin supply chain. Civica Rx is a nonprofit pharmaceutical company formed by a group of health care systems that contracts with generic drug manufacturers to produce drugs in short supply, including heparin (Marsa, 2020). Civica Rx and its manufacturing partner Hikma were not affected by the most recent swine flu outbreaks because their supply of raw materials was sourced from a geographic location different from where the outbreak occurred (CivicaRx, 2019).

selves, prevents the market from rewarding quality manufacturers, and causes supply disruptions and shortages (FDA Drug Shortages Task Force, 2020). The committee's examination of quality-related shortages highlights important observations that must be included in thinking about how to make medical product supply chains safer and more resilient: *For nearly a decade, analyses have found that quality problems are responsible for a majority of the drugs that go into shortage. As a result, there have been repeated calls for a robust and mature quality management system to ensure consistent and reliable drug manufacturing and quality performance. However, there is still no such system and the quality problems persist. Purchasers of medical products lack access to sourcing and quality information, which limits their ability to incorporate supply chain resilience when making contracting, purchasing, and inventory decisions.*

Counterfeit Medical Products

Counterfeiting, or the proliferation of substandard or falsified medical products, is also a challenge with a globalized supply chain. The complex, and at times circuitous, distribution routes that medical products follow from manufacturer to patient can lead to unregistered/unlicensed, substandard, and falsified (SF) medicines entering the market (The PEW Health Group, 2011). Diverted, stolen, or counterfeited medical products may make their way to American consumers from both domestic and foreign sources (The PEW Health Group, 2011). The American market is particularly vulnerable to the entrance of SF medical products during shortages, when wholesalers and distrubtors may exchange products multiple times, complicating the tracability of the products and raising concerns about the authenticity and quality of the medical products being sold (Rockefeller et al., 2012).

Counterfeiting in the global supply chain is more than a safety issue; it can become a national security issue if individuals introduce counterfeit drugs into the supply chain with the intention to cause harm (Marucheck et al., 2011). For instance, if a counterfeit drug contains contaminated components, it can cause serious harm beyond the lack of therapeutic effect (Bos, 2009). While the World Health Organization's (WHO's) Global Surveillance and Monitoring System[3] for SF medical products maintains a database of suspected and validated SF reports, the data cannot be extrapolated to country-specific prevalence because regulatory authorities are not always willing, able, or incentivized to report the incidents (NASEM, 2021). One option to address counterfeiting used for pharmaceuticals is serialization, whereby individual drug units are assigned unique identification numbers. This allows

---

[3] WHO Global Surveillance and Monitoring System is available at https://www.who.int/who-global-surveillance-and-monitoring-system (accessed January 19, 2022).

for tracking the product, authenticating the product within the distribution chain, as well as identifying counterfeits (Pascu et al., 2020). However, in order for such a system to be successful for globalized supply chains, coordination between international health authorities, such as the World Health Organization, and regional or national authorities is crucial to maintaining the integrity and transparency of supply chains (Pascu et al., 2020).

Inability to Ramp Up Production

Manufacturers' inability to quickly ramp up production is a factor that compounds capacity disruptions. Manufacturers may face multiple barriers to ramping up production in response to intermittent supply disruptions (NASEM, 2021). For most companies, maintaining standing capacity to ramp up production rapidly is neither logistically nor financially feasible. Generic drug manufacturing, in particular, is a low-margin business that does not allow for idle capacity. If a competitor experiences a supply disruption or demand surge, there will likely be insufficient excess capacity available for other manufacturers to increase production to fill the gap, as was the case during a 2010 propofol shortage (FiercePharma, 2010; Jensen and Rappaport, 2010; Woodcock and Wosinska, 2013).

Additional factors that limit the ability of manufacturers to ramp up production can include operational and regulatory risks as well as packaging and labeling capacity (Jung, 2020). Operational delays may include limits on production, constraints on plant or shipping capacity, and problems with transportation and distribution. Particularly if the disruption is caused by a disaster or public health emergency, operational risks could include human resource deficits (e.g., absenteeism), restrictions of work shift capacity that limit output, or constraints in certain parts of supply chains (e.g., cold-chain storage), especially if multiple manufacturers are attempting to ramp up production to meet demand signal fluctuations (Jung, 2020). Among the potential regulatory risks that manufacturers may face when increasing production are facility inspection delays for new products, generics, and biosimilars, which can lead to longer approval times, as well as inspection requirements following importation (Jung, 2020). The packaging and labeling needed to contain, transport, distribute, and administer products often relies on foreign sources for components, such as resin-based bottles and films, paper cartons and labels, and stainless steel needles. If those components are not consistently available, it can contribute to disruptions in the supply of the finished product (Jung, 2020). Furthermore, decisions to manufacture a new product or ramp up production of an existing product can force companies to make production trade-offs if they are already operating at full capacity, as many generic manufacturers do.

Manufacturers may also have other reasons not to increase their manufacturing capacity during a shortage. For example, after the 2009 H1N1 influenza pandemic, when the mask manufacturer Prestige Ameritech ramped up production during the emergency, they were left with excess product and financial problems when demand suddenly disappeared. Consequently, the company was initially reluctant to ramp up N95 production during the early weeks of the COVID-19 pandemic. The company did eventually install several new mask-making machines and secured investments and multiyear contracts from facilities to make additional masks, which enabled them to ramp up production significantly (Noguchi, 2021).

The above observations lead the committee to conclude that *manufacturers often lack incentives to maintain surge capacity in their supply chains, as it is neither financially nor logistically feasible. This limits the ability of supply chain managers to react to disruptions and leads to shortages.*

Lack of Investment in Modern Technology

The use of outdated technology is common in medical product manufacturing, and it contributes to manufacturers' ability to ramp up production. It also introduces product errors that can subsequently lead to shortages. While other industries typically function at an error rate below 3.4 defects per million opportunities, the pharmaceutical manufacturing industry operates at a rate of around 66,000 defects per million opportunities—owing in part to out-of-date manufacturing processes (Woodcock and Kopcha, 2020). Public and private investment in advanced manufacturing is needed to improve the reliability of medical products and reduce the opportunity for quality defects.

Advanced manufacturing techniques, such as continuous manufacturing, and additive manufacturing, such as 3D printing, can improve product quality and address shortages (FDA, 2021a). However, a survey of medical product manufacturers, conducted by Manufacturing x Digital (MxD) and the International Academy of Automation Engineering (IAAE), found that surveyed manufacturers largely still relied on manual, paper-based processes and were only just beginning to advance to more automated and integrated process stages (MxD and IAAE, 2021).

The committee concludes that *advanced manufacturing techniques can improve product quality and reliability, thereby addressing frequent causes of shortages. However, medical product manufacturers have little incentive to harden supply chains through updated techniques, processes, and controls that promote reliability and quality in medical products.* The medical product industry will likely require additional incentives to spur investment in updated manufacturing technologies that promote reliability. Namely, health systems will need information regarding products' manufacturing processes to provide manufacturers the incentive to invest in quality.

Lean Inventory Management

Lean inventory management practices can lead to capacity reductions and increase the risk of medical product shortages. It is common practice among manufacturers, distribution centers, and health care organizations to use a just-in-time (JIT) inventory management system (Fox and McLaughlin, 2018). In many cases, JIT leads to smaller inventory levels across the supply chain, which, as illustrated in Figure 4-3, reduces the time it takes for a shortage to reach patients and thereby makes shortages more likely to occur. Lean practices are an example of policies that optimize profits under normal conditions but can also make supply chains less able to respond to disruptions and emergencies. A lack of transparency of inventory practices across supply chain actors and regulators further compounds these challenges (NASEM, 2018). Lean systems are especially vulnerable during major disruptions caused by a natural disaster or public health emergency (NASEM, 2020). The committee therefore concludes that *market forces incentivize lean inventory management in medical product manufacturing and ordering, which limits the ability of the health care system to withstand shortages and increases the likelihood that shortages will affect patients.*

Regulatory Barriers

In 2020, the FDA Drug Shortages Task Force found that logistical and regulatory challenges can make market recovery difficult following a supply disruption (FDA Drug Shortages Task Force, 2020). Furthermore, as drug supply chains have become more complex, it has become increasingly difficult for manufacturers to respond to shortages because of additional regulations involved, gaps in API procurement, and FDA application requirements for new market entry (FDA Drug Shortages Task Force, 2020). If U.S. medical product supply chains depend heavily upon a few manufacturers, and one manufacturer exits the market, there can be a significant time lag before a new manufacturer can enter the market and increase the available supply. FDA is taking steps to bring greater efficiency to the generic drug review process and respond to shortages. For example, when a shortage is reported, FDA can expedite review of new production lines or new raw material sources. The agency can also consider extending the expiration date for a product experiencing shortage if expired stock is available (FDA, 2013) and thereby increase the available supply. FDA has also taken steps to expedite the development and marketing of generic drug products. For example, in 2019 the agency announced a process to expedite U.S. Pharmacopeial Convention small molecule monograph updates (FDA, 2019b). However, the approval of a new manufacturer can still take 1 to 2 years (FDA, 2021a; Sullivan, 2018).

Other forms of regulation can also lead to unintended capacity reductions in medical product supply chains. In 2019, the firm Sterigenics closed a sterilization plant after the Illinois Environmental Protection Agency prohibited the firm from using the carcinogen ethylene oxide in its sterilization process because of the resulting chemical emissions from the plant (Goldberg, 2019). Closure of the plant severely reduced the total medical device sterilization capacity in the United States. The closure caused several devices to go into shortage (Crotti, 2019) and FDA warned that widespread shortages were possible (Maxwell, 2019). At the time of the closure, about 50 percent of devices requiring sterilization used ethylene oxide (Maxwell, 2019), and only 2 percent of those had an alternate validated sterilization method available for use (Lim, 2019). FDA is now working to advance innovation in ways to sterilize medical devices using lower levels of ethylene oxide and other currently available agents, and it is funding research into alternative sterilization techniques (FDA, 2020b).

Natural and Man-Made Disasters

In addition to causing demand surges, natural and manmade disasters can also cause capacity reductions. The past three decades have seen drug shortages result from natural disasters, either by affecting product availability, damaging production facilities, and/or creating unexpected demands for drugs needed to treat the injured (Fox et al., 2009). In 2017, for example, Hurricane Maria severely disrupted the production of medical use saline (NASEM, 2020). At the time, the majority of saline produced for the U.S. market was manufactured by a single firm, Baxter International, at three facilities in Puerto Rico. Hurricane Maria disrupted power at these facilities in September 2017, and power was not completely restored until January 2018. The 4-month supply disruption resulted in widespread saline shortages at hospitals in the United States throughout 2018 (NASEM, 2020). See Box 4-2 for a case study on saline, which illustrates the vulnerabilities created by concentrated production (even when that production is located on U.S. territory), how hoarding exacerbated the shortage, and the importance of being able to tap the global supply chain for backup supplies in an emergency.

COORDINATION FAILURE

A coordination failure leads to shortages of medical products when total supply is available to meet demand, but circumstances prevent the supply from being matched to the demand. Examples of coordination failures include disruption in transportation and delivery, geopolitical issues, and lack of transparency and information sharing. In addition to exacerbating shortages, coordination failures can also inhibit response and recovery.

Disruption in Transportation and Delivery

Particularly in emergency conditions, supply may be available but is unable to reach the people who need it because of challenges in transportation and delivery. This happens frequently in hurricanes and other natural disasters. When Hurricane Maria hit Puerto Rico in 2017, there was extensive damage to the electrical grid, roads, airports, and fuel supplies, disrupting delivery of raw materials and components to Baxter International's saline production facilities, halting their production lines and causing a shortage (AEP, 2018). Bottlenecks in shipping have caused widespread delays during the COVID-19 pandemic. The cost of a shipping container has quadrupled since 2020 (Page, 2021), and ports have been backed up, unable to load and unload items waiting to be shipped (Page, 2021). A survey of medical technology manufacturers revealed that over 70 percent of firms had experienced delays in their semiconductor supply chains (Murray and Bradley, 2021). Semiconductors are in high demand across many industries, and as a result, manufacturers are competing for the same supply. The Advanced Medical Technology Association appealed to the secretary of the Department of Commerce to help medical device manufacturers gain priority access to the limited supply (AdvaMed, 2021). Many medical products such as vaccines must be kept in temperature-controlled environments from the time they leave the production facility to the time they are delivered to patients. This poses particular challenges in transportation and delivery to rural and remote locations. This challenge was evident during the distribution of certain vaccines against COVID-19, but it has also been an ongoing challenge in delivering medical products around the globe for many decades (Lloyd and Cheyne, 2017; UNICEF, n.d.).

Geopolitical Issues

Geopolitical risks can arise because of the consequences of national politics or societal disruption and have the potential to prevent supply from reaching demand and causing a shortage. Political crises often occur due to the economic consequences of the domestic political milieu, legislative actions, or the instability of governments and other institutions, such as political transitions, corruption, policy shifts, inadequate law enforcement, societal conflict, and "buy national" policies (Cline et al., 2019, 2020). Foreign sources of supply could also become unavailable, not because of a deliberate strategic choice on the part of the government, but because that government's own ability to maintain order within its territory is somehow threatened. Societal disruption can arise when groups such as nongovernmental organizations, trade unions, and consumer bodies develop a collective political identity and engage in activism or activities—such as boycotts, protests, supply disruptions, or corporate espionage—that can affect manufacturing firms who are operating both nationally and transnationally (Cline et al., 2019, 2020).

Trade restrictions, a heavy reliance on foreign manufacturing in certain product classifications and areas, including APIs, and the inability to get foreign supply to the United States have been related to shortages during the COVID-19 pandemic (Mullen, 2020). Geopolitical tensions may also arise when a country limits access to raw or finished materials as a matter of deliberate strategic choice, as observed following the U.S. use of the Defense Production Act, thereby limiting access to materials. The drug supply chain is also increasingly vulnerable to cyberattacks by malicious geopolitical actors. These cybersecurity vulnerabilities justified the military's involvement in Operation Warp Speed as an effort to prevent the sabotage of critical infrastructure (Florko, 2020).

Extensive reliance on foreign sources for medical products, their key components, or even transportation could leave the United States vulnerable to the geopolitical and trade decisions of those nations. When seen through the lens of national security, other foreign actors could use these market concentrations to put undue influence on American policy makers when negotiating bilateral and multilateral agreements (NASEM, 2021). Although geopolitical issue-driven supply chain disruptions are rare and difficult to identify as the root cause of a shortage, the concern remains among lawmakers, federal agencies, and the private sector (Chalfant, 2017; DoD et al., 2021). Greater situational awareness to anticipate geopolitical shocks could support better recognition and response to emerging concerns.

Lack of Transparency and Information Sharing

Lack of transparency and information sharing is a coordination failure that has ramifications throughout supply chains, and is frequently highlighted as a major shortcoming in the current system. U.S. drug supply chain vulnerabilities are not sufficiently transparent to support timely management of drug shortages, which makes it "nearly impossible" to predict shortages (Schondelmeyer et al., 2020). See Box 4-3 for a case study on heparin, highlighting the dangerous consequences of a lack of transparency in a medical product supply chain. Similarly, there are also issues of transparency in medical device supply chains. For example, Dai and colleagues (2020) examined the past 5 years' financial disclosure of three major PPE manufacturers (3M Company, Honeywell International Inc., and MSA Safety Inc.) and conducted an exhaustive search of 2020 media reports about the PPE supply chain, and found no basic supply chain data, including, for example, the exact domestic versus foreign capacity of N95 masks. Basic PPE supply chain data (e.g., the production quantity in each facility) is treated as confidential and not disclosed to any government agency, the public, or the companies' shareholders.

As will be discussed in Chapter 6, many of the measures needed to address the medical product shortage problem in the United States will require a dramatic increase in transparency at every step of the supply chain, particularly regarding sourcing, quality, volume, and capacity information. Improved transparency and information sharing with FDA and other health authorities provides the means to mitigate and prepare for shortages (Tolomeo et al., 2020). For example, industry stakeholders identified limited market insights into future demand as a major issue in their ability to manage shortages (The PEW Charitable Trusts; International Society for Pharmaceutical Engineering, 2017). Companies reported being reluctant to invest in setting up additional manufacturing capacity to protect against shortages in the absence of accurate information about expected demand—particularly for low-volume, low-margin products. They suggested that insight into future demand could be improved through better management of internal operations such as sales and operations planning and demand forecasting, as well as better practices for sharing information about the market landscape, such as how long other manufacturers are expected to be out of the market.

Drug manufacturers, foreign or domestic, that wish to sell products in the United States must register with FDA and report limited information on what products are manufactured at specific facilities.[4] However, manufacturers are not required to report information such as the fraction of product produced at any given facility or the fraction of an API sourced from a particular supplier. The Coronavirus Aid, Relief, and Economic Security Act (CARES Act) improved upon previous reporting requirements by requiring manufacturers to report the amount of drug manufactured.[5] However, many gaps remain in FDA's ability to collect and analyze data in a timely manner to react to sudden disruptions and shortages (The White House, 2021). It is therefore not possible for FDA to identify when a supply chain is dangerously concentrated or otherwise vulnerable to disruption (The White House, 2021). It is also important to note that although FDA has these limited data from drug manufacturers, the agency receives very little information from medical device manufacturers on supply chain and shortages.

Transparency is an issue for regulatory agencies, manufacturers, and consumers as medical product supply chains become more global and the supply chain networks become more complex. Regardless of supply chain type (e.g., global versus domestic), there is little insight into the where and how of medical product manufacturing. In many cases, the specific factory,

---

[4] Information given by testimony of Janet Woodcock (House Committee on Energy and Commerce, 2019).
[5] CARES Act, 15 U.S.C. § 116-136.

or even the country in which the drug is produced, is kept confidential as proprietary information. Manufacturers are also hindered by lack of transparency into foreign sources of API and other components. A disruption that affects a single API manufacturer could create a major problem by halting production across multiple finished dosage form (FDF) manufacturers. If a manufacturer needs to find a new API source—either to increase production or because of a disrupted supply from another API source—it can be challenging to find a foreign API source that complies with global regulatory requirements (FDA Drug Shortages Task Force, 2020). FDA compiles lists of approved API suppliers and recently inspected API manufacturing facilities.[6] However, the agency does not provide a centralized source of information about API suppliers. Consumers have even less information about the sources of drugs and devices. In the case of prescription drugs sold in the United States, labels are not required to disclose the identity or location of the API or FDF manufacturer (Conti et al., 2020). Regulations regarding country of origin that apply to other imported products are not typically enforced by U.S. Customs for prescription drug imports (Schondelmeyer et al., 2020).[7] This undermines the ability of both purchasers and policy makers to analyze data to identify and mitigate supply chain vulnerabilities (Schondelmeyer et al., 2020).

Although it is widely accepted that better visibility across the supply chain into manufacturers' sources, locations, and volumes of raw materials, APIs, and finished products could help to prevent and mitigate supply disruptions, many manufacturers are reluctant to provide that information (NASEM, 2021). Barriers to increasing transparency in manufacturers' supply chains include

- competition among manufacturers;
- lack of (accurate) data collection;
- concerns about privacy and confidentiality such as proprietary and trade secrecy concerns on the part of industry;
- concerns about counterfeiting;
- lack of incentive structures;

---

[6] "API facilities are included in FDA Inspections Classification Database, which includes final classifications for surveillance inspections of all API facilities in the human pharmaceutical program. This database includes results of FDA inspections and where FDA has made use of an inspection conducted by a capable inspectorate under the mutual recognition agreement (MRA). API facilities not currently supplying the U.S. market would not be included in this database. Furthermore, the database does not list the products being made at the facilities" (FDA Drug Shortages Task Force, 2020).

[7] "Country of origin" is defined as "the country of manufacture, production, or growth of any article of foreign origin entering the United States" (Code of Federal Regulations. Title 19, Part 134, Subpart A, Section 134.1, Country of Origin Marking, General Provisions, Definitions. April 1, 2011).

- potential risk to shareholders;
- lack of data collection mechanisms and supporting infrastructure, including guidance on what data are needed and the tools needed to make the data accessible to the people that need them;
- interest in maintaining security of sources; and
- complexity and multiplicity of components (NASEM, 2021).

The committee concludes that *a lack of transparency in medical product supply chains has led to limited empirical evidence regarding best strategies for addressing supply chain issues. The current practice of keeping medical product supply chains confidential conflicts with public health needs and puts the public's health at risk. Improving the public's access to data that are important to their health and well-being is critical.*

EFFECTS OF MEDICAL PRODUCT SHORTAGES

Shortages of medical products have pervasive consequences that extend from the individual patient level through health care facilities, manufacturers, and suppliers (FDA Drug Shortages Task Force, 2020). For patients, shortages can potentially lead to poor clinical outcomes that are caused by substitutions, medical errors, treatment delays, or even lack of treatment if no alternative is available (Fox et al., 2014; Phuong et al., 2019; Tucker et al., 2020). Health care facilities across the United States must also contend with the effects of increasingly frequent product shortages that impose a variety of costs, from higher drug budgets to lost revenue to additional labor costs required to mitigate those effects (Kaakeh et al., 2011). During periods of shortage, manufacturers and suppliers of critical medical products may face intense pressure to compensate for supply chain disruptions, but they are often unable to ramp up production to meet unpredicted surges in demand (Ventola, 2011).

Effects on Patients

Effect on Clinical Outcomes and Patient Safety

Medical product shortages can affect patients in myriad ways, from poor clinical outcomes to other detrimental experiences that affect their quality of life. A 2019 global scoping review synthesized literature on the economic, clinical, and humanistic effects of drug shortages on patient outcomes in the United States and other countries (Phuong et al., 2019). The review found that during times of shortages, clinical outcomes associated with the effects of shortages included increases in drug errors, adverse events, and mortality. Drug shortages at health care facilities can undermine the quality of patient outcomes through delays in inpatient medication treatment, delays or cancellations of outpatient infusions, delays in immunization, and delays in medical procedures (Vizient, 2019). When a heparin shortage occurred in 2008, elective surgeries were canceled to conserve supply in an attempt to reduce demand for the product (Zhu et al., 2019) (see Box 4-3 for more on heparin shortages). Facilities faced with shortages may need to ration drugs, devices, and other medical products that are in short supply based on patient characteristics and clinical evidence, potentially giving rise to difficult ethical decisions about how to prioritize patients (Fox and McLaughlin, 2018; Grimm, 2020; Hantel, 2014).

Drug shortages can have potentially devastating effects on individual patients, particularly those who depend on the medications for lifesaving treatment. A 2013 survey of U.S. oncology pharmacists found that in 2011, frequent shortages of oncology drugs contributed to delays and changes in chemotherapy regimens, as well as increasing the risk of medication errors and adverse outcomes (McBride et al., 2013). In 2019, Teva Pharmaceuticals, one of two manufacturers of vincristine—used to treat a variety of pediatric cancers—stopped production for economic reasons; the remaining manufacturer, Pfizer, was unable to cover the unmet demand (Caruso, 2020). For high-risk patients living with chronic conditions, shortages can cause sudden treatment interruptions that quickly escalate into acute emergency situations that require them to move from their homes to acute care settings for treatment (NASEM, 2021). In some cases, shortages can leave patients with no treatment options at all. For instance, shortages of lidocaine can make it unavailable for treating patients undergoing anesthesia and sedation with propofol—which can cause a burning sensation on induction—leading to pain and agitation for the patient (FDA Drug Shortages Task Force, 2020).

Medical device shortages can have equally devastating effects on patients. During the COVID-19 pandemic, hospitals did not have enough mechanical ventilators to meet the demand (Jacobs et al., 2020). These shortages prompted many U.S. hospitals to develop triage protocols to decide which patients would receive ventilation—a decision of who lives and who dies for patients with severely compromised breathing (Kerr and Schmidt, 2021; Truog et al., 2020). Other hospitals resorted to placing multiple patients on the same ventilator (Bernstein and Cha, 2020). This comes with increased risk to patients and increased challenges to clinical care (FDA, 2021c). Twenty-six states provided guidance to providers on how to allocate ventilators in the case of a severe shortage (Piscitello et al., 2020).

Effect of Substitutions and Alternatives

Drug shortages can result in poor outcomes for patients—especially those who are most vulnerable—when their substitutes are less efficacious, have a worse adverse-event profile, or require a less common or more difficult dosing regimen (Fox and McLaughlin, 2018). A 2017 survey found that 71 percent of providers could not provide patients with a treatment of choice because of drug shortages, and almost half of those providers believed that their patients received a less effective treatment as a result (Institute for Safe Medication Practices, 2018). A retrospective cohort study reported that during the 2011 hospital-level norepinephrine shortage in the United States, patients admitted with septic shock who were treated with an alternative vasopressor (e.g., phenylephrine) in hospitals affected by the shortage had higher in-hospital mortality compared to those treated in hospitals during periods when the first-line norepinephrine treatment was not in shortage (Vail et al., 2017). In another example, a 2016 shortage of bleomycin—a palliative treatment for patients with cancer—warranted the use of alternative regimens that required inpatient treatment, which is more stressful for patients and families, increases the risk of patients' nosocomial exposure to pathogens, and is more costly (FDA Drug Shortages Task Force, 2020).

Effect of Medication Errors

Drug shortages can undermine patient safety in a host of ways. For example, they can contribute to medication errors when pharmacies are required to change their practices around how drugs are prescribed, prepared, or dispensed (Fox and McLaughlin, 2018). According to a survey of hospital pharmacy staff about the effect of drug shortages on outcomes for hospitalized patients from March 2011 to March 2012, 16 medications in short supply were each involved in more than one report of patient harm, including prolonged disease duration, disease progression, injuries, and death (Institute for Safe Medication Practices, 2012). Patient harms reported in the survey fell into four general categories:

1. Inadequate treatment because the alternative medication provided was not the drug of choice,
2. Medication errors when an alternative drug or form/strength of drug was used as a substitute,
3. Omission of vital medication (nontreatment), and
4. Errors in attempts to compound unavailable drugs (Institute for Safe Medication Practices, 2012).

Effect on Patients' Experiences

Shortages can negatively affect other types of patient experiences, as well. The 2019 scoping review by Phuong and colleagues found that patients were more likely to report increased out-of-pocket costs during shortages. Patient outcomes affected by shortages included patient complaints, frustration, and anger, as well as increased travel time (Phuong et al., 2019). According to a 2013 survey of pharmacy directors, 38 percent of respondents reported patient complaints caused by drug shortages at their institutions (McLaughlin et al., 2013). For the health care providers who care for patients, drug shortages can also lead to burnout, stress, and frustration; these are the secondary effects of shortages, and they negatively affect providers' ability to deliver high-quality care to patients (NASEM, 2021).

Patients are typically unaware of the risks and realities of shortages (NASEM, 2021). However, a 2015 survey focused on the patient perspective regarding the effects of drug shortages in the United States and Canada, finding that about three-quarters of respondents reported wanting to be notified about drug shortages that could affect their care—prior to elective surgery, for example (Hsia et al., 2015).

Effect on Researchers and the Conduct of Clinical Trials

Drug shortages can also undermine clinical trials for novel therapeutics in cases where the drug that is the current standard of care is unavailable. These unforeseen drug shortages may necessitate substitutions and result in deviations from the study protocol. Shortages of oncology drugs affected the conduct of clinical trial research at 44 percent of represented institutions in the 2013 survey of U.S. oncology pharmacists (McBride et al., 2013). For instance, drug shortages can substantially delay patient enrollment in clinical trials. One oncology trial enrolled less than 60 percent of the expected number of patients because of a shortage of one of the drugs in the comparison arm (Goozner, 2012).

Shortages of medical supplies are another threat to clinical trials and drug research and development. A series of supply chain disruptions in early 2021 precipitated a global shortage of pipette tips—disposable plastic tips commonly used in the conduct of biomedical research (Sheridan, 2021). The shortage forced research institutions to begin contemplating which studies to prioritize and threatened to prompt delays in clinical research.

Effect on Health Systems

Medical product shortages have a near-universal effect on all types of health care facilities and most of their personnel, from clinicians and pharmacists to buyers and facility administrators. For example, severe shortages of PPE at the onset of the COVID-19 pandemic endangered health care workers (WHO, 2020). Vizient conducted a study across more than 6,000 U.S. facilities,[8,9] all of which reported being affected by drug shortages and more than half of which reported having managed a minimum of 20 shortages during the 6-month survey period (Vizient, 2019). At the facility and hospital level, critical medical product shortages are associated with substantial costs that affect budgets, resources, and the ability to provide high-quality and efficient care (Shaban et al., 2018).

For facilities, the direct and indirect costs of drug shortages include increased drug budgets, lost revenue from canceled treatments and procedures, greater need for pharmacy and technician employees, and lost productivity owing to reallocation of pharmacy resources (Vizient, 2019). According to the survey, critical drug shortages cost facilities an estimated $360 million per year for the additional labor required to mitigate the effects of shortages on patient care (Vizient, 2019). Further, to manage the effects of drug shortages, U.S. hospitals are estimated to spend an additional 8.6 million personnel hours per year.

The effects of drug shortages have been documented at private-sector health care facilities as well as government health systems. A 2018 study investigating the effects of drug shortages on the U.S. Department of Veterans Affairs (VA) health care system found that—similar to the private sector—drug shortages are a major barrier to patient care for the larger facilities within the VA system, affecting both quality and efficiency of care, as well as increasing staff workloads and institutional operational costs (Shaban et al., 2018).

The example of the medical oxygen shortages encountered in California in December 2020 and January 2021 depict the broad effect of medical product shortages on health care facilities. Aside from the effects on COVID-19 patients and other individuals with respiratory conditions that require the use of medical oxygen, the oxygen shortage caused patient intake backlogs, reduced the capacity of ambulances to transport patients, tested hospitals' aging oxygen infrastructure, and precipitated the need for makeshift field hospitals (Nirappil and Wan, 2021). The effects of this shortage rippled outward as hospital's low oxygen supply forced them to turn away patients, crippling the ambulances that were unable to find hospitals accepting patients, and exacerbating the shortage of portable oxygen tanks. This, in turn, further stressed

---

[8] Vizient is a company that partners with health care organizations throughout the United States to help improve health care performance by providing data, insights, and purchasing power to their members. For more information see https://www.vizientinc.com/what-we-do.

[9] Including nonacute facilities and health systems; academic medical centers; self-governed children's hospitals; small-, medium- and large-sized hospitals; critical access hospitals; behavioral facilities; long-term care facilities; specialty hospitals; and ambulatory care facilities.

ambulances in addition to delaying the discharge of COVID-19 patients who would otherwise be able to leave the hospital with a portable oxygen tank, thus furthering hospitals' oxygen shortages.

Effects on Manufacturers and Suppliers

During medical product shortages, manufacturers and suppliers may receive purchase orders substantially above historical levels and come under pressure to ramp up supply quickly. However, this degree of agility is challenging and may be infeasible for many of them, depending on the cause of the shortage. For example, manufacturers that are reliant on single sources of key components may have no recourse to expand production sufficiently to meet the demand. Drug manufacturers may be unable to source an API at all (e.g., because it is not being produced), or they may be dependent upon an API that is not available or is shipped in insufficient quantities to the finished dosage manufacturer to meet demand.

Ramping up and expanding production also tends to be very capital and time intensive, without a guaranteed return on that investment. As previously described, N95 manufacturer Prestige Ameritech was left with a surplus of product and financial instability when demand abruptly fell after ramping up production during the 2009 H1N1 outbreak (Noguchi, 2021).

A serious concern that faces hospitals, health care facilities, and other purchasers of medical products are rogue distributors that operate in the gray market (Rockefeller et al., 2012). These distributors charge exorbitant sums of money for products that are in shortage, and knowingly or unknowingly sell counterfeit or substandard medical products. Gray market distributors often seize on the uncertainty in the supply chain once a shortage arises and health care facilities can no longer reliably purchase products from their normal suppliers. However, even compliant distributors may need to increase their prices when upstream supply chain disruptions increase the price of raw materials (Sheridan, 2021).

CONCLUDING REMARKS

Although it can be difficult to identify the cause of a specific medical product shortage owing to the lack of transparency throughout supply chains, the root causes of shortages can generally be classified into one of three categories: demand surges, capacity reductions, and coordination failures. No matter the root cause, medical product shortages can have devastating effects on patients by undermining the ability of the health care system to provide high-quality care. Some supply chain resilience measures, such as stockpiling inventory, provide protection against a broad range of disruptions, while others, such as improving oversight of quality assurance systems, reduce the risk of very specific types of disruptions. To select the appropriate elements of a cost-effective strategy for increasing the resilience of critical medical product supply chains, a framework is needed for systematically enumerating and evaluating options. This is the subject of the next chapter.

REFERENCES

AdvaMed (Advanced Medical Technology Association). 2021. *AdvaMed response to the Department of Commerce's request for public comments on risks in the semiconductor supply chain.* https://www.advamed.org/wp-content/uploads/2021/11/AdvaMed-Response-to-the-Department-of-Commerce.pdf (accessed February 15, 2022).

AEP (Analytic Exchange Program). 2018. *Public-private analytic exchange program (AEP).* https://www.dhs.gov/sites/default/files/publications/2018_AEP_Threats_to_Pharmaceutical_Supply_Chains.pdf. (accessed November 2, 2021).

AMA (American Medical Association). 2020. *Advocacy resource center - recently enacted medical liability immunity statutes related to COVID-19.* https://www.ama-assn.org/system/files/2020-12/medical-liability-immunity-statutes-chart.pdf (accessed December 7, 2021).

Ammar, M. A., G. L. Sacha, S. C. Welch, S. N. Bass, S. L. Kane-Gill, A. Duggal, and A. A. Ammar. 2021. Sedation, analgesia, and paralysis in COVID-19 patients in the setting of drug shortages. *Journal of Intensive Care Medicine* 36(2):157-174. https://doi.org/10.1177/0885066620951426.

Armour, S., and T. M. Burton. 2018. *Hospitals wrestle with shortage of IV bags, linked to hurricane.* https://www.wsj.com/articles/hospitals-wrestle-with-shortage-of-iv-bags-linked-to-hurricane-1515349271 (accessed October 25, 2021).

Bernstein, L., and A. E. Cha. 2020. A New York hospital is treating two patients on a device intended for one. *The Washington Post*, March 29, A08.

Bos, J. 2009. Globalization of the pharmaceutical supply chain: What are the risks?–the FDA's difficult task. *Society of Actuaries* 23-26.

Bradsher, K., and L. Alderman. 2020. The world needs masks. China makes them, but has been hoarding them. *The New York Times*, March 14, B05.

Brunell, N. 2020. *What happened to California's medical supply stockpile for a pandemic.* https://spectrumnews1.com/ca/la-west/health/2020/04/08/what-happened-to-california-s-big-medical-supply-stockpile-for-a-pandemic (accessed October 25, 2021).

Butler, D., J. Eilperin, and T. Hamburger. 2020. "No offense, but is this a joke?" Inside the underground market for face masks. *The Washington Post*, May 18.

California ACEP (American College of Emergency Physicians). 2021. *COVID-19 PPE resources.* https://californiaacep.org/page/COVID-19_PPE (accessed December 6, 2021).

Callaway Kim, K., M. Tadrous, S. L. Kane-Gill, I. J. Barbash, S. D. Rothenberger, and K. J. Suda. 2021. Changes in purchases for intensive care medicines during the COVID-19 pandemic: A global time series study. *Chest* 160(6):2123-2134. doi:10.1016/j.chest.2021.08.007.

Caruso, C. 2020. Oncology drug shortages persist. *Cancer Discovery* 10(1):6.

Caspi, H. 2015. *Non-sterile saline enters hospital supply chain, sickens 40.* https://www.healthcaredive.com/news/non-sterile-saline-enters-hospital-supply-chain-sickens-40/353333/ (accessed October 25, 2021).

Cavallo, A., E. Cavallo, and R. Rigobon. 2014. Prices and supply disruptions during natural disasters. *Review of Income and Wealth* 60:S449-S471.

CBS News. 2017. *IV bags in short supply after Hurricane Maria disrupted production in Puerto Rico.* https://www.cbsnews.com/news/iv-bags-in-short-supply-after-hurricane-maria-disrupted-production/ (accessed October 25, 2021).

CBS News. 2018. *Protective masks fly off store shelves in wildfire-ravaged California.* https://www.cbsnews.com/news/fires-in-california-protective-masks-high-demand-camp-fire-bay-area/ (accessed October 21, 2021).

CDC (Centers for Disease Control and Prevention). 2021a. *Personal protective equipment: Questions and answers.* https://www.cdc.gov/coronavirus/2019-ncov/hcp/respirator-use-faq.html (accessed December 6, 2021).

CDC. 2021b. *Strategies for optimizing the supply of n95 respirators.* https://www.cdc.gov/coronavirus/2019-ncov/hcp/respirators-strategy/index.html (accessed October 26, 2021).

Cha, A. E. 2007. *Pig disease in China worries the world.* https://www.washingtonpost.com/wp-dyn/content/article/2007/09/15/AR2007091501647.html (accessed October 25, 2021).

Chalfant, M. 2017. *Lawmakers worry cyberattacks could cause drug shortages.* https://thehill.com/policy/cybersecurity/351797-lawmakers-worry-cyberattacks-on-health-industry-could-produce-drug (accessed October 21, 2021).

Chaudhuri, S. 2020. Coronavirus prompts hospitals to find ways to reuse masks amid shortage. *The Wall Street Journal,* March 31.

Childs, B. 2019. *Re: FDA-2018-n-3272, identifying the root causes of drug shortages and finding enduring solutions; public meeting; request for comments,* edited by S. Gottlieb. Premier. https://www.premierinc.com/downloads/FDA-Drug-Shortage-Task-Force_Premier-Comments_FINAL.PDF (accessed December 16, 2021).

CivicaRx. 2019. *Civica Rx and Hikma announce shipments of heparin and seven other essential injectable medicines.* https://civicarx.org/civica-rx-and-hikma-announce-shipments-of-heparin-and-seven-other-essential-injectable-medicines/ (accessed October 25, 2021).

Clark, D. B. 2021. Inside the chaotic, cutthroat gray market for N95 masks. *The New York Times Magazine,* November 17, 2020.

Cline, M., J. Shames, and C. Rickert-McCaffrey. 2020. *How to manage political risk in a post-pandemic world.* https://riskcenter.wharton.upenn.edu/lab-notes/how-to-manage-political-risk-in-a-post-pandemic-world/ (accessed December 20, 2021).

Cline, M. K., W. Henisz, S. Behrendt, K. P. Lawless, and R. Abdurakhim. 2019. *Political risk and corporate performance: Mapping impact.* Ernest & Young and The Wharton School. https://riskcenter.wharton.upenn.edu/wp-content/uploads/2019/09/EY-Geostrategic-Business-Group_Impact-of-Political-Risk_Academic_Draft.pdf (accessed December 20, 2021).

Conti, R. M., Berndt, E. R., Kaygisiz, N. B., Shivdasani, Y. 2020. We still don't know who makes this drug. *Health Affairs Blog.* https://www.healthaffairs.org/do/10.1377/hblog20200203.83247/full/ (accessed December 20, 2021).

Crotti, N. 2019. *More device shortages pegged to sterilization plant shutdown.* https://www.medicaldesignandoutsourcing.com/more-device-shortages-pegged-to-sterilization-plant-shutdown/ (accessed October 21, 2021).

Dai, T., G. Bai, and G. F. Anderson. 2020. PPE supply chain needs data transparency and stress testing. *Journal of General Internal Medicine* 35:2748-2749. https://doi.org/10.1007/s11606-020-05987-9.

DoD (U.S. Department of Defense), HHS (U.S. Department of Health and Human Services), DHS (U.S. Department of Homeland Security), and VA (U.S. Department of Veterans Affairs). 2021. *National strategy for a resilient public health supply chain,* edited by Department of Health and Human Services, Department of Defense, Department of Homeland Security, Department of Commerce, Department of State, Department of Veterans Affairs, and The White House Office of the COVID-19 Response. Washington, DC. https://www.phe.gov/Preparedness/legal/Documents/National-Strategy-for-Resilient-Public-Health-Supply-Chain.pdf (accessed October 29, 2021).

Edney, A. 2020. Hurricane season could threaten saline solution production. *Bloomberg.* https://www.bloomberg.com/news/articles/2020-07-16/hurricane-season-could-threaten-saline-solution-production (accessed October 25, 2021).

Evans, J., and J. Meisenheimer. 2020. COVID-19—suffocating the global medical supply chain while breathing life into its future. *Site Selection Magazine*, April.
Evstatieva, M. 2021. *U.S. Companies shifted to make N95 respirators during COVID. Now, they're struggling.* https://www.npr.org/2021/06/25/1009858893/u-s-companies-shifted-to-make-n95-respirators-during-covid-now-theyre-struggling (accessed October 25, 2021).
Fairclough, G., and T. M. Burton. 2008. *China's role in supply of drug is under fire.* https://www.wsj.com/articles/SB120354600035281041 (accessed October 25, 2021).
Fareed, J., W. Jeske, and E. Ramacciotti. 2019. Porcine mucosal heparin shortage crisis! What are the options? *Clinical and Applied Thrombosis/Hemostasis* 25:1076029619878786.
Farrell, N. M., B. D. Hayes, and J. A. Linden. 2021. Critical medication shortages further dwindling hospital resources during COVID-19. *The American Journal of Emergency Medicine* 40:202-203.
FDA (U.S. Food and Drug Administration). 2013. Strategic plan for preventing and mitigating drug shortages. Silver Spring, MD: FDA. https://www.fda.gov/media/86907/download (accessed December 20, 2021).
FDA. 2017. *Entry screening systems and tools.* https://www.fda.gov/industry/import-systems/entry-screening-systems-and-tools#screened (accessed January 19, 2022).
FDA. 2019a. *FDA encourages reintroduction of bovine-sourced heparin.* https://www.fda.gov/drugs/pharmaceutical-quality-resources/fda-encourages-reintroduction-bovine-sourced-heparin (accessed October 25, 2021).
FDA. 2019b. *FDA in brief: FDA announces new efforts to expedite generic drug development and marketing to improve patient access to medicines.* Silver Spring, MD: FDA. https://www.fda.gov/news-events/fda-brief/fda-brief-fda-announces-new-efforts-expedite-generic-drug-development-and-marketing-improve-patient (accessed December 16, 2021).
FDA. 2020a. *Current good manufacturing practice (CGMP) regulations.* https://www.fda.gov/drugs/pharmaceutical-quality-resources/current-good-manufacturing-practice-cgmp-regulations (accessed July 22, 2021).
FDA. 2020b. *Ethylene oxide sterilization for medical devices.* https://www.fda.gov/medical-devices/general-hospital-devices-and-supplies/ethylene-oxide-sterilization-medical-devices#actions (accessed October 21, 2021).
FDA. 2021a. *Activities report of the generic drugs program | GDUFA II quarterly performance.* https://www.fda.gov/industry/generic-drug-user-fee-amendments/activities-report-generic-drugs-program-gdufa-ii-quarterly-performance (accessed October 22, 2021).
FDA. 2021b. *FAQs on shortages of surgical masks and gowns during the COVID-19 pandemic.* https://www.fda.gov/medical-devices/personal-protective-equipment-infection-control/faqs-shortages-surgical-masks-and-gowns-during-covid-19-pandemic (accessed December 6, 2021, 2021).
FDA. 2021c. *Using ventilator splitters during the COVID-19 pandemic—letter to health care providers.* https://www.fda.gov/medical-devices/letters-health-care-providers/using-ventilator-splitters-during-covid-19-pandemic-letter-health-care-providers (accessed October 21, 2021).
FDA Drug Shortages Task Force. 2020. *Drug shortages: Root causes and potential solutions.* https://www.fda.gov/drugs/drug-shortages/report-drug-shortages-root-causes-and-potential-solutions (accessed December 16, 2021).
FiercePharma. 2010. *Teva to stop making propofol.* https://www.fiercepharma.com/manufacturing/teva-to-stop-making-propofol (accessed December 16, 2021).
Florko, N. 2020. New document reveals scope and structure of Operation Warp Speed and underscores vast military involvement. *STAT*, September 28.
Fox, E. R., and M. M. McLaughlin. 2018. ASHP guidelines on managing drug product shortages. *American Journal of Health-System Pharmacy* 75(21):1742-1750.

Fox, E. R., A. Birt, K. B. James, H. Kokko, S. Salverson, and D. L. Soflin. 2009. ASHP guidelines on managing drug product shortages in hospitals and health systems. *American Journal of Health-System Pharmacy* 66(15):1399-1406.

Fox, E. R., B. V. Sweet, and V. Jensen. 2014. Drug shortages: A complex health care crisis. *Mayo Clinic Proceedings* 89(3):361-373.

Fry, E. 2015. There's a national shortage of saline solution. Yeah, we're talking salt water. Huh? https://fortune.com/2015/02/05/theres-a-national-shortage-of-saline/ (accessed October 25, 2021).

GAO (Government Accountability Office). 2010. *FDA response to heparin contamination.* http://www.gao.gov/new.items/d1195.pdf (accessed December 16, 2021).

Goldberg, S. 2019. *Sterigenics to close suburban Chicago plant.* https://www.modernhealthcare.com/safety/sterigenics-close-suburban-chicago-plant (accessed October 21, 2021).

Goodnough, A. 2020. Some hospitals are close to running out of crucial masks for coronavirus. *New York Times*, March 9.

Goozner, M. 2012. Drug shortages delay cancer clinical trials. *Journal of the National Cancer Institute* 104(12):891-892.

Grimm, C. A. 2020. *Hospital experiences responding to the COVID-19 pandemic: Results of a national pulse survey March 23–27, 2020.* U.S. Department of Health and Human Services, Office of Inspector General.

Hantel, A. 2014. A protocol and ethical framework for the distribution of rationed chemotherapy. *Journal of Clinical Ethics* 25(2):102-115.

Hantel, A., M. Siegler, F. Hlubocky, K. Colgan, and C. K. Daugherty. 2019. Prevalence and severity of rationing during drug shortages: A national survey of health system pharmacists. *JAMA Internal Medicine* 179(5):710-711.

Herper, M. 2001. Cipro, anthrax and the perils of patents. *Forbes*, October 17.

Hopp, W. J. 2008. *Supply chain science.* New York: McGraw-Hill Irwin.

Hsia, I. K., F. Dexter, I. Logvinov, N. Tankosic, H. Ramakrishna, and S. J. Brull. 2015. Survey of the national drug shortage effect on anesthesia and patient safety: A patient perspective. *Anesthesia & Analgesia* 121(2):502-506.

Hufford, A. 2020a. 3M CEO on N95 masks: 'Demand exceeds our production capacity'. *The Wall Street Journal*, April 2.

Hufford, A. 2020b. Why are N95 masks so important? *The Wall Street Journal*, June 1.

Hufford, A., and M. Evans. 2020. Coronavirus outbreak strains global medical-mask market. *The Wall Street Journal*, February 6.

Institute for Safe Medication Practices. 2012. *A shortage of everything except errors: Harm associate with drug shortages.* ISMP. https://www.ismp.org/resources/shortage-everything-except-errors-harm-associated-drug-shortages (accessed Feburary 12, 2021).

Institute for Safe Medication Practices. 2018. *Drug shortages continue to compromise patient care.* https://www.ismp.org/resources/drug-shortages-continue-compromise-patient-care (accessed March 1, 2021).

IOM (Institute of Medicine). 2009. *Guidance for establishing crisis standards of care for use in disaster situations: A letter report*, edited by B. M. Altevogt, C. Stroud, S. L. Hanson, D. Hanfling and L. O. Gostin. Washington, DC: The National Academies Press.

Jacobs, A. 2021. Can't find an N95 mask? This company has 30 million that it can't sell. *The New York Times*, February 10.

Jacobs, A., N. E. Boudette, M. Richtel, and N. Kulish. 2020. Amid desperate need for ventilators, calls grow for federal intervention. *The New York Times*, March 25.

Jacobsen, J. 2020. *3M responds to Trump's invocation of Defense Production Act to obtain N95 masks.* https://www.kare11.com/article/news/health/coronavirus/pres-trump-invokes-defense-production-act-to-obtain-n95-masks-from-3m/89-d3c72df1-a9d2-445f-93af-b49291b14a0f (accessed October 25, 2021).

Jensen, V., and B. A. Rappaport. 2010. The reality of drug shortages — The case of the injectable agent propofol. *New England Journal of Medicine* 363(9):806-807.

Jung, A. 2020. *COVID-19: Risks and resiliency in the drug supply chain.* https://www.ey.com/en_us/strategy-transactions/covid-19-risks-and-resiliency-in-the-drug-supply-chain (accessed January 5, 2021).

Kaakeh, R., B. V. Sweet, C. Reilly, C. Bush, S. DeLoach, B. Higgins, A. M. Clark, and J. Stevenson. 2011. Impact of drug shortages on U.S. health systems. *American Journal of Health-System Pharmacy* 68(19):1811-1819.

Kerr, W., and H. Schmidt. 2021. COVID-19 ventilator rationing protocols: Why we need to know more about the views of those with most to lose. *Journal of Medical Ethics* 47(3):133-136.

Khazan, O. 2020. *Why we're running out of masks.* https://www.theatlantic.com/health/archive/2020/04/why-were-running-out-of-masks-in-the-coronavirus-crisis/609757/ (accessed October 25, 2021).

King, R. 2020. *HHS defends falling short of PPE goals on Strategic National Stockpile as some shortages linger.* https://www.fiercehealthcare.com/hospitals/hhs-defends-falling-short-ppe-goals-strategic-national-stockpile-as-some-shortages-linger (accessed October 25, 2021).

Kishimoto, T. K., K. Viswanathan, T. Ganguly, S. Elankumaran, S. Smith, K. Pelzer, J. C. Lansing, N. Sriranganathan, G. Zhao, Z. Galcheva-Gargova, A. Al-Hakim, G. S. Bailey, B. Fraser, S. Roy, T. Rogers-Cotrone, L. Buhse, M. Whary, J. Fox, M. Nasr, G. J. Dal Pan, Z. Shriver, R. S. Langer, G. Venkataraman, K. F. Austen, J. Woodcock, and R. Sasisekharan. 2008. Contaminated heparin associated with adverse clinical events and activation of the contact system. *New England Journal of Medicine* 358(23):2457-2467.

Langreth, R., and C. Koons. 2017. *This simple liquid is suddenly in short supply.* https://www.bloomberg.com/news/articles/2017-11-14/this-simple-lifesaving-liquid-is-suddenly-in-short-supply (accessed October 25, 2021).

Le, P., L. Grund, J. Marwa, W. Ojo, J. Otts, Jr., and F. Arab. 2018. Combating substandard and counterfeit medicines by securing the pharmaceutical supply chain: The Drug Supply Chain Security Act (DSCSA) of 2013. *Innovations in Pharmacy* 9(2):1-11.

Lee, J. 2014. *Growing IV saline shortage has providers scrambling during bad flu season.* https://www.modernhealthcare.com/article/20140123/NEWS/301239970/growing-iv-saline-shortage-has-providers-scrambling-during-bad-flu-season (accessed October 25, 2021).

Lim, D. 2019. *Ethylene oxide plant closures put us on 'cusp of a major medical logistical failure'.* https://www.medtechdive.com/news/ethylene-oxide-plant-closures-place-united-states-on-cusp-major-medical-logistical-failure/566922/ (accessed October 21, 2021).

Linskey, A., J. Dawsey, I. Stanley-Becker, and C. Janes. 2020. As feds play 'backup,' states take unorthodox steps to compete in cutthroat global market for coronavirus supplies. *The Washington Post*, April 11.

Lloyd, J., and J. Cheyne. 2017. The origins of the vaccine cold chain and a glimpse of the future. *Vaccine* 35(17):2115-2120.

Manufacturing x Digital (MxD) and the International Academy of Automation Engineering (IAAE). 2021. Analysis of the advantages of and barriers to adoption of smart manufacturing for medical products. Food and Drug Administration. https://www.fda.gov/media/152568/download (accessed January 27, 2022).

Marsa, L. 2020. *Tackling dangerous drug shortages.* https://health.usnews.com/health-care/patient-advice/articles/tackling-dangerous-drug-shortages (accessed October 25, 2021).

Marucheck, A., N. Greis, C. Mena, and L. Cai. 2011. Product safety and security in the global supply chain: Issues, challenges and research opportunities. *Journal of Operations Management* 29(7):707-720.

Maxwell, Y. L. 2019. *FDA warns of potential medical device shortage due to sterilization woes.* https://www.tctmd.com/news/fda-warns-potential-medical-device-shortage-due-sterilization-woes (accessed October 21, 2021).

Mazer-Amirshahi, M., and E. R. Fox. 2018. Saline shortages—Many causes, no simple solution. *New England Journal of Medicine* 378(16):1472-1474.

McBride, A., L. M. Holle, C. Westendorf, M. Sidebottom, N. Griffith, R. J. Muller, and J. M. Hoffman. 2013. National survey on the effect of oncology drug shortages on cancer care. *American Journal of Health-System Pharmacy* 70(7):609-617.

McCarthy, C. P., M. Vaduganathan, E. Solomon, R. Sakhuja, G. Piazza, D. L. Bhatt, J. M. Connors, and N. K. Patel. 2020. Running thin: Implications of a heparin shortage. *Lancet* 395(10223):534-536.

McLaughlin, M., D. Kotis, K. Thomson, M. Harrison, G. Fennessy, M. Postelnick, and M. H. Scheetz. 2013. Effects on patient care caused by drug shortages: A survey. *Journal of Managed Care Pharmacy* 19(9):783-788.

Mentzer, J. T., W. DeWitt, J. S. Keebler, S. Min, N. W. Nix, C. D. Smith, and Z. G. Zacharia. 2001. Defining supply chain management. *Journal of Business Logistics* 22(2):1-25.

Mullen, R. 2020. COVID-19 is reshaping the pharmaceutical supply chain. *Chemical and Engineering News* 98(16):10.

Murray, B., and S. Bradley. 2021. *The semiconductor chip shortage hits medtech: Strategies to build resilient supply chains.* https://www.advamed.org/2021/09/23/the-semiconductor-chip-shortage-hits-medtech-strategies-to-build-resilient-supply-chains/ (accessed October 21, 2021).

NASEM (National Academies of Science, Engineering, and Medicine). 2018. *Medical product shortages during disasters: Opportunities to predict, prevent, and respond: Proceedings of a workshop—in brief,* edited by A. Nicholson, L. Runnels, C. Giammaria, L. Brown, and S. Wollek. Washington, DC: The National Academies Press.

NASEM. 2020. *Strengthening post-hurricane supply chain resilience: Observations from Hurricanes Harvey, Irma, and Maria.* Washington, DC: The National Academies Press.

NASEM. 2021. *The security of America's medical product supply chain: Considerations for critical drugs and devices: Proceedings of a workshop—In brief,* edited by A. Nicholson, E. Randall, L. Brown, C. Shore, and B. Kahn. Washington, DC: The National Academies Press.

Nirappil, F., and W. Wan. 2021. Los Angeles is running out of oxygen for patients as COVID hospitalizations hit record highs nationwide. *The Washington Post*, April 28.

Noguchi, Y. 2021. *Why N95 masks are still in short supply in the U.S.* Washington, DC: NPR. https://www.npr.org/sections/health-shots/2021/01/27/960336778/why-n95-masks-are-still-in-short-supply-in-the-u-s (accessed December 16, 2021).

Paavola, A. 2017. *4 ways the FDA is addressing the saline bag shortage.* https://www.beckershospitalreview.com/supply-chain/4-ways-the-fda-is-addressing-the-saline-bag-shortage.htm (accessed October 25, 2021).

Page, P. 2021. *Container shipping prices skyrocket as rush to move goods picks up.* https://www.wsj.com/articles/container-ship-prices-skyrocket-as-rush-to-move-goods-picks-up-11625482800 (accessed October 22, 2021).

Palmer, E. 2019. *B. Braun commits $1B to expand in face of IV fluid shortages.* https://www.fiercepharma.com/manufacturing/b-braun-commits-1b-to-expand-face-iv-fluid-shortages (accessed October 29, 2021).

Parshley, L. 2020. *The mask shortage is forcing health workers to disregard basic coronavirus infection control.* https://www.vox.com/2020/4/3/21206726/coronavirus-masks-n95-hospitals-health-care-doctors-ppe-shortage (accessed October 25, 2021).

Pascu, G. A., G. Hancu, and A. Rusu. 2020. Pharmaceutical serialization, a global effort to combat counterfeit medicines. *Acta Marisiensis-Seria Medica* 66(4):132-139.

Patton, D. 2021. *Analysis: African Swine Fever inflicts renewed toll on northern China's hog herd.* https://www.reuters.com/business/healthcare-pharmaceuticals/african-swine-fever-inflicts-renewed-toll-northern-chinas-hog-herd-2021-04-01/ (accessed October 25, 2021).

The PEW Charitable Trusts and International Society for Pharmaceutical Engineering. 2017. *Drug shortage: An exploration of the relationship between U.S. market forces and sterile injectable pharmaceutical products—Interviews with 10 pharmaceutical companies.* PEW and ISPE. https://www.pewtrusts.org/-/media/assets/2017/01/drug_shortages.pdf (accessed October 25, 2021).

The PEW Health Group. 2011. *After heparin: Protecting consumers from the risks of substandard and counterfeit drugs.* https://www.pewtrusts.org/en/research-and-analysis/reports/2011/07/12/after-heparin-protecting-consumers-from-the-risks-of-substandard-and-counterfeit-drugs (accessed October 25, 2021).

Phuong, J. M., J. Penm, B. Chaar, L. D. Oldfield, and R. Moles. 2019. The impacts of medication shortages on patient outcomes: A scoping review. *PLoS ONE* 14(5):e0215837.

Piscitello, G. M., E. M. Kapania, W. D. Miller, J. C. Rojas, M. Siegler, and W. F. Parker. 2020. Variation in ventilator allocation guidelines by US state during the Coronavirus Disease 2019 pandemic: A systematic review. *JAMA Network Open* 3(6):e2012606.

Ranney, M. L., V. Griffeth, and A. K. Jha. 2020. Critical supply shortages—the need for ventilators and personal protective equipment during the COVID-19 pandemic. *New England Journal of Medicine* 382(18):e41.

Raymond, N. 2019. *U.S. Closes IV solution shortage antitrust probe, Baxter says.* https://www.reuters.com/article/us-baxter-intl-antitrust-idUSKCN1QB25K (accessed October 25, 2021).

Rockefeller, J. D., T. Harkin, and E. E. Cummings. 2012. *Shining light on the "gray market": An examination of why hospital are forced to pay exorbitant prices for prescription drugs facing critical shortages.* https://www.commerce.senate.gov/services/files/AFA98935-2FF5-4004-88DC-BE70D1C22B5D (accessed December 16, 2021).

Sacks, C. A., A. S. Kesselheim, and M. Fralick. 2018. The shortage of normal saline in the wake of Hurricane Maria. *JAMA Intern Medicine* 178(7):885-886.

Sathya, D. 2021. *How the N95 masks shortage evolved to a supply-demand disconnect.* https://getusppe.org/how-the-n95-masks-shortage-evolved-to-a-supply-demand-disconnect/ (accessed October 24, 2021).

Schondelmeyer, S. W., J. Seifert, D. J. Margraf, M. Mueller, I. Williamson, C. Dickson, D. Dasararaju, C. Caschetta, N. Senne, and M. T. Osterholm. 2020. Part 6: Ensuring a resilient us prescription drug supply. In *COVID-19: The CIDRAP viewpoint*, edited by J. Wappes. Minneapolis, MN: Regents of the University of Minnesota. https://www.cidrap.umn.edu/sites/default/files/public/downloads/cidrap-covid19-viewpoint-part1_0.pdf (accessed December 16, 2021).

Scutti, S. 2018. *IV bags in short supply across US after Hurricane Maria.* https://www.cnn.com/2018/01/16/health/iv-bag-shortage/index.html (accessed October 25, 2021).

Senate Committee on Finance. 2020. *COVID-19 and beyond: Oversight of the FDA's foreign drug manufacturing inspection process: Congressional testimony of Judith A. McMeekin.* June 2. https://www.fda.gov/news-events/congressional-testimony/covid-19-and-beyond-oversight-fdas-foreign-drug-manufacturing-inspection-process-06022020 (accessed January 25, 2022).

Shaban, H., C. Maurer, and R. J. Willborn. 2018. Impact of drug shortages on patient safety and pharmacy operation costs. *Federal Practitioner for the Health Care Professionals of the VA, DoD, and PHS* 35(1):24-31.

Sheridan, K. 2021. *How blackouts, fires, and a pandemic are driving shortages of pipette tips—and hobbling science.* https://www.statnews.com/2021/04/28/pipette-tips-shortage/ (accessed April 30, 2021).

Socal, M. P., J. M. Sharfstein, and J. A. Greene. 2020. Critical drugs for critical care: Protecting the US pharmaceutical supply in a time of crisis. *American Journal of Public Health* 110(9):1346-1347.

Sullivan, T. 2018. *FDA under pressure to speed up generic approvals.* https://www.policymed.com/2017/04/fda-under-pressure-to-speed-up-generic-approvals.html (accessed October 25, 2021).

Szajek, A., E. Gray, D. Keire, B. Mulloy, A. A. Hakim, C. Chase, M. Da Luz Carvalho Soares, D. Cairatti, J. Hogwood, P. Mourão, and T. S. Morris. 2015. *Diversifying the global heparin supply chain: Reintroduction of bovine heparin in the United States?* https://www.pharmtech.com/view/diversifying-global-heparin-supply-chain-reintroduction-bovine-heparin-united-states (accessed October 25, 2021).

Tolomeo, D., K. Hirshfield, and D. L. Hustead. 2020. Engage with health authorities to mitigate & prevent drug shortages. In *ISPE Special Reports.* ISPE. https://ispe.org/pharmaceutical-engineering/july-august-2020/engage-health-authorities-mitigate-prevent-drug (accessed October 25, 2021).

Truog, R. D., C. Mitchell, and G. Q. Daley. 2020. The toughest triage—Allocating ventilators in a pandemic. *New England Journal of Medicine* 382(21):1973-1975.

Tucker, E. L., Y. Cao, E. R. Fox, and B. V. Sweet. 2020. The drug shortage era: A scoping review of the literature 2001–2019. *Clinical Pharmacology & Therapeutics* 108(6):1150-1155.

UNICEF. n.d. *What is a cold chain?* https://www.unicef.org/supply/what-cold-chain (accessed October 25, 2021).

Usdin, S. 2009. The heparin story. *International Journal of Risk & Safety in Medicine* 21(1-2):93-103.

Vail, E., H. B. Gershengorn, M. Hua, A. J. Walkey, G. Rubenfeld, and H. Wunsch. 2017. Association between us norepinephrine shortage and mortality among patients with septic shock. *JAMA* 317(14):1433-1442.

van der Meer, J. Y., E. Kellenbach, and L. J. van den Bos. 2017. From farm to pharma: An overview of industrial heparin manufacturing methods. *Molecules* 22(6):1025.

Ventola, C. L. 2011. The drug shortage crisis in the United States: Causes, impact, and management strategies. *Pharmacy and Therapeutics* 36(11):740-757.

Vilanova, E., A. M. F. Tovar, and P. A. S. Mourao. 2019. Imminent risk of a global shortage of heparin caused by the African Swine Fever afflicting the Chinese pig herd. *Journal of Thrombosis and Haemostasis* 17(2):254-256.

Vizient. 2019. Drug shortages and labor costs mesuring the hidden costs of drug shortages on U.S. hospitals. In *Vizient Drug Shortages Impact Report.* Irving, TX: Vizient Inc. https://www.vizientinc.com/-/media/documents/sitecorepublishingdocuments/public/vzdrugshortageslaborcost_fullreport.pdf?la=en&hash=19172F274A8B03817E042C2EF423BED98CDF0401 (accessed December 20, 2021).

Ward, N. 2019. *Crystalloids: An overview.* https://hospitalhealthcare.com/clinical/albumin/2019-focus/crystalloids-an-overview/ (accessed October 25, 2021).

Weber, L. 2018. *Hurricane Maria's effect on the health care industry is threatening lives across the U.S.* https://www.huffpost.com/entry/iv-bag-drug-shortage-puerto-rico-hurricane-maria_n_5ba1ca16e4b046313fc07a8b (accessed October 25, 2021).

Weber, L., and Kaiser Health News. 2020. *State mask stockpiling orders are hurting nursing homes, small clinics.* https://www.nbcnews.com/news/us-news/state-mask-stockpiling-orders-are-hurting-nursing-homes-small-clinics-n1245395 (accessed October 25, 2021).

Wendelbo, M., and C. C. Blackburn. 2018. *A saline shortage this flu season exposes a flaw in our medical supply chain.* https://www.smithsonianmag.com/innovation/saline-shortage-this-flu-season-exposes-flaw-in-our-medical-supply-chain-180967879/ (accessed October 25, 2021).

Weschsler, J. 2001. Bioterrorism threat shines spotlight on drug manufacturing. *Pharmaceutical Technology* 25(12):14-22. https://cdn.sanity.io/files/0vv8moc6/pharmtech/69918b666 16ce9011d3997e5ec39c710fdd68eab.pdf/article-3397.pdf (accessed February 15, 2022).

Westly, E. 2011. *A more modern blood thinner.* https://www.technologyreview.com/2011/10/28/189986/a-more-modern-blood-thinner/ (accessed October 25, 2021).

The White House. 2021. *Building resilient supply chains, revitalizing American manufacturing, and fostering broad-based growth.* Department of Commerce, Department of Energy, Department of Defense, Department of Health and Human Services. https://www.whitehouse.gov/wp-content/uploads/2021/06/100-day-supply-chain-review-report.pdf (accessed October 25, 2021).

WHO (World Health Organization). 2020. *Shortage of personal protective equipment endangering health workers worldwide.* https://www.who.int/news/item/03-03-2020-shortage-of-personal-protective-equipment-endangering-health-workers-worldwide (accessed October 25, 2021).

Woo, J., Wolfgang, S., Batista, H. 2008. The effect of globalization of drug manufacturing, production, and sourcing and challenges for American drug safety. *Clinical Pharmacology & Therapeutics* 83(3):494-497.

Woodcock, J., and M. Wosinska. 2013. Economic and technological drivers of generic sterile injectable drug shortages. *Clinical Pharmacology and Therapeutics* 93(2):170-176.

Woodcock, J., and M. Kopcha. 2020. Quality: The often overlooked critical element for assuring access to safe and effective drugs. HealthAffairs. https://www.healthaffairs.org/do/10.1377/hblog20200311.912049/full/ (accessed October 19, 2021).

Zhu, Y., F. Zhang, and R. J. Linhardt. 2019. Heparin contamination and issues related to raw materials and controls. In *The science and regulations of naturally derived complex drugs.* Cham, Switzerland: Springer. Pp. 191-206.

PART II: MEASURES FOR ENHANCING THE RESILIENCY OF MEDICAL PRODUCT SUPPLY CHAINS

5

A Framework for Resilient Medical Product Supply Chains

As described in Chapter 1, the primary goal of resilient medical product supply chains is to prevent public health and safety from being compromised by shortages of medical products. However, because resources are limited, costs must be considered. Excess spending to enhance resilience of one supply chain may mean inadequate resources for improving resilience of another supply chain or other actions to promote public health and safety. Therefore, the aim must be to find a cost-effective mix of measures to promote a socially desirable level of medical product supply chain resilience.

This chapter presents a framework for increasing the resilience of medical product supply chains. First, the chapter describes a method for determining which medical products are *supply chain critical*, and therefore in need of resilience interventions. Second, the chapter explains a process for determining the level of protection needed for a given product on the supply chain critical list. And third, the chapter shows how to use the framework for systematically enumerating options to enhance supply chain resilience for a given medical product.

The resulting framework is depicted in Figure 5-4, which shows that policies for enhancing medical product supply chain resilience can be classified into four categories: awareness, mitigation, preparedness, and response. Although this framework is described as if it will be used to analyze and remediate each product individually, it can also be used to gain insights into general policies, such as information disclosure requirements, that affect many medical products. The framework will be used in this latter context in Chapters 6–9 to justify several specific recommendations that address the most significant gaps between current and desired protection levels. Taken together, these recommendations form the basis for an integrated strategy to build resilience of critical medical product supply chains.

DEFINING RESILIENCE FOR MEDICAL PRODUCT SUPPLY CHAINS

In Chapter 1, supply chain critical medical products were defined as those that are both medically essential and vulnerable to supply chain shortages. A clear definition of resilience is needed to identify which medical products warrant supply chain resilience interventions. This section refines and quantifies a definition of resilience in medical product supply chains using a standardized procedure that takes into account past data and future forecasts to provide reasonable estimates. This should be adequate for focusing attention on the products for which combined clinical and supply chain risks justify intervention. Toward this end, the subscript (i) is used as a product index in the following definitions:

> H_i = *expected patient harm from a unit of shortage of product* (i). For example, if harm is measured to human health in quality adjusted life years (QALYs), (H_i) represents the average number of QALYs lost because of the unavailability of one unit of product (i). Note that measuring harm only in terms of the effect on human health leaves out other costs, such as health system expenses to shift patients to alternate treatments, but one could in theory include such costs.[1]

> S_i = *expected supply shortage of product* (i) *in any given year.* This value depends on the likelihood, length, and magnitude of a disruption, which could in turn depend on the trigger event that caused the shortage as well as protections (e.g., safety stocks and surge capacity) built into supply chains.

> $R_i = H_i\, S_i$ = *risk defined as expected patient harm due to disruption of product* (i). If (S_i) is defined as the expected shortfall magnitude in the next year and (H_i) is defined in QALYs, then (R_i) represents the annual expected loss of QALYs attributable to disruptions of product (i). The product ($H_i\, S_i$) can also be thought of as the risk level or risk score of expected patient harm.[2]

These definitions allow the total expected harm from all medical products to be expressed as the sum of the individual product risks:

---

[1] Health and financial costs could be combined by attaching a dollar value to QALYs. However, since the model is being used conceptually, rather than computationally, it will focus only on human health for simplicity.

[2] Note that ($H_i S_i$) is mathematical shorthand for the multiplication of (H_i) and (S_i), or ($H_i \times S_i$) (Bergman, n.d.).

$$\text{Total Expected Harm} = \Sigma_i R_i = \Sigma_i H_i S_i \quad \text{(Equation 5-1)}$$

If the supply chain resilience problem is framed as one of reducing total expected harm by as much as possible for a given level of investment, Equation 5-1 indicates that focus should be on products with high $H_i S_i$ values—particularly if they are amenable to inexpensive intervention. Products with high $H_i S_i$ values are of concern because they present substantial clinical and supply chain risks. Therefore, such products should be on the supply chain critical list.

However, there are two reasons why the supply chain critical list should not be limited to the products with the highest $H_i S_i$ values, both of which have to do with the fact that H_i and S_i are expectations. First, the expected value H_i could be low because product i has very few users, even if the medical importance of product i to each user is very great. For example, a drug for treating a rare cancer may be essential for the patients using it, but a shortage might result in the loss of relatively few QALYs because of the small patient population. Leaving such a product off the supply chain critical risk would cause these patients to bear an undue portion of the total risk, violating equity. Furthermore, protecting these patients from harm might be relatively inexpensive because a small stockpile would cover demand for a significant time period. Therefore, it is appropriate to include products that are extremely medically essential on the supply chain critical risk, even if the expected harm from a shortage is low.

Similarly, the expected value S_i could be low because the events that would trigger a shortage are extremely unlikely. Bioterror and nuclear attacks are examples of events that are unlikely but serious. Furthermore, extremely rare events are precisely the ones for which estimating likelihoods is most difficult, which means expectations will be subject to error. For these reasons, the expected outcome is not a very helpful characterization of highly unlikely events with extreme consequences. Products with such unlikely, but large, risks warrant consideration of mitigation measures. However, unlike the case of an essential drug for a small population, where protection costs are likely to be low, the cost of protection against a large but unlikely event could be high because of the volumes of product required. Therefore, the assessment of whether the risks justify the costs of protection will be more nuanced and difficult than when considering essential but small market products.

The conclusion here is that highlighting medical products with high $H_i S_i$ values is a good start to developing a supply chain critical list. But equity and extreme risk considerations must be factored in. Including products that are vital to life and without viable alternatives is important from an equity perspective, while including products that are subject to unlikely but extreme events is important from a security standpoint. For the remainder of this chapter, it will be assumed that these nuanced assessments have been made and that a list of supply chain critical medical products has been generated.

Individual Medical Product Targets

The next step is to determine the socially desirable level of protection needed for each medical product on the supply chain critical list. To do this, a characterization of the *distribution* of shortages a product might face is needed in addition to the expected shortage S_i. If shortages are measured in weeks of supply, such a distribution would look something like Figure 5-1—which depicts the likelihood that a disruption, given that one occurs, will result in a shortage equivalent to n weeks of supply for various values of n. As n grows larger, the probability of a disruption lasting n weeks approaches 1 (or 100 percent). Indeed, if it is assumed that capacity could be repaired, expanded, or replaced within n weeks, then the cumulative distribution will reach 1 (100 percent) at n.

Getting data to construct a shortage distribution like that in Figure 5-1 is nontrivial. Options for obtaining and using such data are described in Appendix C. These include using statistical analysis of past disruptions for products, such as generic drugs, that are prone to routine disruption by process failures, and subjective scenario analysis of disruptions by major emergencies such as pandemics. It is important to note, however, that the goal of such analysis is not precise characterization of shortage distributions. Rather it is to provide a sense of the range of shortage risks a product

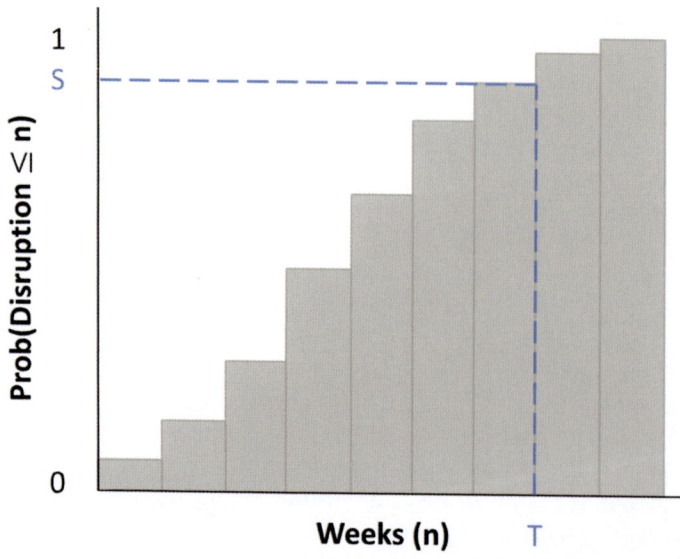

FIGURE 5-1 Cumulative probability distribution of supply disruption time.

faces so that these risks can be addressed in a balanced manner across the medical products on the supply chain critical list.

Figure 5-1 helps describe the fundamental trade-off that must be considered when determining an appropriate protection target. Suppose for the sake of discussion that one is limited to using an inventory stockpile as protection against a supply shortage for a given product. As the weeks of supply (indicated by T) increase in the stockpile, the protection (defined as the probability of having enough stock to offset a shortage and indicated by S) will also increase. The stockpiling cost will increase in proportion to the amount of inventory. However, while the cost of inventory will increase linearly, the protection will increase at a decreasing rate as it gets closer and closer to 100 percent. This in turn implies that the harm (measured in QALYs) avoided becomes increasingly expensive as the protection level increases. In economics terms, investments in supply chain protection will exhibit diminishing returns to scale.

This diminishing returns insight is essential to achieving a balanced supply chain resilience strategy. For example, imagine that there are stocks of two products in the Strategic National Stockpile (SNS) that are clinically similar (i.e., have similar H_i values) and have similar unit costs (and therefore similar costs to carry inventory). However, after evaluating shortage scenarios, it is determined that the stock level of the first product is sufficient to provide a protection level of 75 percent, while the stock level for the second product is enough for a protection level above 99 percent. When this is the case, increasing the stockpile of the first product, while decreasing the stockpile of the second product to keep the cost constant, will increase overall protection. The reason is that the diminishing returns property implies the added investment in the first product stockpile will result in a relatively large increase in the number of QALYs, while the reduced investment in the second product stockpile will result in a much smaller reduction in the number of QALYs.

The point here is not that inventory of one product should literally be sold to buy inventory of another product. Rather, it is that protection targets should be set consistently in a manner that accounts for clinical criticality, product cost, and disruption risks.[3] Appendix C offers additional details on this calculation. But providing a comprehensive manual for setting stockpile

---

[3] Investing in measures to protect against medical supply shortages is directly analogous to buying insurance. Increasing the amount of insurance (i.e., the payout limit) protects us against increasingly unlikely events (e.g., large liability assessments). Just as we reasonably choose different levels of insurance protection against different types of losses (e.g., we might want greater coverage of medical expenses than of property damage), we should set different protection targets for medical products with different implications for health and safety. But when insuring against comparable risks (e.g., liability coverage for different automobiles), protection levels should be consistent. The same is true in a balanced supply chain resilience strategy.

levels is beyond the scope of this report. Therefore, for the remainder of this chapter, it will be assumed that sensible protection targets for the products on the list of supply chain critical medical products have been set. This poses the most important question addressed in this chapter, which is how to systematically identify potential actions for achieving these targets.

MULTILAYERED PROTECTION

The above discussion of protection targets used inventory stockpiling to illustrate the trade-offs involved in investments to protect people from the consequences of medical product shortages. But stockpiling is only one of a wide array of policies that could be used as protection. In order to enumerate options in a systematic way, a framework is needed. To construct one, the committee notes that building resilience into medical product supply chains is an example of a reliability problem. Admittedly, it is a complicated and difficult reliability problem because there are many resilience options available that fit together in intricate ways. There are three major reasons for this:

1. Medical product supply chains are complex systems that involve people, processes, technologies, and policies. Consequently, their resilience can be addressed in many ways by focusing on different aspects of the system.
2. The Redundancy Principle, which states that "independent layers of protection increase the reliability of a system" (Hopp and Lovejoy, 2012), implies that multiple safeguards are useful in achieving a high level of reliability.
3. Interventions to improve resilience can be made at different points in the timeline because disruptive events and their consequences play out over time. Consequently, these interventions can complement one another by addressing public health and safety in a time-phased manner.

James Reason (2000) introduced the Swiss cheese model as a graphical illustration of the Redundancy Principle (Figure 5-2). In this model, slices of cheese represent layers of defense against a hazard causing harm or losses. Just as Swiss cheese has holes, all defense systems (e.g., alarms, warning lights, checklists, and human oversight) are fallible. If a hazard penetrates all the layers of defense (slices of cheese), harm will occur (Box 5-1).

In medical product supply chains, a disruptive trigger event will only result in harm to people if multiple layers of defense fail. For example, if a drug manufacturer has a quality problem that interrupts production (failure of layer 1), there is insufficient inventory in the supply chain (failure of layer 2), there are no other production facilities with additional capacity (failure of layer 3), and health systems have no substitution strategy (fail-

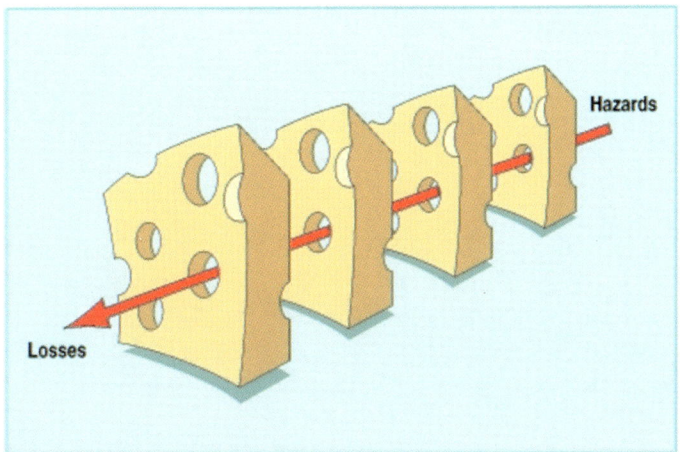

FIGURE 5-2 Swiss cheese model of system failure.
SOURCE: Reason, 2000. Reproduced from *Human error: Models and management*, James Reason, Vol 320, 769, ©2000 with permission from BMJ Publishing Group Ltd.

ure of layer 4), patients could be harmed. Invoking the Swiss cheese model description of the Redundancy Principle, the resilience of this supply chain can be improved by adding more layers of defense (more slices of cheese) or by improving the effectiveness of individual layers (fewer holes).

BOX 5-1
Breakdown Example of a Multilayered Defense System

A tragic example of the breakdown of a multilayered defense system occurred in a Denver hospital in 1996 (see Smetzer and Cohen, 1998, for details). Briefly, an infant was born to a non-English speaking mother with a history of syphilis. Because of the language barrier, hospital staff were unable to confirm status or treatment of the disease and decided to treat the newborn for congenital syphilis. The attending physician ordered penicillin to be administered, but the pharmacist misread the handwritten order and issued a ten-fold overdose. The nurses, concerned that the large dose would require multiple injections, consulted a reference book to see if the antibiotic could be administered intravenously instead of intramuscularly. Again, misreading the handwritten order, they mixed up the drug with another type of penicillin for which intravenous (IV) administration was allowed. The combination of the overdose and the IV delivery resulted in the death of the infant. Even more tragically, an autopsy revealed that the infant did not have congenital syphilis and therefore did not need treatment. Figure 5-3 illustrates how this disastrous outcome was the result of failures in four different systems.

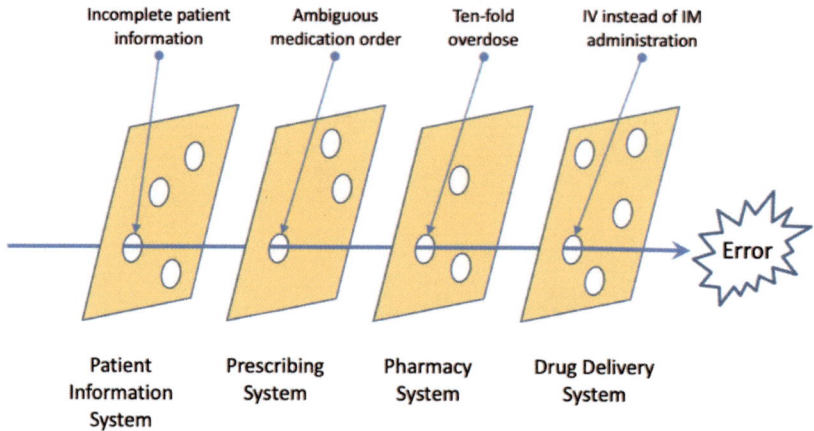

FIGURE 5-3 Swiss cheese model of medication error.
SOURCE: Reason, 1997. Copyright (© 1997) From *Managing the risks of organizational accidents* by James Reason. Reproduced by permission of Taylor and Francis Group, LLC, a division of Informa plc.

It is important to note that additional layers of defense only improve reliability if they are at least partially independent. In the Swiss cheese analogy, an additional slice of cheese whose holes align with those of an existing slice does not add any protection. In a real-world example, adding an additional fill-and-finish plant for a drug will do little to improve reliability if it relies on the same source of active pharmaceutical ingredient (API) supply as all other plants and the API supplier is the main source of disruption risk. For medical product supply chains, which interventions are appropriate, independent, and compatible will depend on both the type of medical product and the disruptive event(s). The implication, therefore, is that different interventions will be appropriate to different medical product supply chains.

THE COMMITTEE'S MEDICAL PRODUCT SUPPLY CHAINS RESILIENCE FRAMEWORK

With the Swiss cheese representation of the Redundancy Principle in mind, the committee developed a framework for enumerating supply chain resilience interventions in a systematic manner. Because the steps that lead to a supply shortage play out over time, it is logical to consider options with respect to their position on the disruption timeline, from preknowledge of risks to postdisruption of medical product supply chains. Figure 5-4 depicts the path from a potential trigger event to public harm and shows the categories of ways to increase the resilience of medical product supply chains.

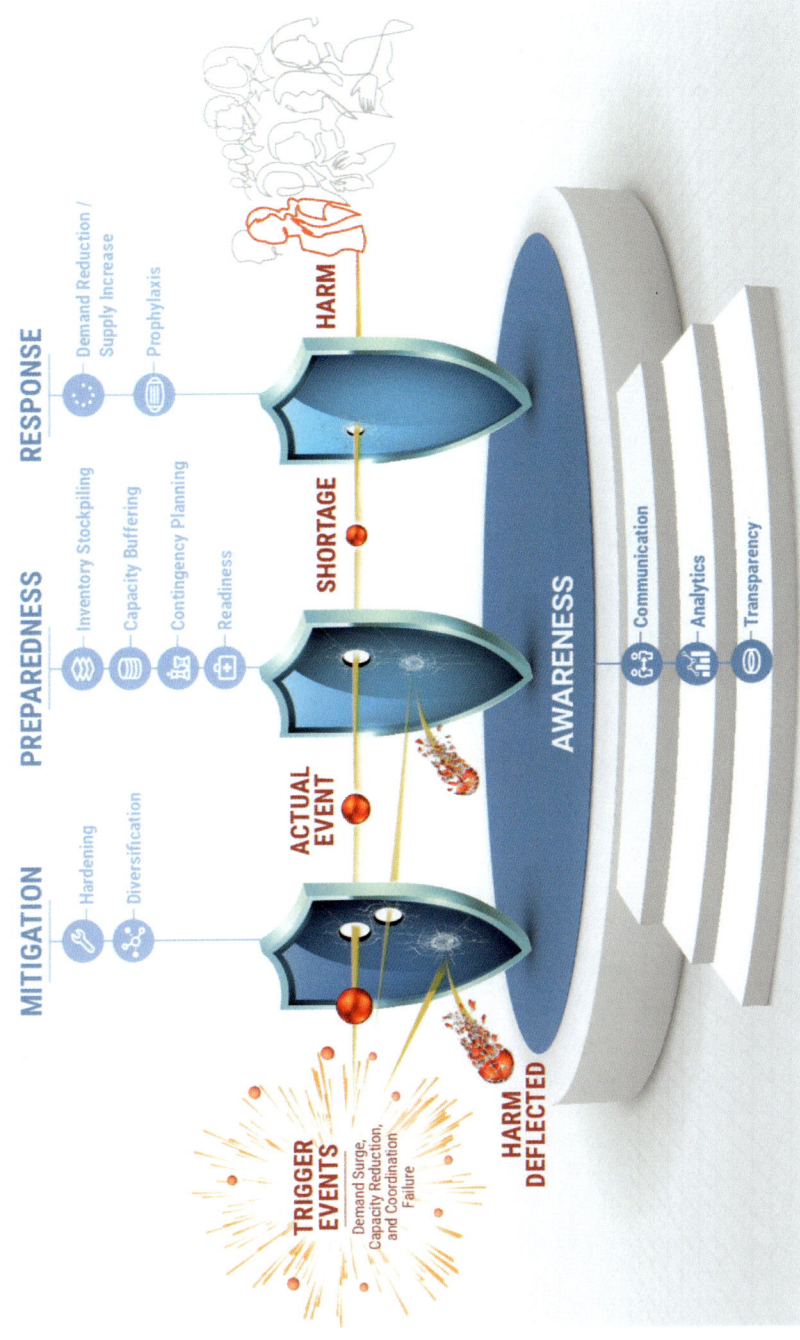

FIGURE 5-4 Medical product supply chains resilience framework: potential trigger events and resilience measures.

Clearly, the medical product supply chain resilience framework depicted in Figure 5-4 is a version of the Swiss cheese model of system reliability. The layers of defense (depicted here as shields, rather than cheese) are specifically related to medical product supply chains. These protective layers are grouped into mitigation, preparedness, and response—the standard phases of emergency response (FEMA, 2021). According to the Federal Emergency Management Agency (FEMA), mitigation takes place prior to an emergency and focuses on "preventing future emergencies or minimizing their effects" (FEMA, 2021). Preparedness measures also take place prior to an emergency and focus on "preparing to handle an emergency" (FEMA, 2021). Response measures take place during an emergency and focus on "responding safely to an emergency" (FEMA, 2021). FEMA also includes a fourth phase, recovery, which includes measures after an emergency. The recovery phase has been omitted here; however, a fourth category of awareness has been added and serves as the support base for the three layers of defense.

The basic sequence in the framework of Figure 5-4 is as follows. A trigger event occurs, which creates a potential event; for example, a fire breaks out in a pharmaceutical plant. Whether this potential event becomes an actual supply chain disruption will depend on the mitigation measures. Therefore, if the sprinkler system functions properly and puts out the fire before heat and flames damage the production process, the harm has been deflected and no disruption occurs. But if the fire is not stopped, and the plant is seriously damaged, production stops and an actual event begins. Whether disruptions become shortages affecting providers and patients depends on the preparedness measures in place. For instance, if there is sufficient inventory of the drug in emergency stockpiles to cover the shortfall until the plant is back online, then patients and providers do not see a shortage; otherwise, a shortage occurs. If that happens, the magnitude of the harm caused will depend on the response measures. Crisis standards of care that prioritize the drug for some patients and provide substitutes for others might reduce the health effects. Finally, mitigation, preparedness, and response measures all depend on awareness measures, which make information available to all decision makers.

Building increased resilience into supply chains depends on each of these four categories of actions, which are described below.

Awareness

As depicted in Figure 5-4, awareness is the foundation for resilience in medical product supply chains. Here, awareness is the possession by the appropriate people of the information needed to assess, mitigate, prepare for, and respond to risks of medical product shortages. This includes information about where medical products come *from*, where in the system medical products *are*, and many other characteristics of medical product supply chains. Without being able to identify and evaluate risks that exist in medical product supply chains, actions cannot be taken to mitigate, prepare for, or respond to them. Hence, the awareness category includes actions that promote understanding of risks and vulnerabilities across the entire medical product supply chain ecosystem from raw material or component suppliers (e.g., makers of ingredients, subassemblies) to producers (e.g., final assembly plants, fill-and-finish facilities), to distributors (e.g., wholesalers), to providers (e.g., health systems, pharmacies, retailers), and finally to patients so the focus and priority can be given to the appropriate resilience efforts.

Awareness measures can be broken into three subcategories: (1) transparency activities that make data available—which includes both surveillance/collection to obtain data and disclosure to make it available; (2) analytics activities that process those data into useful information, which includes compilation, graphical display, statistical analysis, and any other data processing to reveal their meaning; and (3) communication activities, including report writing, database construction and management, and anything else that gets the information into the hands of the people responsible for mitigation, preparedness, and response.

An example of an awareness initiative involving all three subcategories is mapping the supply chains of drugs and devices from production to patient to develop a full picture of the capacity and diversification of production and the profile of inventories across the supply chain. This might reveal that certain drugs or devices have highly limited or concentrated steps that pose risks of disrupting the supply or preventing a response to a spike in demand.

Awareness measures can be promoted at all levels of the supply chain, as well as by the government and third parties that monitor and influence medical supply chains. For example, a potential source of vital information is a hospital pharmacy. This is typically where a health care system would first notice a shortage of a drug. To mitigate a drug shortage within their own hospital, the pharmacy team could inform prescribers of the issue and recommend they use alternative drugs; the team could also contact other suppliers for the product, substitute the prescribed medication, and update their formulary (Shukar et al., 2021). As such, this represents the medical product supply chain resilience framework in a microcosm, with the pharmacy promoting awareness that underpins multiple layers of protective measures.

Mitigation

This category includes actions taken prior to a disruptive event to avoid the event altogether or reduce its magnitude. Mitigation can be divided into two subcategories: (1) hardening activities, that reduce the likelihood or magnitude of disruptive events within stages of the system, and (2) diversification activities, which create parallel versions of stages to reduce the risk of catastrophic failure. In terms of the medical product supply chain resilience framework, hardening strengthens the layers, by reducing the number of penetrating holes in a single shield, while diversification creates more layers of shields. For example, a possible hardening measure for a medical device production process that is prone to interruptions by quality control problems could be product redesign. By reducing the number of components and/or assembly steps, a redesign could reduce opportunities for error (holes in the cheese). An example of a diversification measure for the medical device could be to set up a second production line to share the production load. If one line encounters process problems, the other can continue producing and may even make up some or all of the lost production from the disrupted line.

Mitigation measures do not need to directly address the physical elements of supply chains. For example, regulatory action by the U.S. Food and Drug Administration (FDA) to require better quality process documentation by manufacturers of generic drugs could push manufacturers to scrutinize and improve their processes, thereby reducing the number of quality problems, and hence the number of shortages caused by recalls. FDA (FDA Drug Shortages Task Force, 2020) estimated that quality and process issues are responsible for 62 percent of drug shortages; therefore, steps to reduce these would have a significant effect on both routine drug shortages and shortages during major emergencies. In addition to preventing such shortages, better quality control processes could remediate problems more quickly, thereby reducing the duration of shortages that do occur.

Preparedness

This category includes actions taken prior to a disruptive event that will reduce negative effects on health and safety should an event occur. Preparedness can be grouped into four subcategories, two physical and two virtual. Physical preparedness measures include inventory buffering and capacity buffering, in which actual stock or productive capacity are held in readiness to fill a supply shortfall. Virtual preparedness measures include contingency planning, which establishes plans for dealing with specific scenarios, and readiness, which builds capabilities for dealing with scenarios without specific plans made in advance.

Like the shields in the medical product supply chain resilience framework, the subcategories of the preparedness category can be viewed in terms of their distance from the point where products are used by providers to treat patients. Finished product inventory stockpiling is the closest because, subject to a transport step to move products to the location needed, it is ready to be used by providers. Capacity buffering is an additional step removed, since the product must be made and then shipped to the desired location. Contingency planning to scale up some form of capacity is one more step removed from providers and patients since the plan must be carried out to create the capacity to produce inventory. Finally, a readiness strategy that builds organizational capabilities is yet another step removed. Thinking carefully about the time sequence involved in medical product shortages and in shortage prevention can help in enumerating a broad range of interventions for enhancing supply chain resilience. This observation also highlights the fact that measures that are closer to being ready to use can be accessed more quickly, which, as discussed below, is important in matching different measures as part of a comprehensive resilience strategy.

Inventory Stockpiling and Capacity Buffering

Although inventory stockpiling and capacity buffering are both physical forms of preparedness, they are different in character. Inventory stockpiling involves maintaining a store of medical products, components, or raw materials that are immediately available. Capacity buffering involves maintaining a capability to produce medical products, components, or raw materials. Strictly speaking, a physical capacity buffer refers to ready-to-use production. For example, a medical device manufacturing plant might have the equipment, labor, and components to immediately produce 20 percent more product than its normal volume. If so, then this extra capacity represents a physical buffer that can compensate for a shortage, subject only to the production and delivery lead times.

Inventory stockpiling and capacity buffering also differ with regard to their dependence on one another. While finished goods inventory is ready to be used, inventory held at the intermediate level (components for devices, APIs for drugs) or the raw material level depend on *downstream* capacity to be made into finished products. In contrast, buffer capacity at any level requires *upstream* inventory. For example, the final fill-and-finish stage of drug manufacturing requires API inventory, while API production requires raw material inventory, to carry out their respective manufacturing steps. This mirror-type interdependence—combined with the differences in speed of availability—makes inventory and capacity buffers natural complements, with inventory providing the first line of protection and capacity providing additional layers of protection subject to ramp-up lead times.

Relative Economics of Inventory Stockpiling and Capacity Buffering

In addition to depending on lead times, the right combination of inventory stockpiling and capacity buffering for a given medical product also depends on the relative costs. In general, inventory stockpiling involves a high up-front cost to establish a stockpile and an ongoing maintenance cost to store and rotate it. These costs are incurred regardless of whether the inventory is used or not. Capacity buffering costs are more varied. Since all plants have some excess capacity, they can provide some buffering with no up-front cost or ongoing maintenance cost. Typically, a plant can provide additional buffering by adding labor and/or equipment, with an up-front cost and a longer lead time to ramp up capacity. A production process that can ramp up quickly and efficiently is *scalable*. But whether or not a process is scalable, the production costs (e.g., materials, labor, energy, etc.) for manufacturing products or inputs are incurred only if the extra capacity is needed. This implies that buffer capacity will be more economical than buffer inventory for products or components that are expensive and/or rarely needed.

The characteristics of inventory stockpiling and capacity buffering suggest a natural pairing in which enough inventory is held to cover the lead time to ramp up enough additional capacity to achieve the target protection. For production stages where capacity can be ramped up enough to provide the target protection without excessive up-front costs or lead time this could be a highly effective strategy. But there may be production stages where capacity cannot be ramped up quickly or economically. If so, different buffers may be appropriate for different production stages of the supply chain. For example, suppose a pharmaceutical fill-and-finish plant is capable of ramping up capacity to the level needed to achieve the desired protection target, but the API plant that feeds it would require a very large cost and a very long lead time to increase capacity sufficiently. In this case, holding finished goods inventory to cover the lead time to increase final production, and holding API inventory sufficient to cover the full protection target, may be appropriate. In general, the most economical mix of inventory stockpiling and capacity buffering, as well as the form in which inventory should be held (finished goods, components, raw materials), depends on the details of the manufacturing and supply chain processes for a given medical product. See Box 5-2 for a blueprint for making economic sense of preparedness measures: inventory stockpiling and capacity buffering.

The economics that govern effective use of inventory stockpiling and capacity buffering as protection against medical product shortages to enhance public health also govern the use of these buffers as protection against loss of sales to enhance private profits. Consequently, producers and marketers of medical products maintain buffer inventory and buffer capacity at various levels of their supply chains to ensure business continuity. However, because private profit incentives differ from public health incentives, protection investments by firms may or may not produce socially beneficial outcomes. For example, consider the relatively likely occurrence of short disruptions due to process problems or demand fluctuations. Such disruptions can be

BOX 5-2
Relative Economics of Inventory Stockpiling and Capacity Buffering

The two issues that must be considered in choosing an appropriate balance of inventory and capacity to achieve a protection target volume of X are time and cost. Because capacity requires time to bring online, stockpiles must hold at least enough inventory to cover demand during the lead time to start production from the buffer capacity source. Suppose it is decided to stock a level of inventory that is large enough to cover this lead time and there are Y units of protection left to cover. Whether additional protection should come from inventory or capacity depends on the relative economics.

Suppose the product has an annual unit holding cost of h, a capital cost of K per unit of capacity, and events large enough to exhaust the inventory supply and require activation of the capacity buffer source occur on average every N years. Then the annual holding cost to carry Y units of inventory is hY. The average cost per year to activate the capacity buffer is KY/N. This equation shows that the cost of capacity buffering is less than the cost of buffer inventory if $N > K/h$.

For example, suppose ventilators cost $1,000 to produce and have a carrying cost rate of 25 percent so that h = $250. Further, suppose that it costs $10 million to activate a plant that will produce 10,000 units of emergency product. For the sake of simplicity, this scenario assumes any increases in variable costs for emergency production are factored into the capital cost and that scale economies that reduce unit capital cost as the production volume increases can be ignored. This implies the unit capital cost is K = $10,000,000/10,000 = $1,000. For capacity buffering to be economical, the equation requires that $N > K/h$ = $1,000/$250 = 4 years. That is, unless the events that would require the additional Y units of protection are very common (once every 4 years or less), capacity is more economical than inventory to provide the additional protection.

Note that the likelihood of needing the capacity buffer will depend on how much inventory is held. Stockpiles could hold more than the minimum required to cover the lead time to bring the capacity online. The more inventory that stockpiles hold, the less likely a disruption is to be long enough to exhaust the inventory and require the capacity buffer. This implies that there will always be a maximum amount of inventory that is economical to hold. Above this maximum, it will be more economical to rely on capacity, which may be expensive but will be required so rarely that the average cost is still lower than the cost of inventory.

This model is obviously highly simplified. For example, it does not include ongoing costs to maintain an operable capacity buffer or rotation costs to avoid expiration of stockpiled inventory. These considerations would change the numerical outcome, but not the basic insight that inventory buffering incurs all or most of its costs whether the inventory is used or not, while the majority of the cost of surge capacity is incurred only when it is activated. This implies that inventory is best suited for short, frequent shortages, while capacity is best suited to long, infrequent shortages will not be altered by adding real-world complexity to the model.

covered with modest amounts of inventory that will be tapped relatively often. For high-margin products, holding inventory as protection against losing sales or harming one's brand are easy to justify. Consequently, supply chains for brand-name drugs and patented devices, which have large margins, typically contain inventory stockpiles to protect against variations in supply and demand. They may even contain some form of buffer capacity to protect against larger, less likely disruptions. However, low-margin products, for which cost control is vital, often make use of lean practices that reduce inventory stockpiles to minimal levels.[4] Consequently, even relatively modest disruptions, such as a short-term process problem, can produce supply shortages for these products. This explains why generic drugs account for the majority of routine drug shortages (ASHP, 2018). A high-profile example is vincristine, a chemotherapy drug for childhood cancers, which experienced a severe and prolonged shortage when the primary manufacturer encountered a quality control problem in 2019. The implication is that where profit margins are low, public intervention to spur greater use of inventory stockpiling and/or capacity buffering may be needed to provide socially acceptable levels of protection against medical product shortages.

Buffer Flexibility

As noted above, scalability makes capacity more effective as protection against a supply shortage. Another characteristic that can make both inventory stockpiling and capacity buffering more effective is *flexibility*. A resource is flexible if it can be used to satisfy more than one source of demand. Just as the layers of protection in the medical product supply chain resilience framework need to be independent to reduce risks of a shortage, flexibility is only effective for independent sources of demand. For example, if surges of patients requiring intubation in different regions is perfectly correlated, then resource sharing of ventilators is not helpful. Similarly, if a global pandemic surges demand for N95 masks everywhere at the same time, then reciprocal import/export agreements will be irrelevant. Fortunately, even in widespread events that eventually affect everyone, demand often occurs in waves that are offset in time. This enables flexibility and resource sharing to provide some level of protection. But for major global emergencies, flexibility will not be enough. A combination of inventory stockpiling and capacity buffering will be needed to provide protection in these rare but extreme events.

---

[4] Lean practices are a set of management practices to improve efficiency and effectiveness by eliminating waste. The core principle of these is to reduce and eliminate non-value adding activities and waste (Crawford, 2016).

Contingency Planning and Readiness

In addition to the physical protections of inventory stockpiling and capacity buffering, preparedness measures also include the virtual protections of contingency planning and readiness. The difference between contingency planning and readiness is that a contingency plan addresses a specific scenario, while a readiness measure prepares for a general class of scenarios or a completely unspecified scenario.

Examples of contingency planning include crisis standards of care planning, such as a policy to use N95 masks for up to five shifts, with nightly sterilization between shifts, to address a supply shortage. An example of a contingency plan at a different point in the supply chain would be a contract with an auto manufacturer to assemble ventilators in an emergency. Note that such a plan would provide additional production capacity, albeit with a longer lead time than physical buffer capacity. A contingency plan that identifies supplemental producers for specific supply chain critical medical products and readiness steps, such as sharing supplier and bill-of-material information with these producers, would make ramping up capacity in an emergency faster and more reliable.

Readiness activities are usually in the form of organizational preparation at multiple levels (i.e., top-down, bottom-up). An example of a readiness practice is the establishment of forums for sharing information and ideas. For instance, the Supply Chain Risk Leadership Council (SCRLC) was set up to encourage supply chain managers to discuss awareness and preparedness practices during routine times and to pool expertise to respond during emergency events (SCRLC, n.d.). A similar council could be established specifically for medical product supply chain managers. Training activities to expose individuals and groups to previous emergency events and collaborative exercises to build relationships among them also act as readiness measures. Each of these measures will help to ensure response is quick and effective to whatever scenario arises.

Response

The response category depends on various awareness, mitigation, and preparedness measures and includes actions taken postevent to minimize harm from the shortage and to resolve the shortage. These actions can be subdivided into measures to close the supply gap through (1) reducing the demand or increasing the supply, and (2) prophylaxis measures, which protect human health while the shortage persists. Taken together, response measures seek to return supply chains to normal (or a "new normal") with as little harm as possible to patients.

Measures to reduce demand and increase supply must be implemented at the global and local levels to minimize harm from medical product shortages once they occur. As such, they must deal with both the big picture of global medical product supply chains and the small picture of local distribution and delivery of medical products to the end users (i.e., the last mile of supply chains). These twin approaches are needed to help national supply chains respond to global emergencies and to aid local end users in reducing the effect of shortages on the health of individual patients and communities. International cooperation and coordinated response, such as international agreements or treaties, can help minimize the effects of medical product shortages and strengthen resilience in supply chains.

Examples of prophylaxis measures include the many improvised or inventive ways medical professionals adapted to medical product shortages during the COVID-19 pandemic. One such innovation was the development of an aerosol box that protected health care workers from exhaled aerosols emitted during patient intubation (Begley et al., 2020). In general, prophylaxis activities are front-line, last-mile measures rather than upstream actions as they resolve the immediate issue but do not solve the supply shortage. However, some improvised and inventive activities can have supply chain implications. For instance, use of 3D-printed components to modify ventilators to allow multiple patients to share a single machine was a demand reduction measure during the early days of the COVID-19 pandemic (Ayyıldız et al., 2020; NIH 3D Print Exchange, 2020; Rosen, 2020).

Finally, it should be noted that there is a very close relationship between virtual preparedness measures and response measures. Contingency planning and readiness activities taken prior to a disruptive event can improve the speed and accuracy of response measures. Therefore, in the planning process it makes sense to consider these categories of options in tandem.

Different Taxonomies and Perspectives

There are other taxonomies and perspectives for building resilient medical product supply chains beyond the categories and measures presented in Figure 5-4. Each category can consider interventions that make use of regulations, economics, technology, and so forth. For example, within the preparedness category, capacity buffering measures are identified as potentially attractive options. However, capacity buffering is not something that can be implemented directly. Instead, it needs to be cultivated by a combination of regulatory changes, economic incentives, and technological advances, such as continuous drug manufacturing that would make domestic production and scale-up practical.

Other taxonomies, like one considering options from the perspective of different actors, such as government, private firms, nonprofits, international organizations, and so forth, may also be helpful in thinking through options and helping to evolve an effective resilience strategy for medical product supply chains.

No One-Size-Fits-All Strategy: A Discussion on Cost-Effectiveness and Finding Balance within an Integrated Resilience Strategy

Finally, a fundamental take-away from Figure 5-4 and the logic behind it is that *there is no one-size-fits-all strategy for increasing the resilience of supply chains for all medical products. Different medical product supply chains, different markets, and different risk profiles all require different interventions. The key challenge is to match measures to products in a cost-effective manner.*

At the level of individual medical products, matching appropriate measures to products can be done using the medical product supply chain resilience framework to help select candidate options and then using detailed information about the specific medical product to evaluate the practicality of each option. For medical products identified as supply chain critical, such detailed scrutiny may be warranted. For example, determining the right level of inventory of a given product to hold in the SNS is a policy intervention at the individual product level. The above take-away and the discussion leading to it imply that such a stockpiling decision should take into account the individual characteristics, such as the profit incentive for the market to provide protections, the scalability of the production technology, etc., of the product.

However, it is not possible or practical to make individual analyses of every supply chain critical medical product. Therefore, general purpose regulations and requirements are also needed that enhance supply chain resilience for broad sets of medical products. The implication of the above take-away for this type of policy making is that, where possible, interventions should focus on incentives rather than actions. A useful analogy is the Clean Air Act of 1970, which required use of scrubbers to remove effluents such as sulfur dioxide from the smokestack emissions of power plants. At the time, many economists objected to this requirement, arguing that (1) scrubbers might be a good alternative for some plants but not for others, and (2) the "technology forcing" nature of the requirement removed all incentive for utilities to find more effective ways to control pollution. A better policy would have been to impose an effluent tax that would charge utilities for every pound of effluent they emitted. If the tax was set high enough to make scrubbers more economical than paying the tax, utilities would have incentive to use them. But plants for which other methods (e.g., changes in fuel or process) could reduce pollution more cheaply could use these. And everyone would have incentive to find more efficient means for reducing their effluents. The result would be lower costs, which would translate into lower prices for consumers, and an innovative culture that would promote ongoing progress in pollution control.

Analogously, if policies are adopted that require firms to hold certain amounts of inventory or to adopt certain flexible manufacturing technologies, it is likely that policies that work well to promote supply chain resilience for some products but are highly inefficient or ineffective for other products will be implemented. If instead policies are used that create incentives for supply continuity and emergency readiness, the market will respond by crafting systems appropriate to their supply chains and by innovating to find more efficient and effective ways to enhance medical supply chain resilience.

To make this general recommendation to leverage the market more concrete, the committee forward references two pieces of recommendations. First, in Recommendation 3 (Health System Actions), health systems are encouraged to incorporate quality and supply continuity into their contracts, so that suppliers pay penalties for defects, recalls, and delays that meet specified criteria. The penalties will provide incentive for suppliers to enhance their reliability but leave it to the firms to find the best way to do this. Second, in Recommendation 5 (Capacity Buffering), the committee advocates for publication of "crisis prices" by the federal government that specify premiums to be paid for critical medical products under specified emergency conditions. These provide incentives for firms to find ways to provide "pop-up" capacity for an emergency but leave it to the market to identify which firms will participate and how. In both recommendations, the policies create incentives for firms to enhance medical product supply chain resilience rather than specifying actions that may be suboptimal or become so over time as manufacturing technologies and practices evolve.

In the following sections the medical product supply chain resilience framework is leveraged and general insights and guidelines that may be helpful in identifying incentive-oriented policies to promote supply chain resilience are discussed.

Early Intervention

In general, the earlier that a harm is prevented, the lower the total cost will be to society. In the language of Figure 5-4, mitigation is generally cheaper than preparedness, which is generally cheaper than response. Although all three will be needed to protect the public from harm by medical product shortages during emergencies, it is usually less expensive to avoid disruption events via mitigation measures than to protect people from events that occur through preparedness measures. Similarly, it is usually less costly to avoid public harm through preparedness measures than it is to address that harm through response measures. Furthermore, since awareness is a precursor to mitigation, preparedness, and response, investments in information gathering are particularly cost-effective because they enhance the effectiveness of all other measures.

Clearly, the above observation does not imply that every investment in an early shield (or the awareness foundation) of the medical product supply chain resilience framework is more effective than any investment in a later shield. Foolish investments to collect unnecessary information or to implement ineffective mitigation measures are clearly not better than sensitive and appropriate response measures. The best options early in the timeline, when there is time to plan and prepare, are typically better than the best options later in the timeline, when a crisis is under way. Policies that promote proactive behavior in favor of reactive behavior should not be overlooked.

However, although early interventions are important, they are almost never sufficient on their own. The reason is that many measures exhibit decreasing returns to scale. Each additional increment of protection from a given measure becomes less effective or more expensive. For example, each increment of inventory added to a stockpile becomes less and less likely to be needed, and hence provides fewer and fewer expected health benefits. The cost-effectiveness of inventory investments therefore decreases with scale. Similarly, investments in capacity become less valuable with scale, but they also become more expensive. The first increment of buffer capacity may be very cheap to achieve by simply scheduling overtime. A second increment may be more expensive because additional workers must be hired and trained to staff an additional shift. A third increment may be extremely expensive (and slow to achieve) if additional production facilities are needed. Consequently, as with inventory, the cost-effectiveness of capacity investments decreases with scale. Because of this, the most efficient measures—the low-hanging fruit—should be prioritized in all of the protective layers of the medical product supply chain resilience framework to find the most cost-effective mix of measures for promoting resilience in medical product supply chains.

Virtual Protection

Virtual measures are cheaper but slower than concrete measures. For example, the expected cost of a contingency plan to obtain extra inventory will be less than that of an inventory stockpile because the contingency plan might not need to be implemented, while the stockpile will cost whether or not it is needed. Analogously, general readiness measures that address a broad range of scenarios may be cheaper than many specific contingency plans to address each scenario because more time and expense will be invested to generate concrete plans than to be ready in a general sense.

However, the more concrete the resilience measure is, the more rapidly it can be deployed. For example, inventory is immediately available, while a contingency plan must be carried out before it becomes effective. The implication is that concrete measures are generally best suited for short, frequent disruptions, while virtual measures are better suited for long, infrequent disruptions. As noted earlier, while it may be easy to justify the high up-front cost of inventory stockpiling to cover expected disruptions, it is more pragmatic to rely on capacity buffering to cover large disruptions that are highly unlikely.

Figure 5-5 provides a graphical illustration of how to align resilience measures on different points of the virtual/concrete scale to medical products with different risk profiles. Consistent with the discussion above, the most concrete physical measures of inventory and capacity buffering (along with measures to make them flexible) are suited to products at high risk of supply disruption. Intermediate contingency planning measures, which do not create physical assets but do create explicit plans for specific scenarios, are suited to products having an intermediate risk of disruption. The most virtual measures of response are the options of last resort for dealing with products at low risk of disruption. Finally, the willingness to use a more concrete measure should increase with the medically essential score of a product because the higher cost of human harm justifies more expensive investments to provide faster and more reliable protection. On the other end of the scale, for medical products that are sufficiently nonessential, it may be optimal to do nothing so that resources can be used to secure supplies of more supply chain critical medical products.

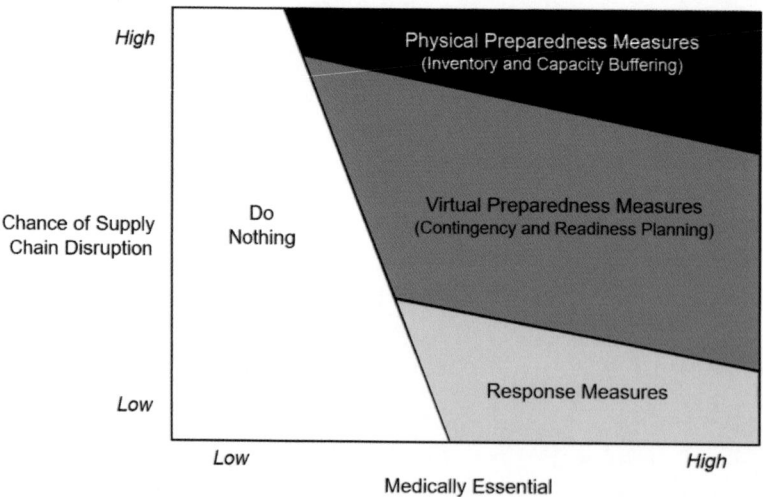

FIGURE 5-5 A layered protection strategy for matching resilience measures to medical products.
SOURCE: Adapted from Hopp, 2008.

Hybrid Strategies

The detailed goal set for this chapter was to be able to cover a shortage of size X_i for each product i on the supply chain critical list. Based on the development and discussion of the resulting medical product supply chain resilience framework, it is clear that it will be more cost-effective to do this with a combination of supply chain resilience measures, rather than with a single measure. A main reason is because the size of the supply disruption is uncertain. By the logic of Figure 5-5, the fast, concrete measures of inventory stockpiling and capacity buffering should be used to cover smaller shortage amounts that are likely to occur, but the slower response measures should be relied on to deal with large but very unlikely shortages. Contingency planning can be used for intermediate cases. The implication is that a layered protection strategy, with inventory to cover the first X_i units of shortage and virtual measures to provide additional coverage if needed, is likely to be a sound approach for most products.

The proper mix of physical and virtual protection depends on lead times. If the time to bring backup capacity online is very short, such as a plant simply scheduling extra shifts, then it would be wasteful to hold a large amount of inventory in a stockpile. Hence, the most cost-effective hybrid strategy for building supply chain resilience of a given medical product will depend on how critical it is, as indicated in Figure 5-5, and also on the characteristics of its supply chain, which influence how quickly capacity can be ramped up. Furthermore, measures in the different layers can be strongly synergistic. For example, measures that promote better process control (a mitigation measure) may be the most cost-effective way to avoid shortages caused by manufacturing quality problems.

CONCLUDING REMARKS AND OVERVIEW OF COMMITTEE RECOMMENDATIONS

To achieve the goal of promoting resilient medical product supply chains that are cost-effective and protect public health in both normal and emergency conditions, all protective layers of the medical product supply chains resilience framework must be used.

In the remaining chapters (Chapters 6–9), the committee articulates seven recommendations within the four protective layers (or shields)—awareness, mitigation, preparedness, and response—of the medical product supply chains resilience framework. While the recommendations may address more than one layer, the list in Box 5-3 shows the recommendations under the layer with which they are primarily aligned. Taken together, the seven recommendations shown below will increase the resilience of medical product supply chains at all four protective layers of

> **BOX 5-3**
> **Summary of Recommendations**
>
> The following points collectively summarize the necessary actions recommended by the committee that are needed to increase the resilience of medical product supply chains:
>
> Awareness
> 1. Public Transparency—Make sourcing, quality, volume, and capacity information publicly available for all medical products approved or cleared for sale in the United States.
> 2. Public Database—Establish a public database for the supply chain information acquired for medical products.
>
> Mitigation
> 3. Resilience Contracting by Health Systems—Deliberately incorporate quality and reliability, in addition to price, in contracting, purchasing, and inventory decisions.
>
> Preparedness
> 4. Stockpiling—Modernize and optimize inventory stockpiling management to respond to medical product shortages at the national and regional levels.
> 5. Capacity Buffering—Cultivate capacity buffering for supply chain critical medical products where such capacity is a cost-effective complement to stockpiling.
>
> Response
> 6. International Treaty—Negotiate an international treaty with other major medical product exporters that rules out export bans on key components of global medical product supply chains.
> 7. Last-Mile Management—Establish a working group to examine last-mile and end user issues regarding medical product supply chains.

the resilience framework. Furthermore, where possible, the committee has articulated ways to address these layers by means of incentives that promote actions to enhance supply chain resilience but leaves specifics to the market to allow the power of market competition and innovation to generate the best available solutions. Given balanced attention and coordination, these recommendations will substantially improve the nation's ability to maintain supplies of medical products and prevent harm during normal and emergency conditions.

REFERENCES

ASHP (American Society of Health-System Pharmacists). 2018. ASHP guidelines on managing drug product shortages. *American Journal of Health-System Pharmacists* 75:1742-1750.

Ayyıldız, S., A. M. Dursun, V. Yıldırım, M. E. İnce, M. A. Gülçelik, and C. Erdöl. 2020. 3D-printed splitter for use of a single ventilator on multiple patients during COVID-19. *3D Printing and Additive Manufacturing* 7(4):181-185.

Begley, J. L., K. E. Lavery, C. P. Nickson, and D. J. Brewster. 2020. The aerosol box for intubation in Coronavirus Disease 2019 patients: An in-situ simulation crossover study. *Anaesthesia* 75(8):1014-1021.

Bergman, G. M. n.d. *Order of arithmetic operations.* https://math.berkeley.edu/~gbergman/misc/numbers/ord_ops.html (accessed November 2, 2021).

Crawford, M. 2016. *5 lean principles every engineer should know.* The American Society of Mechanical Engineers. https://www.asme.org/topics-resources/content/5-lean-principles-every-should-know (accessed November 2, 2021).

FDA (U.S. Food and Drug Administration) Drug Shortages Task Force. 2020. *Drug shortages: Root causes and potential solutions.* https://www.fda.gov/drugs/drug-shortages/report-drug-shortages-root-causes-and-potential-solutions (accessed December 16, 2021).

FEMA (Federal Emergency Management Agency). 2021. *The four phases of emergency management.* https://training.fema.gov/emiweb/downloads/is10_unit3.doc (accessed December 16, 2021).

Hopp, W. J. 2008. *Supply chain science.* New York: McGraw-Hill Irwin.

Hopp, W. J., and W. S. Lovejoy. 2012. *Hospital operations: Principles of high efficiency health care.* Pearson Education. Upper Saddle River, NJ: FT Press.

NIH 3D Print Exchange. 2020. *LRTee: Ventilator splitter.* NIH. https://3dprint.nih.gov/discover/3dpx-013734 (accessed November 3, 2021).

Reason, J. 1997. *Managing the risks of organizational accidents.* Burlington, VT: Ashgate Publishing.

Reason, J. 2000. Human error: Models and management. *BMJ (Clinical Research Edition)* 320(7237):768-770.

Rosen, J. 2020. *Johns Hopkins engineers developing 3D-printed ventilator splitter,* edited by Johns Hopkins University and Office of Communications. Johns Hopkins University. https://releases.jhu.edu/2020/04/02/johns-hopkins-engineers-developing-3d-printed-ventilator-splitter/ (accessed November 3, 2021).

SCLRC (Supply Chain Risk Leadership Council). n.d. *Supply Chain Risk Leadership Council.* http://scrlc.com/about.php (accessed December 9, 2021).

Shukar, S., F. Zahoor, K. Hayat, A. Saeed, A. H. Gillani, S. Omer, S. Hu, Z.-U.-D. Babar, Y. Fang, and C. Yang. 2021. Drug shortage: Causes, impact, and mitigation strategies. *Frontiers in Pharmacology* 12:1772.

Smetzer, J., and M. Cohen. 1998. Lesson from the Denver medication error/criminal negligence case: Look beyond blaming individuals. *Hospital Pharmacy* 33(6).

6

Awareness Measures for Resilient Medical Product Supply Chains

The medical product supply chain resilience framework described in Chapter 5 and reproduced in Figure 6-1 identifies awareness as the foundation for resilient medical product supply chains. Awareness is achieved through transparency (i.e., visible data), analytics (i.e., processes for turning data into information), and communication (i.e., channels for sharing

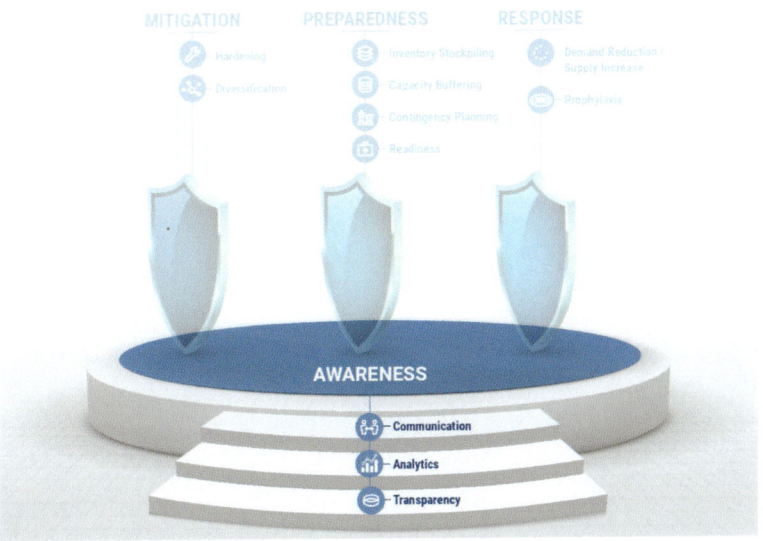

FIGURE 6-1 Medical product supply chain resilience framework: potential awareness measures.

information with the relevant actors in the supply chain). These three parts of awareness are interdependent because without transparency, there is no data on which to perform analytics, and without analytics there is no information to communicate. Therefore, all three elements of awareness are needed to be able to execute the three layers of protection—mitigation, preparedness, and response—in the framework.

Awareness can have substantial effects on supply chain operations, patient safety and end user outcomes, ethical decisions, market competition, and other issues (Woodcock and Wosinska, 2013). Box 6-1 lists a wide range of benefits from information sharing in supply chains (Lotfi et al., 2013).

Unfortunately, as concluded in Chapter 4, *a lack of transparency in medical product supply chains has led to limited empirical evidence regarding best strategies for addressing supply chain issues. The current practice of keeping medical product supply chains confidential conflicts with public health needs and puts the public's health at risk. Improving the public's access to data that are important to their health and well-being is critical.* It is clear that situational awareness across medical product supply chains is lacking, and that the coronavirus disease 2019 (COVID-19) pandemic response has highlighted the haphazard and inconsistent federal approach used to monitor medical

---

BOX 6-1
Benefits of Information Sharing in Supply Chain Management

- Inventory reduction and efficient inventory management
- Cost reduction
- Increased visibility and significant reduction of uncertainties
- Significant reduction or complete elimination of bullwhip effect*
- Improved resource utilization
- Increased productivity, organizational efficiency, and improved services
- Building and strengthening social bonds
- Early problem detection
- Quick response
- Reduced cycle time from order to delivery
- Better tracing and tracking
- Earlier time to market
- Expanded network
- Optimized capacity utilization

SOURCE: Lotfi et al., 2013.

---

* Bullwhip effects are created when supply chain members process the demand input from their immediate downstream member in producing their own forecasts. Demand information can be distorted as it is transmitted up the chain, and small fluctuations downstream can cause progressively larger fluctuations upstream (Lee et al., 1997).

product supply chains. This chapter addresses this problem by describing options for building awareness as part of an integrated resilience strategy. It culminates in two recommendations pivotal to collecting, compiling, and disseminating the data on where and how medical products are made.

TRANSPARENCY

Awareness across the entire medical product supply chain ecosystem requires actions by regulators, suppliers, producers, distributors, and providers. Issues that lead to risks and supply shortages can be spatially and temporally distributed over the supply chain. Without the ability to analyze the dynamics of the entire system, it is not possible to pinpoint problems and identify remedies. Consequently, efforts are needed to collect, compile, and disseminate medical product supply chain data from the various stakeholders to increase end-to-end awareness that will facilitate identification and mitigation of risks. Toward this end, the committee identifies upstream transparency efforts as a critical first step to increasing the resilience of medical product supply chains.

Several countries have already started taking actions toward greater transparency in pharmaceutical supply chains. For example, in New Zealand, the name and location of active pharmaceutical ingredient (API) and finished dosage form (FDF) manufacturers, as well as the product sponsor and marketer in the country, for prescription drug products are collected and made public via a centralized, public access website (Schondelmeyer et al., 2020). Schondelmeyer and colleagues noted that making these data publicly available has not appeared to have commercially harmed manufacturers or marketers.

Data Types to Increase Upstream Transparency

The following are important types of data identified by the committee and others that could be made transparent because of their role in addressing the gaps in understanding where and how medical products are made:

- complete registration and listing requirements,
- sourcing information,
- manufacturing location,
- drug and medical device manufacturing volume and capacity,
- information on increases in demand and reported disruptions, and
- risk-based Site Selection Model score.

Manufacturers and the U.S. Food and Drug Administration (FDA) already have much of these data in their systems, per FDA requirements.

However, these data are not shared with the public or other U.S. government agencies or even regulatory agencies in other countries. Making certain data submitted to the FDA transparent to the public may also warrant certain legislative changes. For instance, it might necessitate a statutory amendment in the form of a change to section 301(j) of the Food, Drug, and Cosmetic (FD&C) Act (21 U.S.C. § 331(j)), which would be required only to the extent that the data that are proposed be disclosed outside the U.S. Department of Health and Human Services (HHS) are deemed as "concerning any method or process which as a trade secret is entitled to protection." In addition, 18 U.S.C. § 1905 (the Trade Secrets Act) would have to be amended to the extent the disclosed information "concerns or relates to … trade secrets, processes, [or] operations … or to the identity [or] confidential statistical data" of any company, unless disclosure of that information is otherwise "authorized by law."

Complete Registration and Listing Requirements

Some foreign medical product manufacturers fail to register their facilities because they do not ship their products directly to the United States. Such entities should be required to report complete registration and listing requirements for each of their products, as also recommended by the recent 100-day review of Executive Order 14017 (The White House, 2021).

Sourcing Information

Supply chain security requires robust reporting of sourcing information—including volume information—by both finished product manufacturers and API manufacturers. For example, drug manufacturers should be required to report all sources of APIs and major excipients, and API manufacturers should report sources of raw materials. At a minimum, drug manufacturers should include the facility FDA Establishment Identifier (FEI) of the sites that processed the API and performed the finish-and-fill operation. In this vein, the 100-day review of Executive Order 14017 recommended the requirement that the labeling of APIs and finished product labeling include original manufacturers (The White House, 2021). Also, when the FDF manufacturer receives an API from multiple sources it should report the percentage of the API it uses that comes from each API source. These data would vastly increase the ability of FDA, health systems, and third parties to identify and remediate pharmaceutical supply chain risks.

Analogous data are needed from manufacturers of medical devices to facilitate supply chain resilience measures. Specifically, device producers should be required to report sources of major components, including percentages of supply for multisourced components. Ideally, suppliers of components would also report their suppliers to facilitate tracing of supply chains. However, where medical device supply chains rely on general electronic and other types of components and materials, it will be increasingly difficult to compel sourcing disclosure under medical product regulatory requirements. At a minimum, device manufacturers should be able to provide information about the top layers of their supply chains. Other means may be needed to identify vulnerabilities in lower tiers.

Manufacturing Location

Visibility into the locations where medical products and their constituent components are manufactured is essential to assessing supply risks and formulating policies to address them. Critical information includes the manufacturing locations for FDFs, APIs, and major excipients for drugs and the major locations of primary manufacturing and final assembly steps for medical devices that are intended for sale in the United States.

FDA's FEI is an existing tool that can be used to more effectively track manufacturing location. FDA assigns FEI numbers to uniquely identify firms associated with FDA-regulated products.[1] Because the FEI number indicates the manufacturing location of each product, researchers can associate location data directly with other key FDA datasets, such as the Inspection Classification Database.[2] The FEI number is also used in FDA's Drug Establishments Current Registration Site, which is updated daily to include all currently registered establishments that "manufacture, prepare, propagate, compound, or process drugs that are distributed in the United States or offered for import to the United States" (FDA, 2020). However, although this platform makes information about all the sites for which a given firm may be approved to manufacture any product publicly available, it does not clearly indicate where a specific product is actually made. For instance, searching for *Pfizer* in this database will yield a list of all of Pfizer's FDA-approved sites, but will not provide information about which products are manufactured in which locations. To be useful to health systems, pharmacies, providers, and consumers the FEI data described in this section must also be linked to individual National Drug Codes. The product specific detail is necessary to assess product risk factors and to predict and respond to medical product shortages.

---

[1] The FEI number is also known as the Firm or Facility Establishment Identifier (https://www.fda.gov/about-fda/fda-data-dashboard/glossary-fda-data-dashboard).

[2] The Inspection Classification Database contains information about inspections conducted by FDA and assessments of regulated facilities; however, it does not include information about inspections conducted by states on behalf of FDA (https://www.fda.gov/inspections-compliance-enforcement-and-criminal-investigations/inspection-classification-database).

Drug and Medical Device Manufacturing Volume and Capacity Information

Drug and medical device manufacturing volume information is another type of data that is essential to risk assessment and can aid in identifying and resolving supply chain bottlenecks. For example, the manufacturer of a FDF of a drug should be required to disclose not only the sources of the API it uses in the FDF, but also (when the FDF manufacturer receives API from multiple sources) the volume of API it receives from each source. Analogously, a device manufacturer should report both sources and volumes from component suppliers.

Information about manufacturing *capacity*—that is, how much the company is actually capable of making, not merely how much they decided to make—is potentially even more valuable than information about manufacturing volume, because companies may have unused capacity that could be used during shortages. The HHS Assistant Secretary for Planning and Evaluation's (ASPE's) economic analysis of shortages identified inadequate capacity as a key driver of shortages after finding that many manufacturers had expanded their number of products without a corresponding expansion of capacity (Haninger et al., 2011).

Information on Increases in Demand and Reported Disruptions

Information from manufacturers about increases in demand and reported disruptions is another category of information that should be transparent (The White House, 2021). A caveat is that manufacturers could experience increased demand for reasons unrelated to shortages, so it is important to coordinate manufacturer-level data about externally driven demand surges. While the reporting of disruptions is already required for lifesaving drugs and devices (see the FD&C Act, sections 506C and 506J),[3] it could be expanded to include increases in demand or extended beyond lifesaving products.

Risk-Based Site-Selection Model Score

Relevant information on drug quality that is included on prescription labeling would enable better decision making on the part of health systems and increase consumer awareness. FDA guidance on package-level standardized numerical identifiers is one step toward implementing mitigation measures to secure drug supply chains (FDA, 2020).

---

[3] Federal Food, Drug, and Cosmetic Act of 1938, 75th Cong. § 506C and 506J, 21 U.S.C. ch.9 § 301 et seq.

In 2005, FDA implemented a risk-based approach to drug facility surveillance to prioritize inspections of the highest-risk facilities, defined as those with the "greatest potential for public health risk should they not comply with established manufacturing quality standards."[4] Facilities are prioritized for inspection using the risk-based Site Selection Model, which evaluates risks related to API and FDF quality that can arise from not following current good manufacturing processes (CDER, 2018).[5] Specific risk factors considered by the Site Selection Model are detailed in Box 6-2.

Within FDA's Office of Pharmaceutical Quality, the Office of Surveillance prioritizes sites for surveillance inspections by entering the names of the facilities selected by the Site Selection Model into the Center for Drug Evaluation and Research's (CDER's) Catalog of Manufacturing Sites, which are sites that are subject to routine inspection,[6] thus producing CDER's Site Surveillance Inspection List (CDER, 2018). This list ranks subject sites by their Site Selection Model score so the highest-risk sites can be prioritized for surveillance inspection by the Office of Regulatory Affairs. Thus, the Site Selection Model provides FDA with a measured indicator of the level of

---

BOX 6-2
FDA's Site Selection Model: Risk Factors

Consistent with Section 510 of the FD&C Act, risk factors considered by FDA's Site Selection Model include

- The compliance history of the establishment
- The record, history, and nature of recalls linked to the establishment
- The inherent risk of the drug manufactured, prepared, propagated, compounded, or processed at the establishment
- The inspection frequency and history of the establishment, including whether the establishment has been inspected pursuant to Section 704 within the last 4 years
- Whether the establishment has been inspected by a foreign government or an agency of a foreign government recognized under Section 809
- Any other criteria deemed necessary and appropriate by the secretary for purposes of allocating inspection resources

SOURCE: https://www.fda.gov/media/116004/download.

---

[4] Information given by testimony of Janet Woodcock (House Committee on Energy and Commerce, 2019).

[5] FD&C Act section 501(a)(2)(B) and related regulations: 21 CFR parts 210 and 211.

[6] CDER's Catalog of Manufacturing Sites includes sites that commercially manufacture a finished pharmaceutical drug product, an in-process material, or an API for a drug intended for human use (https://www.fda.gov/media/116004/download).

manufacturing quality or safety risk associated with a given manufacturing facility that is based on data *only* possessed fully by FDA. This information is not publicly available, and Site Selection Model scores are not divulged to the manufacturers. FDA's Center for Devices and Radiological Health (CDRH) also uses a site-selection, score-based approach to rank medical device manufacturing facilities for site inspections by priority (Mulero, 2018).

ANALYTICS

Data are not information and can be misleading, so mandating data collection and disclosure is only the first step. To enable stakeholders in medical product supply chains to make better decisions, data must be compiled into useful, meaningful forms—such as risk assessments, quality ratings, summary statistics, and other results from analyses.

By comprehensively understanding the risks and vulnerabilities at multiple levels—and from multiple perspectives—of medical product supply chains, it is possible to identify and prioritize mitigation, preparedness, and response actions. The types of data discussed earlier in this chapter could be used by researchers and others to identify risks and vulnerabilities, improve situational awareness and predict potential shortages, conduct research on supply chain resilience, and monitor the effects of increased transparency.

As with risk assessment, making data public could facilitate third-party rating systems. In 2013, Woodcock and Wosinska published recommendations for transparency regarding manufacturing quality as well as an FDA-provided quality rating system for medication manufacturing (see Chapter 6 for an additional discussion on quality as it relates to mitigation measures). FDA's report, *Drug Shortages: Root Causes and Potential Solutions*, provides recommendations for enduring solutions to shortages, including "developing a rating system to incentivize drug manufacturers to invest in quality management maturity for their facilities." To date, FDA has not taken steps to provide a quality rating system (FDA Drug Shortages Task Force, 2020). Manufacturer participation in FDA's Quality Metrics Program is voluntary (FDA, 2021b). Increased transparency is required for a third party to provide a rating system because only FDA currently has access to all of the necessary data.

Third parties could develop their own rating scales for risk and quality using the publicly accessible data if manufacturers of medical products were required to disclose their manufacturing locations and FDA shared the risk-based Site Selection Model scores and the Office of Pharmaceutical Quality scores for facilities that manufacture medical products sold in the United States. As called for by other studies, credible ratings of medical product suppliers will help health systems and group purchasing organizations factor supply chain resilience into their purchasing decisions (see Chapter 7).

This in turn could help to create a market for reliability, which will reduce the ongoing shortage situations in low-margin products.

Making information about medical products' sourcing, manufacturing location, quality, and risk publicly available provides opportunities to use academic researchers and technology firms to devise innovative ways to mine these data for insights. For instance, machine learning and other AI techniques may be very useful in highlighting risks no one was even looking for.

COMMUNICATION

Timely and effective communication among stakeholders in medical product supply chains is important to mitigate, prepare, and respond to medical product disruptions or shortages. Early and accurate communication fosters trust, preempts misinformation, and ensures appropriate expectations with the public and stakeholders. A recent report by the International Society for Pharmaceutical Engineering, *Engage with Health Authorities to Mitigate and Prevent Drug Shortages,* further describes the pathways for a medical product manufacturer to notify and collaborate with health authorities and other stakeholders in medical product supply chains to minimize the effect of medical product disruptions or shortages (Tolomeo et al., 2020).

Meaningful transparency requires shared data to be standardized within interoperable systems if the information is to yield actionable insights (USP, 2020). Establishing a publicly available database to share and summarize critical data for medical products would provide a powerful platform for transforming data into action and will enable health system purchasers to reduce their risk of supply disruptions or enable government officials to determine how and where to spend resources to protect the public health from such disruptions. This publicly available database should be end to end, and could be used to yield meaningful value from the information by a broad range of actors within and beyond FDA, including government, regulators, purchasers, patients, patient advocates, researchers, public health workers, legislators, and international organizations. It could link to external variables, such as weather events and social media, and serve as an "early warning" or "surveillance system" about potential or existing disruptions to medical product supply chains.

The Agricultural Market Information System (AMIS)[7] provides an instructive example of a platform to enhance transparency and policy response for supply chains. AMIS assesses global food supplies and has

---

[7] More information about the AMIS platform is available from http://www.amis-outlook.org/amis-about/en/ (accessed February 2, 2022).

helped to increase transparency and coordination in global food markets to prevent unexpected price hikes and to strengthen global food security. The AMIS Secretariat produces monthly updates of the food market situation and regular food market outlooks, carries out independent data validation, strengthens national capacities for food market assessments, and in the event of instability, coordinates appropriate policy measures (AMIS, 2015).

CURRENT EFFORTS TO INCREASE AWARENESS

Recent reports have called for increased awareness of medical product supply chains through an array of recommendations (see Appendix B). In 2021, a set of reviews pursuant to Executive Order 14017, "America's Supply Chains," included a recommendation for HHS to better track information on pharmaceutical manufacturing facilities and the sourcing of APIs (The White House, 2021). If implemented, this recommendation aimed to improve supply chain transparency on "the sources of drug manufacturing and the quality of the facilities that make them" for the benefit of distributors and purchasers (The White House, 2021).

In the report *National Strategy for a Resilient Public Health Supply Chain* from July 2021, HHS and other agencies outline the goals and objectives of supply chain visibility. Critical to this goal are policies that increase the U.S. government's ability to monitor and manage the supply chain through visibility and engagement. Visibility should be promoted through government-led efforts to maintain the "visibility and analytics needed to anticipate, prevent, mitigate, and respond to supply chain shortages and disruptions." Engagement requires government coordination with partners in both the private sector and state, local, tribal, and territorial governments (DoD et al., 2021).

In 2019, the U.S. Pharmacopeia's (USP's) *Global Policy Position, Key Elements to Building a More Resilient Supply Chain* highlighted the need to enable more transparency and data sharing (USP, 2019). The report calls for increasing transparency across the supply chain by expanding reporting requirements for health care providers and the industry to include indicators of potential or existing drug shortages, as well as requiring manufacturers and ingredient suppliers to monitor and report their ingredient quality and manufacturing capacity. To improve global cooperation, the report recommends that countries' regulators should engage in greater information sharing and establish regulatory recognition and reliance agreements.

In a subsequent 2020 report, USP identified multiple opportunities and benefits for manufacturers, regulators, pharmacies, and health systems to increase transparency in the supply chain (USP, 2020). The report recommended that manufacturers should track and share information about (1) the types and volume of medical products they produce, (2) the sources of their raw ingredients and other essential materials, and (3) their distributors and distribution channels. To mobilize resources and leverage combined regulatory capacity across countries, regulators should (1) have access to information about manufacturers' sites, products, volume, and capacity and (2) share information with other regulatory authorities. To gain greater visibility into the demand for medical products—as well as the supply—pharmacies and health systems should track and share information about (1) electronic health record data about prescriptions, (2) medications dispensed, and (3) drug shortages experienced (USP, 2020).

USP's 2020 report also explores a range of voluntary and mandatory approaches to increase information sharing across medical product supply chains. One voluntary approach is for procurers to put financial incentives in place for manufacturers and distributors to share information. Another is to use public–private partnerships to help balance the need for more information sharing in the industry with the need to protect commercial interests (USP, 2020). However, unless virtually all of the industry stakeholders were willing to participate in voluntary strategies, then complementary mandatory approaches may be required to address critical information gaps in the supply chain. Mandatory approaches include instituting reporting requirements through statutory or regulatory changes. To help alleviate the burden of increased reporting requirements on manufacturers, USP suggests using a risk-based framework that prioritizes reporting requirements for medicines that are essential, at risk of shortage, or subject to quality concerns (USP, 2020). Regardless of which approach—or a hybrid—is used, it is critical to predetermine which information will be collected and how it will be shared.

Federal Efforts

Efforts to increase awareness in medical product supply chains are planned or under way across multiple federal entities within HHS, including FDA (and specifically CDRH) and the ASPR.

FDA Efforts

In March 2021, FDA announced its Data Modernization Action Plan (DMAP) to modernize and strengthen its data practices (Woodcock, 2021). This initiative builds upon FDA's 2019 Technology Modernization Action Plan to update its approach to using technology in its regulatory functions. The DMAP has three broad objectives to improve FDA's practices in collecting, tracking, and using data from an increasingly diverse range of digital sources. The first objective is to identify and execute high-value driver projects for individual centers and FDA. Driver projects are multistakeholder initiatives with measurable value that support innovative solutions and bolster foundational capabilities. The second objective is to develop consistent and repeatable data practices across FDA through investment in the pillars of identification, data curation, governance, and automation. The third objective is to create and sustain a strong talent network that combines the agency's internal strengths with key external partnerships.

FDA has made other efforts to address mounting concerns about the lack of transparency and the need for broader information sharing across the increasingly globalized supply chain for medical products. For instance, manufacturers need greater incentives to engage in more robust quality management systems that extend beyond mere compliance with current good manufacturing practice regulations. To that end, FDA has endorsed the aim of providing more information to purchasers of medical products—and possibly even consumers—about manufacturers' quality management systems (FDA Drug Shortages Task Force, 2020). FDA could support this aim by assigning quality ratings to manufacturing facilities, which companies could choose to disclose to purchasers and the public (CRS, 2020).

FDA also plays a role in supporting improved postmarket surveillance to ensure the quality of medical devices; this could be expanded to capture supply chain information. The agency was required by the Food and Drug Administration Amendments Act[8] and the Food and Drug Administration Safety and Innovation Act[9] to issue regulations to establish a unique device identification (UDI) system to facilitate the rapid identification of medical devices and attributes related to devices' safety and effectiveness. FDA requires that certain information be shared by device labelers for inclusion in the publicly available Global Unique Device Identification Database (GUDID). The UDI system is designed to simplify the integration of device-related information into data systems, but there is no requirement for device makers to provide supply chain information, such as manufacturing location and distribution data. Requiring those companies to disclose certain types of supply chain data on UDI labels and within GUDID could serve to increase transparency (CRS, 2020).

FDA's CDRH has implemented efforts to prevent shortages and strengthen the resilience of the medical device supply chain. The agency maintains a list of shortages of medical devices and exercises its authority granted by the Coronavirus Aid, Relief, and Economic Security Act (CARES Act) to require medical device suppliers to inform FDA of shortages in order to anticipate and mitigate shortages. During the COVID-19 pandemic, regulatory mitigation efforts have included umbrella emergency

---

[8] Food and Drug Administration Amendments Act of 2007, 110th Cong. § 226, 21 U.S.C. § 830.300.

[9] Food and Drug Administration Safety and Innovation Act 2012, 112th Cong., 126 Stat. 993 - 1132, 21 U.S.C. § 301 et seq.

use authorizations, enforcement policy guidance, and expedited 510k applications. CDRH also addresses the effect of shortages in collaboration with partners on the ground, such as health care delivery organizations, to expand access to medical devices during the pandemic emergency period—for example, by making personal protection equipment (PPE) fit-testing less stringent and providing rapid guidance on how to implement temporary alternative or supplemental uses of medical devices and PPE. In conjunction with the Office of the Assistant Secretary for Preparedness and Response (ASPR) and the Strategic National Stockpile (SNS), CDRH assigns priority ratings to devices, components, and raw materials.

Building on the experience during the pandemic and supported by funding from the CARES Act, CDRH is currently in the first stages of building an AI machine-learning platform for data collection and an end-to-end visualization dashboard of the medical device supply chain. This automated surveillance and reporting system will provide data to underpin predictive models for identifying early signals of demand increases and potential disruptions, allowing for stakeholders to be informed and take action to mitigate the effects.

ASPR Efforts

In 2020, ASPR created the Supply Chain Control Tower (SCCT). The SCCT was implemented to provide greater visibility into the supply chains for critical medical products through information gleaned from manufacturers, distributors, providers, and federal entities including the Federal Emergency Management Agency (FEMA) and the SNS (ASPR, 2020). The initiative aims to facilitate end-to-end supply chain visibility for SNS-specific medical products in support of public health preparedness planning and decision making. Its main aims are (1) creating end-to-end visibility on levels of inventory, capacity of manufacturers, flows of distribution, and consumption at points of care; (2) offering insights to inform demand forecasting, scenario modeling, and gap prioritizing; and (3) strengthening responses with information to inform capacity planning and acquisition, targeted distribution, and policy refinement. The program currently aggregates transaction-level commercial distribution data—shared voluntarily and on a near-daily basis by four distributors who represent about 90 percent of the U.S. pharmaceutical distribution market—to track more than 40 different therapeutics. Other key activities of the SCCT program are (1) to integrate weekly reports by approximately 5,000 hospitals concerning their supply of medications for the highest-level acute care patients; (2) to track requests for pharmaceuticals by state, local, tribal, and territorial governments to FEMA or the SNS; and (3) to integrate information from FDA's drug shortages database. Although this infrastructure could be a boon to increasing transparency beyond the supply chains for pandemic-related critical medical products, these voluntary data-sharing platforms will not necessarily be available after the current pandemic concludes.

Legislative Efforts

New legislation is increasing requirements for supply chain transparency. The most prominent is the CARES Act[10] signed into law in March 2020. The CARES Act amended and expanded the FD&C Act to require all registered drug manufacturers, but not device manufacturers, to annually report to FDA the volume of each drug they "manufactured, prepared, propagated, compounded, or processed" for commercial distribution.[11] This information will also be required if requested by FDA following the declaration of a public health emergency. While these volume data are likely to be held by FDA as confidential, making these data available to the public could help to prevent and mitigate supply disruptions.

The Drug Shortage Reporting Section of the CARES Act[12] amends the FD&C Act section concerning notices of manufacturing discontinuation or disruption for critical drugs[13] by expanding the scope of drugs subject to the notification requirement and requiring notification with respect to APIs. Notifications must include additional information on the following:

- The reason for the discontinuance or interruption;
- If an API is a reason or risk factor, the source of the API and alternative sources;
- Whether any associated devices for the preparation or administration of the product is a reason for or risk in the disruption; and
- The expected duration of the disruption.

The Drug Shortage Reporting Section also adds a mandate to the FD&C that manufacturers of critical drugs, APIs, and associated medical devices must develop, maintain, and implement redundancy risk management plans, which are subject to FDA inspection.[14] In addition, the CARES

---

[10] Coronavirus Aid, Relief, and Economic Security Act of 2020, 116th Cong., 134 Stat. 281-615, 15 U.S.C. § Public Law 116-136.

[11] Federal Food, Drug, and Cosmetic Act of 1938, 75th Cong. § 510(k), 21 U.S.C. § 360(j)(3).

[12] Coronavirus Aid, Relief, and Economic Security Act of 2020, 116th Cong. § 3112(e), 15 U.S.C. § Public Law 116-136.

[13] Federal Food, Drug, and Cosmetic Act of 1938, 75th Cong. § 506C, 21 U.S.C. ch.9 § 301 et seq.

[14] Critical drugs are defined as those that are life supporting, life sustaining, or intended for use in the prevention or treatment of a debilitating disease or condition, including those used in emergency medical care or surgery.

Act further amended the FD&C Act annual reporting requirement[15] by adding that registered drug establishments must report the amount of each listed drug manufactured at their locations.

The CARES Act also created new medical device shortage reporting requirements,[16] amending the FD&C Act to now require that manufacturers of certain medical devices notify FDA during or in advance of a public health emergency if they have a manufacturing discontinuance or an interruption that is likely to lead to a meaningful disruption of the U.S. supply.[17] FDA will also send a copy of inspection reports for manufacturers of critical drugs that have been subject to shortages in the last 5 years and for generic drugs with limited competition to the FDA drug shortage team (Berman et al., 2020).

Although FDA was authorized by the CARES Act to begin collecting these various additional data elements in late September 2020, the agency was delayed (FDA, 2021a). FDA did not intend to begin this process until the data can be collected through a system facilitated by an electronic data submission portal, which was just launched in October 2021 (FDA, 2021b).

A number of other legislative actions have been proposed and introduced in recent years to provide U.S. consumers with more visibility into where their medical products are manufactured (CRS, 2020). In its 2019 annual report to Congress, the U.S.-China Economic and Security Review Commission recommended that Congress should enact legislation to require that companies list APIs and countries of origin on product labels[18] or manufacturers' websites.[19] There have been similar proposals to require disclosure of the country of origin of all APIs and inactive ingredients on drug labels, but they have not been enacted.

Industry Efforts

Industry-driven initiatives are also focusing on improving supply chain transparency and broadening data-sharing practices. As part of its Healthcare Supply Chain Collaborative, the Health Industry Distributors Association has created the Supply Chain Visibility initiative to create a more visible health care supply chain by engaging with providers, distributors, manufacturers, group purchasing organizations, and technology compa-

---

[15] Federal Food, Drug, and Cosmetic Act of 1938, 75th Cong. § 510(j), 21 U.S.C. § 360(j)(3).
[16] Coronavirus Aid, Relief, and Economic Security Act of 2020, 116th Cong. § 3121, 15 U.S.C. § Public Law 116-136.
[17] Federal Food, Drug, and Cosmetic Act of 1938, 75th Cong. § 506(j), 21 U.S.C. § Part A.
[18] S. 3757 (116th Congress), §2(c); S. 3633 (110th Congress).
[19] S. 3105 (115th Congress).

nies.[20] The Healthcare Transparency Initiative is a cross-industry collaboration dedicated to improving supply chain transparency and visibility by providing a data platform that connects stakeholders across the supply chain through rapid data transition.[21] The Medical Device Innovation Consortium (MDIC) is a public–private partnership established to work with stakeholders across government and industry to expand access to innovative medical technologies.[22] The MDIC supports building improved transparency into the supply chain for medical devices.

RECOMMENDATIONS

Awareness measures to promote transparency, analytics, and communication are the foundation of any serious effort to increase the resilience of medical product supply chains. Although the public and private measures listed above have made progress in collecting and using data to assess the risks of medical product supply chains, gaps still exist, and the potential power of the U.S. federal government to achieve greater transparency through required disclosure of entities already under its jurisdiction is far from fully realized. The committee recognizes that there are multiple approaches to increasing awareness across the medical product supply chain ecosystem and different types of data that may be important to collect, compile, and disseminate on a routine basis (to enable strategic decision making to mitigate risk) or during a public health emergency (to enable effective response). Toward this end, the committee proposes two concrete recommendations that take a first step toward increasing awareness.

Recommendation 1 (Public Transparency) calls for quality transparency (via risk-based Site Selection Model scores becoming public[23]) and supply chain transparency (via all FEI location data made public for where products are made). These two dimensions of transparency (quality and supply chain) each have different sources. Quality data are currently kept by regulators, but not made transparent to the public or manufacturers and distributors.

---

[20] More information about the Supply Chain Visibility initiative is available from https://www.hida.org/distribution/advocacy/industry-issues/Supply-Chain-Visibility.aspx (accessed July 16, 2021).

[21] More information about the Healthcare Transparency Initiative is available from https://healthcare.resilinc.com/ (accessed July 16, 2021).

[22] More information about the Medical Device Innovation Consortium is available from https://mdic.org/ (accessed July 16, 2021).

[23] Note that quality data for both drugs (https://www.fda.gov/drugs/questions-and-answers-fdas-adverse-event-reporting-system-faers/fda-adverse-event-reporting-system-faers-public-dashboard) and devices (https://www.accessdata.fda.gov/scripts/cdrh/cfdocs/cfmaude/search.cfm) are currently collected after the products have already failed. The committee is proposing process quality data that be used to predict and hopefully prevent shortages and complaints from happening in the first place.

Supply chain data are currently kept by manufacturers, but not made transparent to the public or regulators. Recommendation 1 (Public Transparency) also calls for volume and capacity transparency to further assess risks directly related to medical product supply chains and to evaluate strategies for ameliorating these. Transparency is required both from manufacturers and from regulators so the public can be informed about their medical products and are empowered to act upon these data through data analysis and potentially put public pressure on regulators and lawmakers. This initial step toward public transparency of data regarding where and how medical products are made could facilitate the collection and dissemination of additional medical product supply chain data. Furthermore, public transparency could facilitate information sharing among federal agencies and other regulatory authorities around the world. Currently, some data might be available to some agencies and other regulatory authorities—but not to all. If medical product supply chain data were made publicly available, lack of information sharing and situational awareness would be less of a barrier.

These data will enable mapping of medical product supply chains, identifying vulnerabilities such as supply concentrations, and assessing what medical products are most at risk. To facilitate use of this sourcing and quality information, the committee proposes the complementary Recommendation 2 (Public Database). This database will provide a user-friendly site for the raw data and statistical summaries collected under Recommendation 1 (Public Transparency) and other transparency efforts. This database could be used by government agents, researchers, health care systems, third-party rating services, and others engaged in the analysis of the risks inherent in medical product supply chains. Because the results of analysis such as ratings and risk assessments are likely to be more useful to decision makers than the raw data alone, this database should also contain such results.

Recommendation 1 (Public Transparency). The U.S. Food and Drug Administration (FDA) should take steps to make sourcing, quality, volume, and capacity information publicly available for all medical products approved or cleared for sale in the United States. These steps include

    a. The manufacturer for a pharmaceutical drug should be required to publicly disclose the manufacturing location, in particular the FDA Establishment Identifier (FEI), the city, and the country, for the finished dosage form (FDF), active pharmaceutical ingredient (API), major excipients, and major packaging and delivery devices for all pharmaceutical drugs sold in the United States. API manufacturers shall be required to publicly disclose the sources of raw materials. This information should be made available on the labels for all pharmaceutical drugs and in a publicly accessible database. The National Drug Code should be associated with the primary FEI (where a majority of the volume is manufactured) in the database.

b. FDA should make publicly available their risk-based Site Selection Model scores for all pharmaceutical drug manufacturing facilities that make drugs sold in the United States. FDA should also make public the Office of Pharmaceutical Quality (OPQ) scores. The risk-based Site Selection Model scores for the API and FDF plants (e.g., FEIs) should be made available on the labels for all pharmaceutical drugs and in a publicly accessible database, and the OPQ scores should also be included in this database.

c. The manufacturer for a medical device should be required to publicly disclose the manufacturing location, in particular the FEI, the city, and the country, for the primary manufacturing and final assembly steps for all medical devices and major components sold in the United States. This information should be made available on the labels for all medical devices and in a publicly accessible database. The part number should be associated with the primary FEI (where a majority of the volume is manufactured) in the database.

d. The risk-based Site Selection Model score for the primary manufacturing and final assembly plants (e.g., FEIs) should be made available on the labels for all medical devices and in a publicly accessible database.

e. Sourcing and quality information should be provided as part of the pharmaceutical drug or medical device approval or clearance processes and on an ongoing basis in order to retain a license or clearance to sell in the United States.

f. Drug volume data reported to FDA, as mandated by the CARES Act, should be made available in a publicly accessible database. This requirement should be expanded to include reporting of capacity, in addition to volume, and should be required for medical devices, in addition to drugs.

g. To the extent that amendments to the Trade Secrets Act at 18 U.S.C. § 1905 and to the Food, Drug, and Cosmetic Act at 21 U.S.C. § 331(j) are necessary to permit public disclosure of all the sourcing, quality, volume, and capacity information referenced in this recommendation, Congress should make such amendments.

Recommendation 2 (Public Database). The U.S. Food and Drug Administration (FDA), in cooperation with other U.S. government agencies, should establish a publicly accessible database containing the supply chain information acquired for medical products. FDA, in cooperation

with other U.S. government agencies, should use the information on medical product supply chains it acquires to
   a. Understand better the vulnerabilities of medical product supply chains as a whole.
   b. Perform risk assessments regarding the risks to the total supply of particular medical products in both normal and emergency scenarios.
   c. Coordinate, conduct, and compile research on the resilience of medical product supply chains, including by funding independent research that uses the established database.
   d. Track the ways in which increased transparency, and the prediction of potential medical product shortages through data tracking, support improved supply chain resilience and functionality.
   e. Incentivize the establishment of third-party rating system(s) for risk and quality.

REFERENCES

AMIS (Agricultural Market Information System). 2015. *About AMIS*. http://www.amis-outlook.org/amis-about/en/ (accessed January 25, 2022).

ASPR (Office of the Assistant Secretary for Preparedness and Response). 2020. *Information management division*. ASPR. https://www.phe.gov/about/offices/program/icc/siim/Pages/Information-Management.aspx (accessed December 16, 2021).

Berman, J., M. Buenafe, R. Dandeker, D. Gucciardo, K. Sanzo, and M. Lewis. 2020. CARES Act provisions impact drug, device, and food manufacturers and suppliers. *JDSupra*. https://www.jdsupra.com/legalnews/cares-act-provisions-impact-drug-device-47212/ (accessed October 29, 2021).

CDER (Center for Drug Evaluation and Research). 2018. Understanding CDER's risk-based site selection model. In *Manual of policies and procedures*, edited by Office of Pharmaceutical Quality. Silver Spring, MD: FDA. https://www.fda.gov/media/116004/download (accessed October 29, 2021).

CRS (Congressional Research Service). 2020. *FDA's role in the medical product supply chain and considerations during COVID-19*, edited by V. R. Green, A. Dabrowska, and K. M. Costin. CRS. https://crsreports.congress.gov/product/pdf/R/R46507 (accessed December 16, 2021).

DoD (U.S. Department of Defense), HHS (U.S. Department of Health and Human Services), DHS (U.S. Department of Homeland Security), and VA (U.S. Department of Veterans Affairs). 2021. *National strategy for a resilient public health supply chain,* edited by Department of Health and Human Services, Department of Defense, Department of Homeland Security, Department of Commerce, Department of State, Department of Veterans Affairs, and The White House Office of the COVID-19 Response. Washington, DC. https://www.phe.gov/Preparedness/legal/Documents/National-Strategy-for-Resilient-Public-Health-Supply-Chain.pdf (accessed October 29, 2021).

FDA (U.S. Food and Drug Administration). 2020. *Drug establishments current registration site*. https://www.fda.gov/drugs/drug-approvals-and-databases/drug-establishments-current-registration-site (accessed December 7, 2021).

FDA. 2021a. *Coronavirus Aid, Relief, and Economic Security Act (CARES Act) drug shortage mitigation efforts*. https://www.fda.gov/drugs/drug-shortages/coronavirus-aid-relief-and-economic-security-act-cares-act-drug-shortage-mitigation-efforts#Creating%20Risk%20Management%20Plans%20for%20Drugs (accessed October 29, 2021).

FDA. 2021b. *Frequently asked questions regarding the quality metrics site visit and feedback programs.* https://www.fda.gov/drugs/pharmaceutical-quality-resources/frequently-asked-questions-regarding-quality-metrics-site-visit-and-feedback-programs (accessed January 1, 2022).
FDA Drug Shortages Task Force. 2020. *Drug shortages: Root causes and potential solutions.* https://www.fda.gov/drugs/drug-shortages/report-drug-shortages-root-causes-and-potential-solutions (accessed December 16, 2021).
Haninger, K., A. Jessup, and K. Koehler. 2011. *Economic analysis of the causes of drug shortages,* edited by ASPE's Office of Science and Data Policy. Washington, DC: HHS. https://aspe.hhs.gov/reports/economic-analysis-causes-drug-shortages-0 (accessed October 20, 2021).
House Committee on Energy and Commerce. 2019. *Securing the US drug supply chain: Oversight of FDA's foreign inspection program: Congressional testimony of Janet Woodcock.* December 10. https://www.fda.gov/news-events/congressional-testimony/securing-us-drug-supply-chain-oversight-fdas-foreign-inspection-program-12102019 (accessed December 10, 2021).
Lee, H. L., V. Padmanabhan, and S. Whang. 1997. The bullwhip effect in supply chains. *Sloan Management Review* 38:93-102.
Lotfi, Z., M. Mukhtar, S. Sahran, and A. T. Zadeh. 2013. Information sharing in supply chain management. *Procedia Technology* 11:298-304.
Mulero, A. 2018. *FDA pilots new site selection process for inspections of device facilities.* RAPS. https://www.raps.org/news-and-articles/news-articles/2018/5/fda-pilots-new-site-selection-process-for-inspecti (accessed October 29, 2021).
Schondelmeyer, S. W., J. Seifert, D. J. Margraf, M. Mueller, I. Williamson, C. Dickson, D. Dasararaju, C. Caschetta, N. Senne, and M. T. Osterholm. 2020. Part 6: Ensuring a resilient us prescription drug supply. In *COVID-19: The CIDRAP viewpoint,* edited by J. Wappes. Minneapolis, MN: Regents of the University of Minnesota. https://www.cidrap.umn.edu/sites/default/files/public/downloads/cidrap-covid19-viewpoint-part1_0.pdf (accessed December 16, 2021).
Tolomeo, D., K. Hirshfield, and D. L. Hustead. 2020. Engage with health authorities to mitigate & prevent drug shortages. In *ISPE Special Reports.* ISPE. https://ispe.org/pharmaceutical-engineering/july-august-2020/engage-health-authorities-mitigate-prevent-drug (accessed October 25, 2021).
USP (United States Pharmacopeia). 2019. *Key elements to building a more resilient supply chain.* https://www.usp.org/sites/default/files/usp/document/our-impact/covid-19/global-policy-supply-chain.pdf (accessed October 29, 2021).
USP. 2020. *Increasing transparency in the medicines supply chain.* https://www.usp.org/sites/default/files/usp/document/about/public-policy/increasing-transparency-medicine-supply-chain.pdf (accessed October 29, 2021).
The White House. 2021. *Building resilient supply chains, revitalizing American manufacturing, and fostering broad-based growth.* Department of Commerce, Department of Energy, Department of Defense, Department of Health and Human Services. https://www.whitehouse.gov/wp-content/uploads/2021/06/100-day-supply-chain-review-report.pdf (accessed October 25, 2021).
Woodcock, J. 2021. *FDA's data modernization action plan: Putting data to work for public health.* FDA. https://www.fda.gov/about-fda/reports/data-modernization-action-plan#:~:text=Specifically%2C%20an%20FDA%20Data%20Strategy%20will%20focus%20on,state-of-the-art%20tools%20to%20enhance%20and%20promote%20public%20health (accessed October 29, 2021).
Woodcock, J., and M. Wosinska. 2013. How to prevent drug shortages yet sustain quality. *Cleanroom Technology* 21(4):27-28.

7

Mitigation Measures for Resilient Medical Product Supply Chains

As discussed in Chapter 4, medical product shortages in the United States are a routine occurrence in clinical care, despite efforts to decrease their frequency and blunt their effects. These shortages have profound effects on the health care system, including increased risks to patients, increased health care costs, and threats to clinical research. Routine shortages ultimately affect the health care system's ability to function effectively during both routine operations and public health emergencies. Making medical product supply chains more resilient during routine conditions will make them more resilient during public health emergencies.

Mitigation measures play a critical role in preventing and minimizing disruptive events that can trigger shortages (Figure 7-1). As described in the conceptual framework (Chapter 5), mitigation measures include (1) hardening measures that reduce the likelihood or magnitude of disruptive events within stages of the system, by promoting quality and reliability, and (2) diversification measures that create redundant processes and product sources to reduce the risk of catastrophic failure.

This chapter discusses specific actions key stakeholders can take to harden and diversify the day-to-day medical product supply chains, and culminates in a recommendation for actions that health systems[1] can take to increase the resilience of these supply chains. Given the prevalence of

---

[1] For the purposes of this report, the flow of goods, manufacturer to wholesaler to purchaser, applies just as much to community pharmacies and other purchasers of medical products as it does to health systems. The committee chose to focus on where the most severe medical product shortages occur and where its recommendations could make the most impact, which primarily occur in health system settings (Fox et al., 2014).

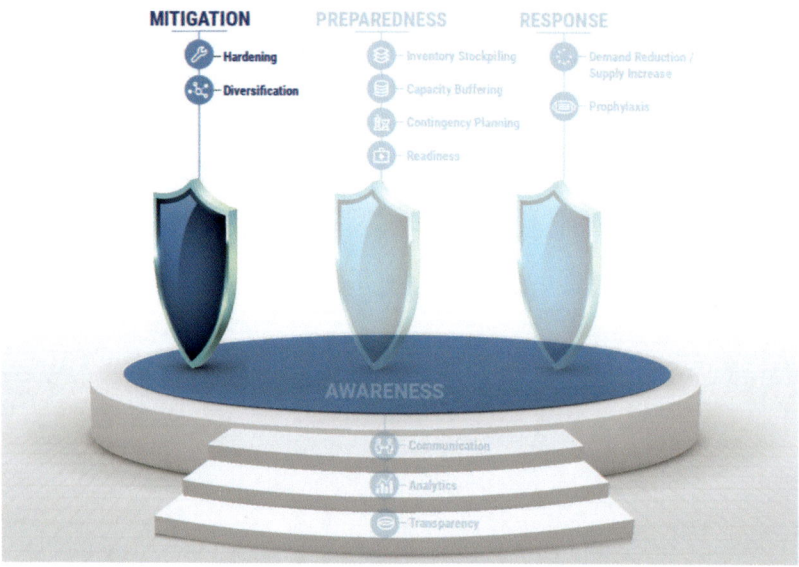

FIGURE 7-1 Medical product supply chain resilience framework: potential mitigation measures.

chronic drug shortages in U.S. hospitals and the enormous consequences these have for patients and health systems alike (Fox et al., 2014), this chapter focuses on mitigation measures for drug products where their implementation can make the most impact. However, many of the described measures may be generalizable across all medical products.

INCENTIVES FOR QUALITY AND RELIABILITY

In most markets, shortages are self-correcting because consumers are willing to pay higher prices when a product is in short supply. Higher prices then attract more suppliers, and more supply rectifies the shortage. However, this often does not occur in markets for medically necessary drugs. In medical product markets, consumer demand for services is largely unaffected by changes in price, because consumers typically purchase drugs and services through health insurance contracts that have prenegotiated rates, and there is a high barrier for new manufacturers to enter a market (FDA, 2012). Therefore, the interests of medical product suppliers and manufacturers, which align with maximizing profits and minimizing costs, can lead to insufficient supply and inadequate quality of medical products causing supply shortages (NASEM, 2018b).

In 2020, the U.S. Food and Drug Administration (FDA) Drug Shortages Task Force noted that there is a "lack of incentives to produce less profitable drugs," which is more often the case for older generic drug manufacturers that face intense price competition and contracting practices that incentivize the lowest price possible. Without information on the quality of medical products, consumers at both the individual and health-system levels are unable to exert their purchasing preferences for high-quality products and industry has little incentive to implement costly updates to manufacturing processes and facilities.

Additionally, the incentives health systems have to manage their supply chain are misaligned with those of manufacturers, and particularly with those of patients. For example, inpatient diagnosis-related group reimbursements do not incentivize the purchase of high-quality products; rather, they incentivize health systems to purchase the lowest cost products for inpatient use, effectively making generic medications distinguishable from each other only by price (FDA Drug Shortages Task Force, 2020).

Contracts focused on price alone can drive competitor products from the market in a "race to the bottom" pricing structure. This can lead to fewer suppliers, which in turn can weaken the resilience of the supply chain, as no options to fill the void are available if a quality or manufacturing issue occurs (FDA Drug Shortages Task Force, 2020).

The committee notes that *the market incentivizes health systems to purchase medical products at the lowest cost, and on a just-in-time basis. These incentives increase the risk of shortages caused by supply chain disruptions, such as deviations in product quality or manufacturing problems, and conflict with the interest of patients.*

HARDENING DAY-TO-DAY MEDICAL PRODUCT SUPPLY CHAINS

Over the past decade, stakeholders have developed sophisticated practices, policies, guidance, and tools to lessen the number of drug shortages, which peaked in 2011 (FDA, 2020), and to ensure medical products meet standards for quality (see Box 7-1). The committee acknowledges this extensive and ongoing related work; therefore, this section builds upon current efforts and highlights ways to bolster current mitigation measures, particularly for generic drug products.

To mitigate routine medical product shortages and their effect on clinical care, manufacturers, suppliers, and health systems must improve existing processes throughout medical product supply chains. This hardening of medical product supply chains requires that manufacturers reliably produce quality medical products, and that health systems purchase these higher quality products for the patients they serve. Reorienting the market to value the quality and reliability of medical products, rather than cost alone, can realign incentives for manufacturers and patients and promote hardening of medical product supply chains.

> **BOX 7-1**
> **Resources for Addressing Medical Product Shortages and Quality Concerns**
>
> **ASHP Drug Shortage Resources**
> The American Society of Health-System Pharmacists (ASHP) collects shortage resources that are available to the public as well as health care providers (ASHP, 2021). The webpage, which is updated regularly, tracks pharmaceutical product shortages and provides evidence-based recommendations for alternative agents and strategies to mitigate patient harm.
>
> **Cleveland Clinic Drug Quality Dashboard**
> This interactive dashboard tracks all pharmaceutical products purchased by the hospital system (Cleveland Clinic, 2017; Hegwer, 2017). It lists drugs by their National Drug Code description and ranks them in descending order according to their annual impact, based on current use throughout the hospital system, operational region, and facility site. The tool can filter by specific products and manufacturers to help identify where changes (e.g., price, manufacture) are originating and coordinates them with product uses.
>
> **FDA Drug Shortage Website and Database**
> The FDA website provides resources for the latest of drug shortage information about specific products, including a searchable database for the status of specific products and a list of products whose use-by dates have been extended (FDA, 2021).
>
> **ISPE Drug Shortage Assessment and Prevention Tool**
> The International Society for Pharmaceutical Engineering (ISPE) tool provides pharmaceutical manufacturers with methods to identify inconsistencies across the pharmaceutical manufacturing supply chain (ISPE, 2020). It enables manufacturers to mitigate problems before they arise, evaluate risk in current processes, and prepare for or manage any potential drug shortage, including drug-quality issues.
>
> ISPE has nearly a decade's worth of publicly available reports that offer recommendations, tools, and prevention plans to mitigate or manage drug shortages across the pharmaceutical manufacturing industry (ISPE, 2021).

Implementing a Drug-Quality Rating System

The FDA Drug Shortages Task Force recommended the implementation of a quality rating system to introduce greater transparency into the quality management systems behind the drugs that consumers purchase (FDA Drug Shortages Task Force, 2020). This rating system would measure the quality management maturity of medical product manufacturing facilities, and reward those that implement robust quality systems with a higher rating.

This system would go beyond the minimum quality standards set by current good manufacturing practices (CGMPs), by rewarding manufacturers that detect and address key vulnerabilities, and implement continuous system improvement. Critically, all manufacturers of medical products and their constituent parts must be required to participate in such a rating system. FDA and pharmaceutical companies alike have expressed concerns that they have less control of and transparency into contract manufacturing organizations, sometimes being barred from entering sites to conduct inspections (The PEW Health Group, 2011). A quality rating system would offer consumers increased transparency into the quality of medical products and give purchasers the ability to distinguish between products based on their quality (see Chapter 6 for a discussion on transparency, quality and the need for a third-party rating system).[2] In providing this transparency, the market will adapt to reward facilities that have a more mature quality system than their competitors.

In the absence of the quality rating system that the Drug Shortages Task Force recommends as an enduring solution to drug shortages, health systems can put pressure on suppliers to share more information on the quality of a product. For example, health systems could insist that group purchasing organizations (GPOs) investigate manufacturers for quality and include minimum quality standards in contracts negotiated on their behalf. At a minimum, health systems should know which company manufactured the medications they are purchasing and the manufacturing location, to enable additional research into FDA inspections and warning letters. This information is also essential for ensuring a more rapid removal of contaminated products from inventory when FDA MedWatch warnings are incomplete (FDA, 2017).

Accreditation organizations play an important role in ensuring quality at health care centers in addition to allowing health systems to participate in the Medicare and Medicaid programs. Currently, the Centers for Medicare & Medicaid Services (CMS) grants authority to public state survey agencies and private accreditation organizations—such as The Joint Commission (TJC) and the Accreditation Commission for Health Care—to verify that health care facilities receiving Medicare reimbursement comply with Medicare conditions of participation (CMS, 2021). These organizations evaluate health care facilities based on accreditation standards that meet or exceed Medicare conditions, and survey activities to verify compliance with CMS policy and regulations. Some accreditation organizations publish the results of their evaluations, which are available to the public to review (TJC, 2021). Guidelines pursuant to Medicare conditions of participation already

---

[2] This quality rating system would distinguish based on maturity of the quality system, which indirectly relates to product quality. However, it is not a product quality assessment. This latter assessment would come from testing the product itself or certification of compliance.

consider a health care facility's processes to alleviate medication shortages as a factor in accreditation (CMS, 2020). When a quality rating system for medical products becomes available, CMS could incorporate—under Interpretive Guidelines §482.25(b)(9)—a metric based on the quality and reliability of the drug supply that a facility purchases, as well as shortages that negatively affect patient care. Doing so would incentivize health care facilities to procure medical products with high-quality ratings.

Incorporating Quality by Design

Quality by design (QbD) can provide manufacturers a competitive edge by improving efficiencies, especially for manufacturers of generic products. Using QbD concepts also promotes flexibility in sourcing material and the overall adaptability of supply chains (Crowley and McCrossen, 2016). Moreover, QbD may be particularly attractive to manufacturers, as its implementation offers a return on investment by decreasing the likelihood of batch failures, and it reduces the need for controls over intermediates and final products, saving the manufacturer time and money (Zacché, 2020). Furthermore, any measures that incentivize quality, such as third-party ratings and incorporation of quality into purchasing contracts, will increase the attractiveness of QbD to manufacturers.

QbD can help medical product manufacturers to supply products that reliably meet high-quality standards, thus reducing the number of shortages triggered by quality and manufacturing failures. QbD as a concept posits that quality can be built into the medical product through the processes used to develop the product (Yu et al., 2014). QbD aims to improve product quality by implementing clinically based quality specifications and increasing the understanding and control of manufacturing processes. Risk management, root cause analysis, and postapproval change management are additional tools used to achieve QbD. FDA's CGMP regulations incorporate elements of a QbD approach, emphasizing the transfer of product knowledge and understanding from the development phase to the ongoing manufacturing and any postdevelopment changes or optimization (FDA, 2006). The implementation of QbD approaches throughout medical product development and manufacturing would promote the use of measurable quality standards based on the clinical performance of the product. Moreover, QbD facilitates postapproval modernization and optimization through a comprehensive understanding of the product and related manufacturing processes.

Purchasing for Unexpected Events

Health systems often attempt to maximize inventory turnover because of a lack of space and to reduce carrying costs. Purchasing on a just-in-time basis places health systems at risk of shortages caused by short-term interruptions—such as weather delays in deliveries—and provides little cushion to prepare a management plan when longer-term shortages occur because of quality or manufacturing problems. Just-in-case purchasing aims to have sufficient product available in case of interruptions to normal supply or demand (Barocas et al., 2021).

Purchasing medical products on a just-in-case basis builds reliability and resiliency into the supply chain. However, because holding excess supply in stockpiles can be costly for health systems, incentives may be necessary to encourage just-in-case purchasing. Including availability of stockpiles for supply chain critical products as a metric under CMS's Hospital Value-Based Purchasing Program[3] could incentivize health systems that bill Medicare and Medicaid to convert to just-in-time purchasing. Additionally, much as the U.S. government invests in the Strategic National Stockpile, just-in-case purchasing in the private sector may require public investment (Barocas et al., 2021). Federal, state, territorial, tribal, or local governments may consider reimbursing health systems that invest in purchasing practices that ensure that excess inventory is retained to respond to unexpected events.

DIVERSIFICATION OF MEDICAL PRODUCT SUPPLY CHAINS

The consolidation and geographic concentration of raw material suppliers in medical product supply chains poses risks to the ability of manufacturers further down the supply chain to secure basic supplies to make their own products (NASEM, 2018a). Similarly, consolidation among manufacturers of low-margin products such as generic drugs, due to extreme price competition, has been a factor in many of the routine shortages that have occurred in recent years (FDA Drug Shortages Task Force, 2020). In some markets, diversification happens naturally. For example, if transportation costs are high for a product, it may be economical to produce it close to the point of use, which leads to many production locations around the world. However, for generic drug product manufacturing, incentives often induce production in the single lowest cost location, which leads to concentration, not diversification of product sourcing, and increases the risk of drug shortages.

Increasing sourcing diversity promotes the resilience of medical product supply chains by ensuring that manufacturers and purchasers have backup capabilities in the event of a disruption (i.e., parallel sourcing of a medical product component from more than one supplier). However, independence

---

[3] For more information, see https://www.cms.gov/Medicare/Quality-Initiatives-Patient-Assessment-Instruments/Value-Based-Programs/HVBP/Hospital-Value-Based-Purchasing (accessed January 24, 2022).

of sources is crucial to diversification strategies because it reduces risks of simultaneous failure. Promoting competition based on the quality and reliability of medical products provides incentives diversification, which can help counteract the market forces that have led to excessive consolidation of medical product manufacturers.

Active pharmaceutical ingredient (API) and raw material suppliers, medical product manufacturers, GPOs and distributors, and health systems all have a responsibility to improve diversification across medical product supply chains. Each of these stakeholders can facilitate diversification through different measures. For example, API and raw material suppliers can increase the geographic diversity of their operations, and health systems can build diversity into their supply chains by contracting with multiple suppliers for a given product. The ways in which diversification can protect supply continuity are complex. Regulation, incentives, and technology are available options to promote the diversification of a concentrated market, a few of which are highlighted below.

Diversifying Sourcing and Manufacturing Practices

Diversity in the location and firms in which raw materials, APIs, device components, and final products are manufactured can help to protect patients from shortages, but such diversity also provides benefits for manufacturers who would otherwise need to stop production until they are again able to acquire the needed material.

To be effective, a diversified market must have independent manufacturers and suppliers. An optimally diversified supply chain would use facilities in different locations operated by separate organizations. A supply chain with manufacturing facilities in the same location is vulnerable to localized events, such as natural disasters. A supply chain with manufacturing facilities in multiple locations, but run by the same company, is vulnerable to disruptions in company operations. Additionally, diversification is needed across the supply chain. For example, if a manufacturer maintains multiple final assembly plants around the world, but relies on a single supplier for a critical component, the entire supply chain remains vulnerable to a disruption if that one component goes into shortage.

Some manufacturers have begun to ensure diversity in their supply of raw materials to safeguard against stoppages and shortages when a supplier experiences a disruption (NASEM, 2018a). However, independently vetting suppliers for quality and reliability can be a costly and time-consuming process for manufacturers. Transparency and rating measures, like those discussed in Chapter 6, could help buyers recognize manufacturers with geographic diversification and give buyers reason to pay a reliability premium for the additional protection it provides.

Diversifying Purchasing Practices

Distributors, GPOs, and health systems can contribute to the diversification of medical product supply chains by purchasing from several suppliers of the same product. While this may lead to hoarding and duplicate orders during a crisis, it more importantly builds resilience into supply chains by providing alternative sources of medical products when a particular supplier experiences a disruption.

Furthermore, the reimbursement policies by payers may also incentivize health systems to overemphasize cost. For instance, bundled payments by diagnosis-related group reimbursement do not reimburse health systems for higher prices paid to suppliers with higher reliability. If health systems accurately account for the costs involved in finding substitutes for drugs in shortage, they will still have an incentive to pay a premium for more reliable supplies. Nevertheless, because of the intricacies of reimbursement plans, Medicare and private payers can contribute to improved resilience by considering the effect of their policies on the incentives for health systems to choose from a variety of reliable high-quality suppliers for drugs and devices. There is an opportunity for future research and pilot programs to determine the specific policy updates, which public and private payers can implement, to incentivize purchasing that rewards and promotes diversification. Because rating systems and accreditation organizations can influence health systems, these organizations can similarly promote resilience by crediting health systems with robust supply assurance systems as part of their rating and ranking processes.

Contracting

Most health systems belong to a GPO that provides access to a variety of contracts (O'Brien et al., 2017). State procurement codes often require a request for proposal (RFP) process if not using a GPO. These RFPs can be time consuming and impractical for accessing lifesaving products in a health system. Some health systems make individual contracts for specific products but most lack the resources to conduct RFPs and negotiate contracts for thousands of products.

To mitigate shortages, health care systems that do conduct RFPs can consider contracting with multiple suppliers for any particular medical product that is at a high risk of shortage. Alternatively, health systems that use GPOs could demand that contracts ensure sourcing from a diverse array of suppliers for high-risk medical products. These purchasing strategies not only help to protect health systems from experiencing shortages when supply from one source is disrupted, but promote competition between medical product manufacturers to provide a more reliable supply.

Many contracts do not require a committed purchase volume nor do they include failure-to-supply provisions (Gonsalkorale et al., 2012). However, newer subscription-type contracting opportunities are becoming available in which health systems make a long-term (e.g., 5-year) commitment to purchase a specific product at a specific volume. If purchase commitments are not realized, the health system faces a penalty. Similarly, if suppliers are unable to supply the health system with the products they ordered, the supplier incurs a penalty. This type of contracting adds resilience to many areas of medical product supply chains. The manufacturer has an assured volume of purchases for an extended period of time, allowing investments in the quality of production. The health systems receive a reliable supply of a critical product at a consistent price, and can devote fewer resources to developing shortage management plans for these products. Contracts that include long-term commitments can likewise counter the risk of just-in-time purchasing by providing health care systems with a more reliable supply that is therefore resilient to short-term disruptions.

One example of this model is Civica Rx.[4] Civica Rx produces or procures generic drugs for over 50 health care systems, including the U.S. Department of Veterans Affairs and the U.S. Department of Defense (Dredge and Scholtes, 2021). The company, run as a nonprofit 501(c)(4) organization, utilizes a business model that is unique within the health care sector and strives to create more efficient and more equitable health care solutions for patients. By securing bulk orders from its various members, Civica Rx is able to offer lower drug prices spread out across its members. The scale and duration of Civica Rx's contracts also enables the company to invest in larger stockpiles, better positioning it to weather short-term disruptions. Other companies that use similar models to provide low-cost generic drugs that are vulnerable to shortage include ProvideGx and the Mark Cuban Cost Plus Drug Company.[5,6]

Weighing Cost and Quality

Most purchasing is based on cost, with some consideration to contract compliance. In many cases, electronic purchasing programs guide buyers to purchase the product with the lowest cost. Automatic substitution programs from distributors—in which a lower-cost product is substituted for the ordered product—can also force purchases based on cost alone. Such programs are to be avoided as they can direct purchasers to buy products from manufacturers with a history of poor quality or shortages. Purchasers must also remember that managing a drug shortage has associated costs

---

[4] For more information, see https://civicarx.org/about/ (accessed October 21, 2021).

[5] For more information, see https://www.premierinc.com/providegx (accessed October 21, 2021).

[6] For more information, see https://markcubancostplusdrugcompany.com/ (accessed October 21, 2021).

(Vizient, 2019). Responding to a shortage with product substitutions, additional labor, and delays in care is expensive to health care facilities. Before purchasing a lower-cost product from a new supplier, health systems can research the quality and reliability of the manufacturer or supplier. FDA publishes quality and production problems associated with drugs via MedWatch,[7] as well as for devices via MAUDE (the Manufacturer and User Facility Device Experience database).[8] Health systems, as well as patients, can also be vigilant about monitoring for product quality, reporting all defects to FDA and the manufacturer.[9] Additionally, health care facilities must attempt to avoid purchases from suppliers with consistent levels of poor quality, regardless of FDA equivalence ratings.

RECOMMENDATION

Given that a high percentage of medical product shortages are the result of process disruptions caused by quality problems, particularly for generic drug products, incorporating information on drug quality and reliability into the contracting, purchasing, and inventory decisions of health systems is an opportunity to reduce the likelihood and magnitude of drug shortages. However, such a mitigation strategy requires overcoming the "cost only" inertia in current health system purchasing systems, as well as other barriers.

Drug shortages impose costs on health systems, so there are incentives for health systems to choose suppliers with reputations for quality and reliability. Previous reports have issued recommendations that call for manufacturers to adopt updated manufacturing processes that would improve the quality and reliability of medical products (see Appendix B). The subsequent recommendation builds on these reports, by tasking health systems with actions, that when taken together with manufacturers and suppliers, can build robust mitigation measures into medical product supply chains.

Recommendation 3 (Resilience Contracting by Health Systems). Health systems should promote a more resilient market for medical products by deliberately incorporating quality and reliability, in addition to price, in their contracting, purchasing, and inventory decisions. When quality ratings for medical products are available, accreditation organizations for health systems should use the ratings of the products

---

[7] For more information, see https://www.fda.gov/safety/medwatch-fda-safety-information-and-adverse-event-reporting-program (accessed October 21, 2021).

[8] For more information, see https://www.accessdata.fda.gov/scripts/cdrh/cfdocs/cfmaude/search.cfm (accessed October 21, 2021).

[9] For more information, see https://www.fda.gov/consumers/consumer-updates/how-report-product-problems-and-complaints-fda (accessed October 21, 2021).

sourced by health systems in their evaluations and ratings, as well as the frequency of shortages experienced at a health system that negatively affected patient care. Specifically,

    a. Health systems should fortify their contracts with medical product suppliers by including failure-to-supply penalties for contracts requiring a committed purchase or purchase volume, preferentially awarding contracts to suppliers that can demonstrate superior quality and reliability, awarding contracts to multiple suppliers of the same medical product, and requiring these same standards in contracts that are negotiated by group purchasing organizations on their behalf.

    b. Health systems should budget to adequately reward select groups of products (e.g., low-cost, low-margin, off-patent, small molecule) if guarantees are met for higher quality and assured supply levels.

    c. Health systems and medical product wholesalers should routinely enter into emergency purchasing agreements for a specified list of emergency supplies or products that guarantees product delivery in the event of an unexpected supply demand or a substantial supply disruption. They should have a good understanding of the supplier's ability to meet demand, considering commitments to other buyers.

REFERENCES

ASHP (American Society of Health-System Pharmacists). 2021. *Shortage resources.* https://www.ashp.org/drug-shortages/shortage-resources (accessed November 7, 2021).

Barocas, J., C. Gounder, and S. Madad. 2021. Just-in-time versus just-in-case pandemic preparedness. *Health Affairs Blog.*

Cleveland Clinic. 2017. *Inpatient pharmacy leaders lower costs with dashboard tool.* https://consultqd.clevelandclinic.org/inpatient-pharmacy-leaders-lower-costs-dashboard-tool/ (accessed October 15, 2021).

CMS (Centers for Medicare & Medicaid Services). 2020. *State operation manual: Appendix A: Survey protocol, regulations and interpretive guidelines for hospitals.* https://www.cms.gov/Regulations-and-Guidance/Guidance/Manuals/downloads/som107ap_a_hospitals.pdf (accessed October 20, 2021).

CMS. 2021. *FY 2019 report to Congress (RTC): Review of Medicare's program oversight of accrediting organizations (AOs) and the Clinical Laboratory Improvement Amendments of 1988 (CLIA) validation program.* https://www.cms.gov/files/document/qso-21-12-ao-clia.pdf (accessed October 20, 2021).

Crowley, P., and S. McCrossen. 2016. *Quality by design for generic products: Opportunities and challenges.* https://www.europeanpharmaceuticalreview.com/article/46471/quality-design-generic-products-opportunities-challenges/ (accessed November 8, 2021).

Dredge, C., and S. Scholtes. 2021. The health care utility model: A novel approach to doing business. *New England Journal of Medicine Catalyst Innovations in Care Delivery.* doi:10.1056/CAT.21.0189.

FDA (U.S. Food and Drug Adminstration). 2006. *Guidance for industry: Quality systems approach to pharmaceutical CGMP regulations.* https://www.fda.gov/media/71023/download (accessed October 19, 2021).

FDA. 2010. *Standards for securing the drug supply chain: Standardized numerical identification for prescription drug packages.* https://www.fda.gov/regulatory-information/search-fda-guidance-documents/standards-securing-drug-supply-chain-standardized-numerical-identification-prescription-drug (accessed November 9, 2021).

FDA. 2012. A review of FDA's approach to medical product shortages. In *National drug shortages: Trends and FDA response*, edited by R. T. Stephens and G. Cook. Hauppauge, NY: Nova Science Publishers. Pp. 75-124.

FDA. 2017. *FDA updates on 2017 Burkholderia cepacia contamination.* https://www.fda.gov/drugs/drug-safety-and-availability/fda-updates-2017-burkholderia-cepacia-contamination (accessed October 15, 2021).

FDA. 2020. *Drug shortages for calendar year 2020.* https://www.fda.gov/media/150409/download (accessed October 11, 2021).

FDA. 2021. *Drug shortages.* https://www.fda.gov/drugs/drug-safety-and-availability/drug-shortages (accessed January 13, 2022).

FDA Drug Shortages Task Force. 2020. *Drug shortages: Root causes and potential solutions.* https://www.fda.gov/drugs/drug-shortages/report-drug-shortages-root-causes-and-potential-solutions (accessed December 16, 2021).

Fox, E. R., B. V. Sweet, and V. Jensen. 2014. Drug shortages: A complex health care crisis. *Mayo Clinic Proceedings* 98(3):361-373.

Gonsalkorale, R., E. Beracochea, V. Dias, S. Gregoire, and J. D. Quick. 2012. Ch 39: Contracting for pharmaceuticals and services. In *MDS-3: Managing access to medicines and health technologies*, edited by M. Embrey. Arlington, VA: Management Sciences for Health. https://msh.org/wp-content/uploads/2013/04/mds3-ch39-contracting-mar2012.pdf (accessed December 21, 2021).

Hegwer, L. R. 2017. *Cleveland clinic saves $22m in pharmacy costs by developing dashboard tool.* HFMA. https://www.hfma.org/topics/article/53608.html (accessed October 15, 2021).

ISPE (International Society for Pharmacoepidemiology). 2020. *Drug shortage assessment & prevention tool.* ISPE. https://www2.ispe.org/imis/ItemDetail?iProductCode=DRUGSHORTDLUS (accessed October 15, 2021).

ISPE. 2021. *Drug shortages publications & tools.* ISPE. https://ispe.org/initiatives/drug-shortages/publications-tools (accessed October 15, 2021).

NASEM (National Academies of Sciences, Engineering, and Medicine). 2018a. *Impact of the global medical supply chain on SNS operations and communications: Proceedings of a workshop*, edited by A. Mack. Washington, DC: The National Academies Press.

NASEM. 2018b. *Medical product shortages during disasters: Opportunities to predict, prevent, and respond: Proceedings of a workshop—in brief*, edited by A. Nicholson, L. Runnels, C. Giammaria, L. Brown, and S. Wollek. Washington, DC: The National Academies Press.

O'Brien, D., J. Leibowitz, and R. Anello. 2017. *Group purchasing organizations: How GPOs reduce healthcare costs and why changing their funding mechanism would raise costs.* FTC (Federal Trade Commission). https://www.ftc.gov/system/files/documents/public_comments/2017/12/00222-142618.pdf (accessed November 2, 2021).

The PEW Health Group. 2011. *After heparin: Protecting consumers from the risks of substandard and counterfeit drugs.* https://www.pewtrusts.org/en/research-and-analysis/reports/2011/07/12/after-heparin-protecting-consumers-from-the-risks-of-substandard-and-counterfeit-drugs (accessed October 25, 2021).

TJC (The Joint Commission). 2021. *Quality check and quality reports.* https://www.joint-commission.org/about-us/facts-about-the-joint-commission/quality-check-and-quality-reports/ (accessed October 20, 2021).

Vizient. 2019. Drug shortages and labor costs: Measuring a hidden cost of drug shortages on U.S. hospitals. In *Vizient Drug Shortages Impact Report.* Irving, TX: Vizient Inc. https://www.vizientinc.com/-/media/documents/sitecorepublishingdocuments/public/vzdrugshortageslaborcost_fullreport.pdf?la=en&hash=19172F274A8B03817E042C2EF423BED98CDF0401 (accessed December 20, 2021).

Yu, L. X., G. Amidon, M. A. Khan, S. W. Hoag, J. Polli, G. K. Raju, and J. Woodcock. 2014. Understanding pharmaceutical quality by design. *The American Association of Pharmaceutical Scientists Journal* 16(4):771-783.

Zacché, M. 2020. The advantages of a 'quality by design' approach in pharma drug development. *PharmaManufacturing.* https://www.pharmamanufacturing.com/articles/2019/the-advantages-of-a-quality-by-design-approach-in-clinical-and-commercial-pharma-development/ (accessed November 8, 2021).

8

Preparedness Measures for Resilient Medical Product Supply Chains

As described in the previous two chapters, awareness and mitigation measures can reduce the size and prevalence of supply disruptions. They are practical and cost-effective strategies for avoiding shortages caused by routine process control problems. However, major supply disruptions and demand surges caused by natural disasters, pandemics, or biological threats are much more difficult to avoid. Manufacturing problems will constrain supply, emergencies will spike demand, and all manner of events—predictable and unpredictable—will lead to imbalances of supply and demand for critical medical products. Therefore, to address these, a balanced supply chain resilience strategy must also contain preparedness measures that shield the public from harm when these events occur.

Preparedness includes actions taken prior to a disruptive event that will reduce the negative effects on health and safety if the event occurs. As described in the medical product supply chain resilience framework in Chapter 5, preparedness measures can be grouped into four subcategories, two physical and two virtual (Figure 8-1). Physical preparedness measures include inventory stockpiling and capacity buffering, in which stock or productive capacity are held to fill a supply shortfall. Virtual preparedness measures include contingency planning, which establishes plans for dealing with specific scenarios, and readiness, which builds capabilities for dealing with scenarios without specific plans made in advance. Each of these categories is vital to an integrated resiliency strategy. Additionally, in the discussion that follows, the committee covers how the measures in the different categories can be complementary, and their selection as preparedness measures must consider this complementarity.

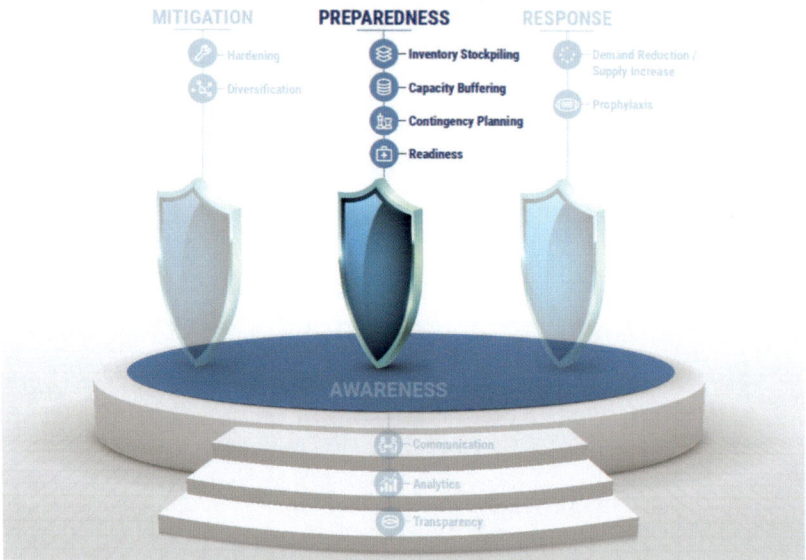

FIGURE 8-1 Medical product supply chain resilience framework: potential preparedness measures.

Some of the preparedness measures the committee recommends represent market interventions by the government. Medical product supply chains need these interventions because, as discussed in Chapter 4, medical product supply chains are typically optimized for routine conditions, with regular lead times and predictable levels of variability in demand and supply. Producers of medical products achieve this by taking steps to ensure supply can regularly meet demand, and thereby protect their revenue streams. Producers also control costs with various measures including lean production and supply chain practices. Lean medical supply chains are effective in serving patients and producing profits under routine conditions but are often ill equipped to respond to disruptions that are outside of the normal variability in supply or demand (HIDA, 2020). As the committee noted in Chapter 4, products with low profit margins are particularly likely to have supply chains that are vulnerable to failures in emergency situations because manufacturers lack any financial incentives to build in protections. When this is the case, outside interventions are needed to induce preparedness measures that meet the public need for public health and safety, rather than only the private sector's incentives to maximize profits.

Box 8-1 provides an overview of how to set a protection target for a given product and how to select and combine preparedness measures to achieve it. More details on this process are given in Chapter 5. In this chapter, the committee elaborates on this process in discussing the issues of execution and coordination within each preparedness category. These discussions provide the motive and inform the two preparedness recommendations that focus on inventory stockpiling and capacity buffering.

BOX 8-1
Overview of Roadmap for Selecting Preparedness Measures

1. **Determine the protection target.** Using the awareness measures (Chapter 6), evaluate various scenarios that could create medical product shortages and determine the number of medical products necessary to offset most shortages. This is the protection target (for a given product i, this target can be X_i units.).

2. **Evaluate current protection measures and determine what, if any, additional preparedness measures are needed.** Using the protection target (X_i) as a reference, evaluate existing mitigation (Chapter 7) and preparedness measures for a more refined view of X_i. For instance, mitigation policies promoting better quality and process controls may reduce both the magnitude and duration of a supply shortage. Similarly, manufacturers may maintain spare capacity and distributors may hold safety stocks (preparedness measures) as part of their normal business continuity practices.

3. **If additional preparedness measures are needed, ensure that the possible distribution of disruptions has been considered before new preparedness measures are implemented.** While the sizes of supply chain disruptions are uncertain, small, consistent disruptions are more likely to occur than large, infrequent ones. Using a layered strategy of different preparedness measures will be cost-effective to cover different parts of X_i. For example, inventory might be kept on hand to cover short, frequent disruptions, while contingency plans might be made to cover long, infrequent disruptions.

4. **When implementing additional preparedness measures, start with the physical measures (inventory and capacity buffering) prior to the virtual ones (contingency planning and readiness).** The physical measures can generally be implemented faster than the virtual ones. However, they tend to also be more expensive. Therefore, firms must think about how much immediately available inventory is needed to cover a shortage before additional capacity can be brought online, and then consider how much capacity can be provided before contingency plans and readiness responses can be executed.

5. **Troubleshoot the implemented preparedness measures to scale and coordinate the measures in the various categories.** For instance, after noting the lead times necessary to bring on various types of additional capacity, it may be necessary to revise the amount of inventory needed to meet demand while capacity is ramping up.

INVENTORY STOCKPILING

The most basic form of inventory stockpiling is holding physical stock in a state of readiness in preparation for a supply shortfall. Manufacturers, distributors, and health care systems all hold inventories of drugs and devices as protection against normal variations in supply and demand. However, these inventories are typically inadequate to protect against an unusual disruption of supply or an unanticipated surge in demand. Therefore, the federal government holds additional physical stock of critical medical products known as medical countermeasures (MCMs) in the Strategic National Stockpile (SNS). In theory, this is an excellent protection measure. With a reasonable estimate of the protection volume X_i for a given product i, then a stock level of X_i is one way to provide the appropriate amount of protection (see Box 8-1). However, it is not the only option, and other forms of preparedness should be considered to find the right balance of measures to improve resilience. Furthermore, there are real-world issues with holding inventory that this chapter will evaluate.

Holding inventory is more complicated in practice than in theory. In reality, problems with forecasting demand, monitoring stock levels, rotating stock to prevent expiration, and other practical details can prevent inventory stockpiles from providing the intended level of protection in an emergency. For example, a recent analysis of the SNS noted that the lack of transparency into medical product supply chains caused a lack of strategic forecasting leading up to the coronavirus disease (COVID-19) pandemic. This analysis also found that a lack of technology to monitor demand further hindered setting appropriate stock levels. Such problems led to inadequate supplies in the SNS, including for personal protective equipment (PPE), which had been depleted during the H1N1 pandemic and was not adequately restocked before the COVID-19 pandemic struck (Klein, 2020; Reinhard and Brown, 2020).

The SNS and other public inventories can improve the effectiveness of their stocks by applying evidence-based approaches to managing their inventories. For example, calculating optimal inventory levels can prevent hoarding and overstock. These calculations take into account the demand rate, order lead time, setup cost, proportional order cost, and inventory holding cost to determine the optimal amount of inventory to have on hand (Nahmias and Olsen, 2021). Using such data-driven models can help provide cost-effective protection against shortages, discourage hoarding, and respond to normal variations in supply and demand. In addition, strategic stockpiling helps to buffer the system against variations outside the normal range of routine disruptions discussed earlier.

The Public Health Emergency Medical Countermeasures Enterprise (PHEMCE) develops the SNS Annual Review. These reviews provide policy guidance to the Office of the Assistant Secretary for Preparedness and

Response (ASPR) and the SNS for budget formulation and procurement of MCMs. Innovations in how the SNS is maintained are a major lever of PHEMCE, and a recently released National Academies report and a recent White House report both call for a root cause assessment of SNS lessons learned from COVID-19 and other past public health emergencies (DoD et al., 2021; NASEM, 2021a). While the SNS's budget is limited by the funds it receives from Congress, a recent National Academies report on examining PHEMCE highlighted multiple options, including public–private partnerships, that could be implemented to improve national preparedness and response. Specifically, these options could assist with "key stockpiling decisions [including] what, how much, where, and how to stock; how to allocate limited resources; and how to resupply" (NASEM, 2021a).

Vendor-Managed Inventory and Consignment Inventory

Decentralization is a common industry approach for dealing with some of the complexities of inventory management. Rather than a single actor (e.g., the health system or the retailer) making all inventory management decisions and incurring the cost of inventory holding, stocking decisions and partial related costs are relegated to other actors—suppliers—with superior knowledge and experience with specific products. Two approaches for this type of decentralization are vendor-managed inventory (VMI), in which suppliers are responsible for controlling inventory levels, and consignment inventory (CI), in which suppliers own and maintain physical stock (Lakra and Bedi, 2014).

An example of VMI is Walmart's policy of allowing suppliers to manage inventories in its warehouses (Greenspan, 2019). Suppliers make use of stock level, point-of-sale data from Walmart, and their experience base (e.g., knowledge of demand seasonality) to calculate the appropriate volume of warehouse stock levels.

To use VMI, the product supplier, such as a medical device or drug manufacturer, takes full responsibility for maintaining an agreed-upon inventory level of the product or its components at the end user's location (e.g., hospital or pharmacy). For example, a hospital seeks to ensure that a given medical product is always in stock. Under a VMI model, the supplier would determine a reorder point that would provide sufficient stock to ensure this level of service, as well as an efficient replenishment quantity that would balance the costs of shipping and holding inventory. Each time the reorder point is reached, the vendor is notified and ships the replenishment quantity to the hospital. With the correct systems in place to monitor the hospital's consumption, such as the vendor being on site checking supply levels or the hospital regularly sending usage reports to the vendor, patterns can be identified, and the product stock levels can be adjusted as needed.

A VMI model can help end users in health care achieve improved patient care and service, reduced demand uncertainty, and reduced inventory costs. However, since VMI systems rely on the vendor/supplier to keep track of the actual number products or units in stock, health systems have a reduced visibility of future inventory, leading to an increased risk of a shortage within a health system and a decreased resilience of the supply chain. Therefore, prior to using a VMI approach, a careful risk assessment must be done to determine how the health system will handle an emergency response situation.

Consignment inventory (CI) is another useful tool to improve the management of medical product inventories. An example of CI is Amazon's use of drop shipping, in which online orders are filled from stocks owned and held by suppliers (Amazon, 2021). Under a CI system, a supplier maintains an end user's promised inventory either at the supplier's site or some other location. The end user purchases the inventory only when they use it. The government and health care systems could use a CI approach to free up working capital, reduce overall supply expenses, and keep products that are expensive and difficult to acquire at the ready. However, a major drawback for end users with a CI system is the lack of direct management, oversight, control, and transparency over inventory; products may become misplaced, damaged, expired, or go to competing nearby facilities. This can lead to increased costs associated with expired or unusable products. Furthermore, a particular unit of product can be promised to several customers without any of them really knowing how many units are being stored against what kind of risk. These problems can become particularly acute during emergencies that cause a sudden surge in demand, resulting in a lower than planned level of protection. For either a VMI or CI model to work between suppliers and end users, it is critical for there to be trust between parties, an understanding of performance capability, clear and frequent communication, and transparency (Sumrit, 2020).

Options for the Strategic National Stockpile

Health systems can make use of VMI and CI to manage inventory effectively during normal routine conditions. While stockpiling is already part of the national preparedness strategy, primarily in the form of the SNS, the exclusive authority vested in that federal function is problematic (Fitzpatrick, 2020; NASEM, 2021a). To make the SNS more effective than it was during COVID-19, the SNS can model how health systems manage inventory. The SNS must refine and improve the ways it holds its inventory as protection against a supply shortage or demand surge. In particular, one problem in the SNS that VMI or CI could address is product expiration. While all drugs and medical devices have expiration dates set by the manufacturer, their actual shelf life, if stored properly, can be much longer (AMA, 2001; Lyon et al., 2006). A federal initiative called the Shelf Life Extension Program was developed in the 1980s to defer and reduce the replacement costs of federal stockpiles of critical medical products by extending useful shelf lives through periodic U.S. Food and Drug Administration (FDA) stability testing and strict environmental controls (Khan et al., 2014; Lyon et al., 2006). Yet, replenishing stockpile products postexpiration is challenging since this can occur long after the events that necessitated their use passed. During the interim, public and political support for large government expenditures to store medical products that may never get used can wane. This was the case after the response to the H1N1 influenza pandemic in 2009. During H1N1, the SNS distributed large quantities of emergency medical supplies, but Congress never appropriated funding to replace the items used in that effort (Quinn, 2020; Rule, 2020). Therefore, when states and other agencies began requesting assistance from the SNS in March 2020 for response to COVID-19, the medical products remaining from the H1N1 response were deemed past their shelf life and unable to be used (Lieb and Dil, 2020; Rule, 2020). The lack of local control and oversight of government-held stockpiles was a serious impediment to flexible responses to the pandemic.

Using VMI or CI strategies where inventory is located adjacent to a manufacturing facility or distribution warehouse would shift rotation and expiration date problems to vendors with detailed product knowledge. This would be particularly valuable for short shelf life products where frequent rotation is necessary. Under a VMI or CI system, new stock would be delivered to the warehouse, spend a specified amount of time in stock, and be shipped out through normal supply channels in first in, first out fashion. This would provide protection for a duration equal to the amount of time the product is kept in stock and would eliminate the excess material handling due to shipping product in and out of a separate SNS facility to manage expiration dates. It would also vastly simplify the SNS management duties of the government.

Note that VMI and CI systems that put responsibility for stocking and rotation in the hands of individual vendors with detailed knowledge of their products will benefit the SNS regardless of whether the stock is owned by the government and held in public facilities (VMI) or owned and stocked by vendors (CI). However, because vendors lack profit incentives to maintain these stocks, accountability measures are still needed. The logical way to achieve this is for the government to pay vendors for the cost of stockpiling products and to monitor vendor performance, perhaps via periodic audits. Unlike the Walmart and Amazon examples where retailers can evaluate suppliers on their ongoing performance, emergency scenarios occur rarely by definition. Therefore, waiting for an emergency to evaluate a stockpile is too late. It must also be stressed that there is no one-size-fits-all strategy.

The key is to analyze product and/or supply chain risk with respect to the medical product supply chain resilience framework (see Figure 8-1) and decide on the most appropriate protection level and strategy.

An additional measure for effective stockpiling would be to push more responsibility for inventory management to the state and local levels. Local health officials and health systems have much better knowledge about inventory usage patterns, distribution plans to rotate stock, and how to align communications and activities needed to make VMI more robust. This gives them the advantageous position to forecast emergency demand, to monitor stock levels, and to allocate and release inventory regionally. These same local officials would also serve as powerful advocates for the replenishment of critical stocks, which might prevent failures to rebuild stockpiles after an emergency, as happened with PPE and other products after the H1N1 pandemic (Quinn, 2020; Rule, 2020). Therefore, a reasonable strategy for the SNS and the National Stockpiling Strategy is to have a national program with regional stockpiles and national guidelines, similar to what is currently in place. However, some central planning, funding/incentives, and oversight must be retained because independent planning will overlook opportunities for resource sharing, such as shipping ventilators from one region to another as relative needs shift during an event.

Without information, VMI, CI, and regional stockpiles cannot function. To manage stockpile inventories, stakeholders—hospitals, health departments, first responders, suppliers—need information about surges in demand and remaining supplies. To evaluate the inventory implications of disruptions, planners need information about prevention and mitigation measures, such as mask reuse and resource sharing. For example, if crisis standards call for N95 masks to be reused X times instead of once, then total demand will be $1/X$ the forecast of uses during the emergency. Finally, stakeholders need inventory data about what medical products are available and where. Because such information has national security concerns, technology is needed to preserve security while providing transparency. The use of blockchain as a data synchronizer,[1] as well as predictive analytics, have been proposed as ways to help forecast demand more effectively and therefore inform stockpiling practices (Bhaskar et al., 2020).

CAPACITY BUFFERING

Economically, capacity buffering can be a cost-effective alternative or supplement to inventory buffering when protecting against shortages. Inventory buffers require the production and storage of products in advance.

---

[1] Blockchain is a shared, fixed ledger that facilitates the process of recording transactions and tracking assets in a network. Assets can be tangible or intangible. Tracking and trading on a blockchain network can reduce risks and costs for all network members.

This is advantageous during sudden shortages as inventory is immediately available. However, inventory stockpiles simultaneously incur both the fixed and variable costs of manufacturing (i.e., facilities/equipment and material/labor, respectively), along with the costs of storage. Capacity buffers, alternatively, rely on having the production capability prepared and manufacture the products only if the additional supply is needed. See Box 8-2 for an example of capacity buffering in action.

While this necessitates lead time to activate the capacity and to produce the needed products, with the fixed-cost investments up front, the overall cost between fixed and variable manufacturing is split (Huang et al., 2016). See Chapter 5 for an additional discussion on the economics of inventory stockpiling and capacity buffering.

It is important to note that, as described in Chapter 5, any strategy for creating capacity will only work if sufficient supplies of ingredients and components are also available. This implies that capacity buffers are needed at all stages of the supply chain or that there are adequate inventory stockpiles of ingredients or components. The latter option is what many firms do via assemble-to-order strategies. For example, Dell Computer stocks components such as central processing units, memory chips, keyboards, screens, and power supplies, and puts them together to configure specific computers for customers. This type of assemble-to-order strategy allows Dell to be responsive to customers while vastly reducing the cost of the inventory they carry (CFI, 2021).

The combination of technology advances, which make final assembly cost competitive in the United States, and an assemble-to-order strategy could facilitate on-shoring (see Box 8-3). For example, suppose advanced manufacturing makes the fill-and-finish stage of production for a given drug cost competitive in the United States, but active pharmaceutical ingredient

---

BOX 8-2
3M's Use of Capacity Buffering

3M uses capacity buffering as a strategy to respond to demand increases for the medical products it produces. The company has drawn on its capacity buffers for N95 respirator masks in response to Ebola outbreaks, the H1N1 influenza pandemic, and most recently, the COVID-19 pandemic (Gruley and Clough, 2020). As part of deploying its capacity buffers, 3M's respirator facilities began production on machinery that had been kept idle and transitioned their employees to overtime to help meet the sudden increase in demand. The realization that it was difficult to predict exponential demand surges, but that such demand surges were inevitable, prompted 3M to build this capacity buffering into their supply chains.

production remains highly uncompetitive. On-shoring the final step would provide little ability to sustain or ramp up production during an emergency if components are in short supply. But if these critical inputs are stockpiled (perhaps using VMI or CI), on-shored final assembly could be beneficial since it could protect against disruption of imported supplies.

BOX 8-3
Comparing the Economics of On-Shoring and Stockpiling*

Both on-shoring and stockpiling have associated costs. It is important to consider each of these costs before deciding which approach offers appropriate resilience at a lower cost. For example, consider respirator face masks and suppose the total annual spending on imported respirator face masks is $1.2 billion during a respiratory public health emergency, which corresponds to 1.2 billion face masks at $1 each. There are four types of shocks that could cause a supply shortage that should be considered:

1. Worldwide events (e.g., pandemic) that spike total demand above available capacity,
2. Regional events (e.g., epidemic, earthquake, hurricane) that spike domestic demand,
3. Regional events (e.g., earthquake, hurricane) that disrupt international supply (e.g., from China), and
4. Regional events (e.g., earthquake, hurricane) that disrupt domestic supply.

Assuming that the stockpile is large enough to cover the supply shortage until global supply catches up with demand, stockpiling will provide protection against all of these categories. In contrast, on-shoring provides protection against categories 1 and 3, but it is only marginally effective for category 2 and not at all effective for category 4.

For an example of the cost of on-shoring, calculations should include an additional 50 percent added to the cost of producing these domestically, a price premium. This can ignore the fixed cost of moving production to the United States because this would be paid for by the price premium. There is also a cost of undetermined value, Z, that corresponds to the cost of the capacity buffering required to increase production. Given this assumption, the *added* cost is [(0.5 × $1.2 billion) + Z]/year = ($600 million + Z)/year.

For the cost of stockpiling, assume that a 6-month supply (at normal demand levels, 0.5 × $1.2 billion) is enough to weather any of the above disruptions and that the annual holding cost rate (e.g., interest on money tied up in inventory, storage cost, cost of rotating inventory) is 15 percent. Then the *added* cost is 0.15/year × 0.5 × $1.2 billion = $90 million/year. The cost of stockpiling in this scenario is considerably less expensive than the cost of on-shoring. However, these calculations must also consider how many years will elapse before the next respiratory public health emergency. For this reason, the relative cost of on-shoring and stockpiling depends

STRATEGIC RECOMMENDATIONS: PREPAREDNESS

Market Incentives

While useful, the medical product supply chain resilience framework has its limitations. Inventory stockpiles and capacity buffers are an important part of a balanced supply chain resilience strategy. But these are not simple levers that can be engaged directly. Although the government on the cost of capacity buffering and the time between emergencies. In general, as the cost of capacity buffering decreases and the time between emergencies increases, stockpiling becomes a less cost-effective option (see Figure 8-2).

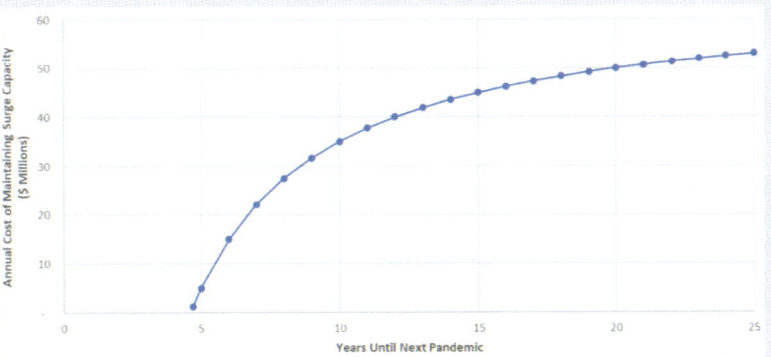

FIGURE 8-2 Cost comparison of stockpiling and on-shoring.
NOTE: Above the line, stockpiling is cheaper. Below the line, on-shoring is cheaper.

Since the above numbers rely on assumptions, sensitivity analyses can test the conclusion. If the value of Z happened to equal $90 million, then on-shoring would never be cheaper than stockpiling, irrelevant of time between emergencies. In fact, stockpiling would be cheaper than on-shoring for all values of X so long as Z was greater than or equal to $65 million. Alternatively, if Z were equal to $5 million, on-shoring would be cheaper than stockpiling if the stockpile had to be maintained for more than 5 years. If Z were $45 million, or half of the annual costs of maintaining the stockpile, then stockpiling would be cheaper as long as X were less than 15 years.

Other products that are manufactured with high levels of automation could narrow the price gap between domestic and international production, or products that have high degrees of spoilage could increase the holding cost rate to the point where on-shoring is cost competitive with stockpiling.

---

* This box references a report commissioned by the Committee on Security of America's Medical Product Supply Chain titled "Where There's a Will: Economic Considerations in Reforming America's Medical Supply Chain," by Phil Ellis (see Appendix D).

can purchase and stockpile supplies of critical medical products, doing this effectively requires regional coordination, engagement of end users, and public–private cooperation, as described earlier and addressed later in Recommendation 4 (Stockpiling). Capacity buffering is even more nuanced because direct government control is problematic, and capacity usually needs to be virtual to be cost-effective.

Although the federal government could set up its own manufacturing facilities to produce needed critical medical products, it would be enormously expensive to hold such capacity idle in anticipation of an emergency. The federal government could also enter selected markets by establishing production facilities to produce generic drugs and simple medical devices. But this fundamental change in the role of government and the workings of the health care system is beyond the scope of this study. Therefore, the most practical approach is to consider options for creating capacity buffers within the current market for drugs and medical devices.

A basic obstacle to the resilience of medical product supply chains is that profit motives of manufacturers and vendors motivate a smaller investment in protection than is optimal from a public health perspective. The gap between privately optimal and publicly optimal investment is most acute where margins are low but medical needs are high. For example, an inexpensive generic drug that is essential to health does not warrant significant private investment to protect revenue streams but does warrant significant public investment to protect health.

On the inventory side, the gap can be bridged with public investment in stockpiles; however, capacity will require a more subtle approach. Ideally, this approach should create incentives for the private sector to create additional capacity buffering but be flexible enough to allow manufacturers or hospitals to find the most efficient ways to do this. As such, incentives should focus on the ends (i.e., production of emergency supplies when needed) rather than the means (i.e., who produces what and how).

A mechanism for inducing more investment for capacity buffering by private firms is to pay for it in the form of "crisis prices." These could be set via auctions in which the federal government takes bids to deliver supplies of specific medical products to supplement stockpile inventories. This is similar to what the government does when the Defense Production Act (DPA) is invoked (FEMA, 2020; Scott, 2020). However, holding open auctions would open the door to innovative entrepreneurs with novel ways of creating capacity buffers. Also, to give firms incentives to make time or money investments to be ready to bid in these auctions, the government should publish, in advance, a list of products eligible for crisis prices, along with information about the events that would trigger an auction. Finally, to prevent fraud, the U.S. government should devise rules, similar to those enacted by other governments like Germany, to prevent firms from inducing or exacerbating a supply shortage only to profit from it (Reese and Chance, 2021).

Determining which products should be included on the crisis-prices list for auctions will require an assessment of risk levels (where risk score is defined as the product of the medically essential score and the disruption likelihood level), as described in Chapter 5. Determining the likelihood of a disruption needs to take into consideration business continuity measures included in firms' risk management plans. This focus should be on high-risk products. But risk alone is not enough to determine which products need increased capacity buffering. A list of products for inclusion on the crisis-prices list with stockpiling policies needs to be constructed. For example, a product for which stockpiling is relatively inexpensive might be best covered entirely by inventory and not included on the list at all. Another product for which stockpiling is expensive might need only enough inventory to cover the anticipated lead time to ramp up capacity.

BUT BUFFER FLEXIBILITY

As discussed in Chapter 5, flexibility makes inventory stockpiling and capacity buffering more effective. For example, resource sharing is a form of inventory flexibility that can significantly reduce the cost of achieving a given level of protection (Song and Song, 2009; Van Mieghem, 2007). Regional inventory stockpiles are inflexible if they can only be used to satisfy demand within the region. If cross-regional sharing is allowed, the stockpiles become flexible because they can satisfy demand in multiple regions. This type of flexibility is valuable when demand can be high in one region and low in another (i.e., regional demand is independent or negatively correlated). A concrete example during the COVID-19 pandemic was the case of ventilators, where there was considerable talk (but much less action) about shifting units between regions because surges of intensive care unit patients occurred at different times in different regions. On a global scale, sharing materials and products across regions is an important element of buffering the capacity of global medical product supply chains. Products with geographically diversified[2] supply chains can be transshipped from low-demand regions to high-demand regions.

Another form of inventory flexibility is substitution. For example, if drug A can be substituted for drug B, then drug A can be used to satisfy two different types of demand. As such, a stockpile of drug A can serve as protection against shortages of both drugs A and B. However, unlike inventory sharing across regions, where the main costs are likely to be transportation and administration, the main cost in substitution could be a decline in clinical effectiveness. Therefore, finding ways to make substitute

---

[2] Note that diversification elevates supply chain protection through both mitigation and preparedness measures prior to and during an event, respectively. Awareness of supply chain diversification is also a vital precursor to understanding the measures for promoting flexibility through diversification.

drugs and devices safely and effectively in advance of an emergency can enhance the flexibility of these products and hence their utility in protecting the public against medical supply shortages.

How to make inventory flexible so it can be used in resource sharing schemes depends on the situation. In some cases, such as the ventilator scenario, it might only require ensuring that the shared items are suitable for all participating health systems (i.e., standards are consistent) and articulating rules for sharing. In other cases, it may also require product modifications. For example, in nonmedical applications, manufacturers design appliances with universal plugs or adapters to make them compatible with the electrical standards of different countries so they can redirect supplies from one country to another to match demand. Because medical products are licensed independently in different countries, this type of flexibility to share supplies across borders may be limited. However, FDA can issue emergency use orders to allow use of medical products approved by other countries, as it did during the COVID-19 pandemic for KN95 masks from China.

As with inventory, flexibility in capacity can take various forms. One of the simplest is cross-training, which makes human capacity flexible so it can shift from producing one product or service to another. Cross-trained workers can be used in medical production facilities to facilitate ramping up capacity for a product with increased demand (e.g., due to an emergency or disruption).

Although labor flexibility can enable use of existing idle capacity (e.g., an unused night shift), further expansion of capacity will also require equipment/manufacturing flexibility. Flexible manufacturing, which makes use of computer and numerically controlled tools and other equipment that can perform multiple functions, along with cross-trained operators, is common in many industries. But in pharmaceutical manufacturing, new technologies such as additive manufacturing,[3] modular manufacturing, single-use manufacturing, and continuous manufacturing[4] are widely touted but still

---

[3] Blockchain technology may facilitate additive manufacturing, an advanced manufacturing technique. Blockchain can verify the authenticity of additive manufacturing product designs when these designs are being shared by a disperse network of global manufacturers (Kurpjuweit et al., 2019). Moreover, blockchain ledgers increase the transparency of the supply chain in a way that meaningfully promotes quality. Quality and identity assessments, performance metrics, input materials, and product ownership can all be logged and tracked across the life cycle of the product—from starting material to delivery of the final product to health care centers (Bhaskar et al., 2020; Kurpjuweit et al., 2019). This technology, if applied correctly, can help reduce the entrance of fraudulent and substandard medical products into the market and protect consumers.

[4] This method of drug manufacturing involves moving pharmaceuticals nonstop within the same facility, eliminating hold times between steps. Material is fed through an assembly line of fully integrated components. This method saves time, reduces the likelihood for human error, and can respond more nimbly to market changes. It can also run for a longer period of time, which may reduce the likelihood of drug shortages (FDA, 2017a).

sparsely used methods for increasing flexibility and scalability.[5] As such, measures that promote the development and use of these advanced manufacturing technologies could help medical product facilities adjust production to meet needs during an emergency. In turn, the ability of such facilities to generate surge capacity more quickly will reduce the amount of inventory that will be needed in stockpiles as protection against a disruption. A 2021 National Academies report on innovation in pharmaceutical manufacturing recommended several actions that the Center for Drug Evaluation and Research (CDER) could implement to improve the uptake of innovative manufacturing technologies (NASEM, 2021b). These included increasing institutional awareness of and expertise in innovative technologies, new mechanisms to approve innovations to existing products, and expanded opportunities for external engagement on the issue.

A number of public–private partnerships have been established to support the development of advanced manufacturing technologies and address their barriers to uptake (FDA, 2021). Manufacturing USA and America Makes are two examples of public–private partnerships that bring together academia, industry, and government to accelerate the innovation and uptake of advanced manufacturing technologies.[6,7] FDA has also taken several steps to promote the implementation of advanced manufacturing. These steps include funding extramural research projects in various aspects of advanced manufacturing, issuing grants to academic institutions and nonprofits to study advanced manufacturing and recommend improvements, and establishing the Additive Manufacturing of Medical Products research facility to improve FDA's technical and regulatory infrastructure. FDA also established the Emerging Technology Program to facilitate industry's adoption of advanced manufacturing, allowing industry to work collaboratively with regulators in addressing potential technical and regulatory barriers (FDA, 2019). In an effort to lower the regulatory barriers that manufacturers face when updating production processes, facilities, and equipment, FDA updated its guidance on the required information on post-approval manufacturing changes in annual reports for drug and biologics in 2014 and 2017, respectively, so changes with minor risk to product quality could be made without prior authorization (FDA, 2014, 2017b).

---

[5] Modular manufacturing is done in a large area with no fixed equipment, allowing for a facility to be broken down into functional building blocks or modules in order to simplify, standardize, verify, and reuse designs as well as actual modules in different implementations (Riley, 2016). Single-use manufacturing uses disposable tools to reduce the risk of product contamination and improve operational efficiency by eliminating the need to sterilize instruments between batches (Parrish, 2018). Continuous manufacturing is done from end to end on a single, uninterrupted production line (Siemens, 2021).

[6] For more information, see https://www.manufacturingusa.com/pages/how-we-work (accessed October 20, 2021).

[7] For more information, see https://www.americamakes.us/ (accessed October 20, 2021).

Another flexible use of capacity is "pop-up capacity," in which new players enter a market to address an emergency shortage. Additionally, pop-up capacity can be used for more routine but not necessarily constant public health emergencies. For instance, during flu season, distilleries in hard-hit areas could be incentivized to produce hand sanitizer, or local businesses accustomed to serving a large volume of customers daily, like a bank or fast-food restaurant, can partner with the local health department to host vaccine clinics (CDPH, 2021; Kaur, 2020).

CONTINGENCY PLANNING AND READINESS

As described in Chapter 5, contingency planning involves mapping out a course of action for responding to a specific scenario, while readiness involves actions that improve the ability to respond to a category of scenarios once the details of the event become known. In contrast to the physical buffers of inventory and capacity, contingency planning and readiness are virtual protections. But they are important parts of the preparedness picture nonetheless because they do not incur the ongoing costs associated with physical assets. As such, they are essential for addressing rare events for which these costs cannot be justified.

Contingency planning can address many factors that influence supply chain resilience, including inventory and capacity. An illustrative example from the COVID-19 pandemic is ventilator production. In April 2020, the DPA was invoked to compel Ford, General Motors, Medtronic, and others to produce ventilators, although most of them had already begun ramping up production (Clark, 2020; Dzhanova, 2020; Vazquez, 2020). Without advance preparation, the auto companies were only able to produce simpler transport ventilators, rather than the intensive care unit ventilators doctors preferred (Bergin, 2020). Furthermore, the on-the-fly supply chain coordination resulted in shortages that led to delays. Despite the good intentions and heroic efforts by medical device and other manufacturers, it seems that they could have ramped up ventilator production more quickly and accurately with some advance planning in place. Additionally, contingency planning and readiness measures can be combined with physical buffering to create capacity on an as-needed basis that could be activated in times of emergency. One approach is "warm basing." This transitional state between the physical and virtual preparedness measures allows for a production facility to remain in a state of partial readiness, with either the physical supplies or trained staff ready to go when the need arises.

A contingency plan that specifies the triggers, mechanisms, and responsibilities of various actors for implementing resource sharing would be one way to promote inventory flexibility. Examples of contingency planning include crisis standards of care (CSC) planning for health systems. Resources on CSC and substitution can be found in Box 8-4.

> **BOX 8-4**
> **Resources for Crisis Standards of Care**
>
> **Crisis Standards of Care (CSC)** are defined as a substantial change in usual health care operations and the level of care it is possible to deliver, which is made necessary by a pervasive (e.g., pandemic influenza) or catastrophic (e.g., earthquake, hurricane) disaster (IOM, 2009).
>
> **ASPR Technical Resources, Assistance Center, and Information Exchange (TRACIE)** provides plans, tools, templates, and other implementable resources to help with preparedness, response, recovery, and mitigation efforts, focusing on CSC (ASPR_TRACIE, 2022).
>
> **The National Academy of Medicine** provides various tools and publications as resources for CSC. These resources have been tailored for health care providers, public officials and emergency planners, and the public plan for the implementation of CSC (NAM, 2022).

Readiness measures can be thought of as organizational preparations at multiple levels (i.e., top-down, bottom-up) allowing for flexibility, dynamic control, and adaptive management during disruptive events (Ivanov and Sokolov, 2012). For these measures to work, partners and stakeholders must be preemptively identified and prepared to act when needed. This is critical to supply chain preparedness.

RECOMMENDATIONS

The COVID-19 crisis served as a stark reminder that holding inventory in stockpiles is more complicated in practice than in theory. In real-world settings, problems with forecasting demand, monitoring stock levels, rotating stock to prevent expiration, and other practical details can prevent inventory stockpiles from providing the intended level of protection in an emergency. Furthermore, as described above, capacity buffering can be a cost-effective alternative or supplement to inventory as protection against shortages. Finally, contingency plans and readiness activities can provide additional levels of protection for rare events that are too costly to buffer with physical inventory and capacity.

Therefore, the committee recommends action related to both inventory stockpiling and capacity buffering. Stockpiling is already part of the national preparedness strategy, primarily in the form of the SNS. Recommendation 4 (Stockpiling) is substantially about refining and improving the ways inventory is held as protection against medical product shortages. Recommendation 5 (Capacity Buffering) complements these steps by advocating measures to develop capacity that can be brought online to supplement inventory stockpiles as needed. Such capacity buffering could be the result of direct contracts, such as advance arrangements to have specific manufacturers provide emergency capacity, as the auto manufacturers did during the pandemic by assembling ventilators. Capacity buffers could also be the result of a list of guaranteed crisis prices that the government would pay for certain products under specified conditions. This would provide incentives for firms to find creative ways to deliver pop-up capacity during emergencies. Finally, the federal government should fund research on advanced manufacturing technologies that make it more economical to locally produce goods and easier to scale up capacity quickly. Both of these would make capacity buffering a more viable preparedness option and hence would facilitate a partial shift away from expensive inventory and toward cheaper capacity.

As noted earlier, on-shoring is often promoted as a means for building medical supply chain resilience via the argument that the more medical products a country produces domestically, the more control it has of supplies during an emergency. By reducing labor costs and promoting flexibility and scalability, the advanced manufacturing technologies advocated in Recommendation 5 (Capacity Buffering) may make on-shoring a good option for some products. Indeed, if technological capabilities permit efficient, small-scale production, then dispersed production in the country of consumption will be the natural market outcome. However, where this is not the case, on-shoring will impose a significant price penalty on an ongoing basis in return for a potentially small advantage during rare emergencies. If many high-income countries pursue on-shoring strategies for many medical products, considerable resources will be spent that could be put to better use addressing other problems. Therefore, on-shoring should be part of an integrated resilience strategy, rather than the option of choice.

> **Recommendation 4 (Stockpiling).** The Office of the Assistant Secretary for Preparedness and Response should take steps to develop strategies to modernize and optimize inventory stockpiling management for the Strategic National Stockpile (SNS) and beyond to respond to medical product shortages at the national and regional levels. These steps include
> a. Consider the recommendations provided in National Academies report, *Ensuring the Effectiveness of the Public Health Emergency Medical Countermeasures Enterprise*, particularly those that focus on adopting a systems approach to managing the SNS.
> b. Analyze risk levels of supply chain critical medical products and the viability of other response strategies (e.g., capacity buffering).
> c. Examine key inventory stockpiling process considerations such as
> - Inventory system visibility.

- Mechanisms and thresholds for the use, sharing, deployment, distribution, and allocation of stockpiled inventory in response to shortages (triggered by both emergencies and routine use) and to prevent product expiration.
- The risks and benefits of stockpiling ingredients or components as opposed to finished goods.
- The risks and benefits of just-in-time production or inventories in larger reserves.
- Funding levels to meet the required inventory levels and management tasks for the regional and national stockpiles as well as incentives for stakeholders for holding inventory.

d. Convene regional and local working groups composed of emergency health planners, clinicians, health care systems, and public health agencies, among others, to discuss and inform expectations for federal SNS support; national and regional stockpile content and pre-deployment positioning; regional supply capabilities and expectations; and roles and responsibilities for key stakeholders.

Recommendation 5 (Capacity Buffering). The Office of the Assistant Secretary for Preparedness and Response (ASPR) and the U.S. Food and Drug Administration (FDA) should take steps to cultivate capacity buffering for supply chain critical medical products where such capacity is a cost-effective complement to stockpiling and as protection against long-lasting supply disruptions or demand surges. These steps include

a. Government investments in capacity buffering should be aimed at all stages of the supply chain and at major public health emergencies.
b. ASPR and FDA should develop and routinely maintain a crisis-prices list of supply chain critical medical products (i.e., medically essential and supply chain vulnerable) and identify which capacity measure is a practical supplement to the stockpiled inventory. Further, ASPR should develop and manage a database to coordinate inventory stockpiling and capacity buffering policies regarding the crisis-prices list.
c. ASPR and FDA should fund research and development for both advanced pharmaceutical and advanced medical technology manufacturing techniques to help make on-shoring more cost-competitive. By making capacity more easily scalable, these technologies would enable firms to respond to the need for capacity buffers more quickly and cost-effectively.
d. ASPR and FDA should create public–private partnerships and support and fund capital and staff investments jointly, to imple-

ment these advanced manufacturing approaches to ensure production capacity. These partnerships will provide a great depth and breadth of expertise and can be leveraged for new economic incentives and regulatory clarity.

    e. ASPR should be responsible for anticipating and assessing public health emergency demand surge for supply chain critical medical products. They should clarify production capacity, identify vulnerabilities in supply chains, and engage producers in developing plans for surge response.

REFERENCES

AMA (American Medical Association). 2001. Pharmaceutical expiration dates. Paper read at American Medical Association Annual Meeting, June 17-21, Chicago, IL.

Amazon. 2021. *Fulfillment by Amazon.* https://sell.amazon.com/fulfillment-by-amazon (accessed November 1, 2021).

ASPR_TRACIE (Assistant Secretary for Preparedness and Response_Technical Resources, Assistance Center, and Information Exchange). 2022. *Topic collection: COVID-19 crisis standards of care resources.* https://asprtracie.hhs.gov/technical-resources/112/covid-19-crisis-standards-of-care-resources/99#plans-tools-and-templates (accessed January 20, 2022).

Bergin, T. 2020. The U.S. has spent billions stockpiling ventilators, but many won't save critically ill COVID-19 patients. *Reuters,* December 2. https://www.reuters.com/article/us-health-coronavirus-ventilators-insigh/the-u-s-has-spent-billions-stockpiling-ventilators-but-many-wont-save-critically-ill-covid-19-patients-idUSKBN28C1N6 (accessed October 14, 2021).

Bhaskar, S., J. Tan, M. L. Bogers, T. Minssen, H. Badaruddin, S. Israeli-Korn, and H. Chesbrough. 2020. At the epicenter of COVID-19: The tragic failure of the global supply chain for medical supplies. *Frontiers in Public Health* 8:821.

CDPH (California Department of Public Health). 2021. *California partners with McDdonald's franchisees across the state for COVID-19 vaccine pop-up clinics.* Sacramento, CA. https://www.cdph.ca.gov/Programs/OPA/Pages/NR21-198.aspx (accessed November 3, 2021).

CFI (Corporate Finance Institute). 2021. *Assemble-to-order.* CFI. https://corporatefinanceinstitute.com/resources/knowledge/strategy/assemble-to-order/#:~:text=Dell%20Technologies%20follows%20an%20assemble-to-order%20business%20model%20for,the%20PC%20is%20assembled%20and%20shipped%20for%20delivery (accessed December 8, 2021).

Clark, D. 2020. Trump invokes Defense Production Act to force GM to make ventilators for coronavirus fight. *NBC,* March 27. https://www.nbcnews.com/politics/donald-trump/trump-invokes-defense-production-act-force-gm-make-ventilators-coronavirus-n1170746 (accessed December 8, 2021).

DoD (U.S. Department of Defense), HHS (U.S. Department of Health and Human Services), DHS (U.S. Department of Homeland Security), and VA (U.S. Department of Veterans Affairs). 2021. *National strategy for a resilient public health supply chain,* edited by Department of Health and Human Services, Department of Defense, Department of Homeland Security, Department of Commerce, Department of State, Department of Veterans Affairs, and The White House Office of the COVID-19 Response. Washington, DC. https://www.phe.gov/Preparedness/legal/Documents/National-Strategy-for-Resilient-Public-Health-Supply-Chain.pdf (accessed October 29, 2021).

Dzhanova, Y. 2020. Trump compelled these companies to make critical supplies, but most of them were already doing it. *CNBC*, April 3. https://www.cnbc.com/2020/04/03/coronavirus-trump-used-defense-production-act-on-these-companies-so-far.html (accessed December 8, 2021).

FDA (U.S. Food and Drug Administration). 2014. *Guidance for industry: CMC postapproval manufacturing changes to be documented in annual reports.* https://www.fda.gov/media/79182/download (accessed October 14, 2021).

FDA. 2017a. *Modernizing the way drugs are made: A transition to continuous manufacturing.* https://www.fda.gov/drugs/news-events-human-drugs/modernizing-way-drugs-are-made-transition-continuous-manufacturing (accessed October 18, 2021).

FDA. 2017b. *Guidance for industry: CMC postapproval manufacturing changes for specified biological products to be documented in annual reports.* https://www.fda.gov/media/106935/download (accessed October 14, 2021).

FDA. 2019. *Emerging technology program.* https://www.fda.gov/about-fda/center-drug-evaluation-and-research-cder/emerging-technology-program (accessed October 20, 2021).

FDA. 2021. *Advanced manufacturing.* https://www.fda.gov/emergency-preparedness-and-response/mcm-issues/advanced-manufacturing (accessed October 19, 2021).

FEMA (Federal Emergency Management Agency). 2020. *Applying the Defense Production Act.* https://www.fema.gov/press-release/20210420/applying-defense-production-act (accessed December 8, 2021).

Fitzpatrick, S. 2020. Why the Strategic National Stockpile isn't meant to solve a crisis like coronavirus. *NBC*, March 28. https://www.nbcnews.com/health/health-care/why-strategic-national-stockpile-isn-t-meant-solve-crisis-coronavirus-n1170376 (accessed January 20, 2022).

Greenspan, R. 2019. *Walmart's inventory management.* Panmore Institute. http://panmore.com/walmart-inventory-management (accessed December 8, 2021).

Gruley, B., and R. Clough. 2020. *How 3M plans to make more than a billion masks by end of year.* https://www.bloomberg.com/news/features/2020-03-25/3m-doubled-production-of-n95-face-masks-to-fight-coronavirus?utm_campaign=news&utm_medium=bd&utm_source=applenews (accessed November 4, 2021).

HIDA (Health Industry Distributors Association). 2020. *Building a more robust supply chain: A public-private framework to create a pandemic response infrastructure.* https://www.hida.org/distribution/advocacy/COVID19/White-Paper-Building-A-More-Robust-Supply-Chain.aspx?utm_source=blueprint-page&utm_medium=web&utm_campaign=medical-supplies-last-mile (accessed December 16, 2021).

Huang, L., J.-S. Song, and J. Tong. 2016. Supply chain planning for random demand surges: Reactive capacity and safety stock. *Manufacturing & Service Operations Management* 18(4):509-524.

IOM (Institute of Medicine). 2009. *Guidance for establishing crisis standards of care for use in disaster situations: A letter report.* Washington, DC: The National Academies Press.

Ivanov, D., and B. Sokolov. 2012. Structure dynamics control approach to supply chain planning and adaptation. *International Journal of Production Research* 50(21):6133-6149.

Kaur, H. 2020. Distilleries are making hand sanitizer with their in-house alcohol and giving it out for free to combat coronavirus. *CNN*, March 19. https://edition.cnn.com/2020/03/16/us/distilleries-hand-sanitizer-coronavirus-trnd/index.html (accessed November 3, 2021).

Khan, S. R., R. Kona, P. J. Faustino, A. Gupta, J. S. Taylor, D. A. Porter, and M. Khan. 2014. United States Food and Drug Administration and Department of Defense shelf-life extension program of pharmaceutical products: Progress and promise. *Journal of Pharmaceutical Sciences* 103(5):1331-1336.

Klein, P. 2020. *America's medical supply crisis* (PBS Frontline Season 2020: Ep. 6). https://www.pbs.org/wgbh/frontline/film/americas-medical-supply-crisis/ (accessed November 3, 2021).

Kurpjuweit, S., C. Schmidt, M. Klöckner, and S. Wagner. 2019. Blockchain in additive manufacturing and its impact on supply chains. *Journal of Business Logistics* 42.

Lakra, P., and P. Bedi. 2014. Topic: The comparative study of consignment and vendor managed inventory with special reference of cost structure. *International Journal of Advancements in Research & Technology* 3(3):142-146.

Lieb, D. A., and C. Dil. 2020. Review: State stockpiles were depleted before the virus. *The Mercury News*, April 23. https://www.mercurynews.com/2020/04/23/review-state-stockpiles-were-depleted-before-the-virus/ (accessed October 14, 2021).

Lyon, R. C., J. S. Taylor, D. A. Porter, H. R. Prasanna, and A. S. Hussain. 2006. Stability profiles of drug products extended beyond labeled expiration dates. *Journal of Pharmaceutical Sciences* 95(7):1549-1560.

Nahmias, S., and T. L. Olsen. 2021. *Production and operations analytics*. 8th ed. Long Grove, IL: Waveland Press.

NAM (National Academy of Medicine). 2022. *Crisis standards of care for the COVID-19 pandemic*. https://nam.edu/112920-crisis-standards-of-care-resources/ (accessed January 20, 2022).

NASEM (National Academies of Science, Engineering, and Medicine). 2021a. *Ensuring an effective public health emergency medical countermeasures enterprise*. Washington, DC: The National Academies Press.

NASEM. 2021b. *Innovations in pharmaceutical manufacturing on the horizon: Technical challenges, regulatory issues, and recommendations*. Washington, DC: The National Academies Press.

Parrish, M. 2018. Product focus: Single-use technologies. Pharma Manufacturing. https://www.pharmamanufacturing.com/articles/2018/product-focus-single-use-technologies (accessed November 2, 2021).

Quinn, M. 2020. What you need to know about the strategic national stockpile. *CBS*, April 7. https://www.cbsnews.com/news/q-a-with-greg-burel-former-director-of-the-strategic-national-stockpile/ (accessed October 14, 2021).

Reese, U., and C. Chance. 2021. Pricing and reimbursement laws and regulations: Germany. In *Global Legal Insights (GLI): Pricing and Reimbursement 2021*. 4th ed., edited by G. Castle. London, UK: Covington & Burling LLP. https://www.globallegalinsights.com/practice-areas/pricing-and-reimbursement-laws-and-regulations/germany (accessed January 11, 2022).

Reinhard, B., and E. Brown. 2020. Face masks in national stockpile have not been substantially replenished since 2009. *The Washington Post*, March 10. https://www.washingtonpost.com/investigations/face-masks-in-national-stockpile-have-not-been-substantially-replenished-since-2009/2020/03/10/57e57316-60c9-11ea-8baf-519cedb6ccd9_story.html (accessed November 3, 2021).

Riley, S. 2016. Modular manufacturing. Pharmaceutical Processing World. https://www.pharmaceuticalprocessingworld.com/modular-manufacturing (accessed November 2, 2021).

Rule, T. 2020. Toward a more strategic national stockpile. *Europe PMC, SSRN*. doi: 10.2139/ssrn.3662799.

Scott, R. E. 2020. Defense Production Act urgently needed for critical medical gear. *The Hill*, March 26. https://thehill.com/opinion/healthcare/489430-defense-production-act-urgently-needed-for-critical-medical-gear#:~:text=to%20use%20the%20Defense%20Production%20Act%20%28DPA%29%20to,of%20medical%20supplies%20is%20a%20job%20for%20governors (accessed December 8, 2021).

Siemens. 2021. Continuous manufacturing. https://new.siemens.com/global/en/markets/pharma-industry/continuous-manufacturing.html (accessed November 2, 2021).

Song, H. U. A., and Y.-F. Song. 2009. Impact of inventory management flexibility on service flexibility and performance: Evidence from mainland Chinese firms. *Transportation Journal* 48(3):7-19.

Sumrit, D. 2020. Supplier selection for vendor-managed inventory in healthcare using fuzzy multi-criteria decision-making approach. *Decision Science Letters* 9(2):233-256.

Van Mieghem, J. A. 2007. Risk mitigation in newsvendor networks: Resource diversification, flexibility, sharing, and hedging. *Management Science* 53(8):1269-1288.

Vazquez, M. 2020. Trump invokes Defense Production Act for ventilator equipment and N95 masks. *CNN*, April 2. https://www.cnn.com/2020/04/02/politics/defense-production-act-ventilator-supplies/index.html (accessed December 8, 2021).

9

Response Measures for Resilient Medical Product Supply Chains

In a sense, response measures are options of last resort, as they depend on various awareness, mitigation, and preparedness measures and include actions taken postevent to minimize harm from the shortage. However, steps can also be taken before an event to facilitate a more effective response after it occurs. Various institutional measures can be implemented to cultivate a general awareness of emergency preparedness actions, enable the right people to talk to one another in a productive manner, provide resources for adapting to medical product shortages, and facilitate steps for reducing harm to people from the shortages while they persist.

As described in Chapter 5 and in the medical product supply chains resilience framework (reproduced in Figure 9-1), response measures include (1) reducing the demand or increasing the supply, and (2) prophylaxis measures, which protect human health while the shortage persists. While international cooperation and coordinated response can help minimize the effect of medical product shortages globally, response measures by front-line clinicians and other medical product end users are essential when mitigation and preparedness measures fail to protect patients from supply chain failures. To address these, this chapter focuses on both the global level, by addressing issues raised by international production of medical products, and the local level, by addressing last-mile issues in medical product delivery. As discussed in Chapter 3, the globalization of the U.S. medical product supply chains brings substantial benefits to American consumers and producers in the form of lower costs, greater access to a diversity of medical products, increased efficiencies, and more innovation. However, the globalization of medical product supply chains also comes with costs and risks, particularly during emergency conditions. These were cast into sharp relief during the coronavirus disease (COVID-19) pandemic, when access to products that are predominantly manufactured abroad was disrupted. The committee concluded in Chapter 3 that *market forces create powerful incentives for medical product supply chains to remain globalized. These global supply chains provide efficiency, innovation, and, in some cases, diversification benefits. However, such global supply chains also pose transparency and coordination challenges. International cooperation can help address these challenges, strengthen the resilience of medical product supply chains, and minimize the effect of shortages. To achieve this, nations and manufacturers must be better equipped to understand and manage the challenges of global medical product supply chains, including issues related to transparency, regulatory authorities, and national security.*

Having the ability to implement response measures and adapt to a current disaster situation or shortage until supply chains have returned to normal is critical to protecting public health and human life. Indeed, it is common for the most difficult and complex part of supply chains to exist in the final delivery and distribution of medical products to end users, so it is logical that disruptions to medical product supply chains often arise in, or are worsened by, problems in the last mile of distribution. This is especially problematic during chaotic emergency situations, such as that experienced during the recent pandemic. Therefore, to protect public health it is vital to be ready to manage this final stage properly in an emergency.

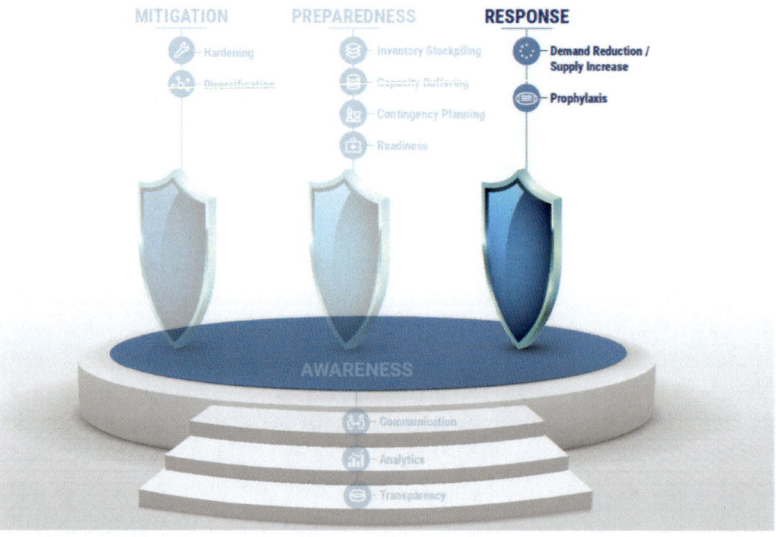

FIGURE 9-1 Medical product supply chains resilience framework: potential response measures.

RESPONSE MEASURES FOR GLOBAL MEDICAL PRODUCT SUPPLY CHAINS

In response to the COVID-19 pandemic, several countries, including the United States, implemented measures that restricted exports of certain medical products, including personal protection equipment (PPE) such as face masks and shields, pharmaceuticals, and medical equipment, such as ventilators. According to a 2020 World Trade Organization (WTO) report, by May 2020, 85 countries and separate customs territories had introduced pandemic-related trade restrictions, such as export bans (WTO, 2020). Roughly half of these measures did not include a specific duration for the trade restriction. While many of the restrictions have since been lifted, as of August 2021, more than 45 countries still have over 70 export restrictions in place, many of which apply to medical products (CRS, 2021). Domestically, U.S. agencies (e.g., U.S. Department of Health and Human Services [HHS], Federal Emergency Management Agency [FEMA]) began using the Defense Production Act (DPA) to place priority ratings on medical supply contracts for agency orders to receive preference over others. Use of the DPA also provided medical supply manufacturers with incentives to expand domestic production of medical supplies to reduce the United States' dependence on foreign sources of supply (GAO, 2020).

WTO rules generally ban export prohibitions and restrictions (WTO, 1994a). However, there are exceptions that allow WTO members to temporarily impose measures "to prevent or relieve critical shortages" of essential products, such as food and medical products, or to protect human, animal, or plant life or health (WTO, 1994a, Article XI). These exceptions give member countries the flexibility to impose trade restrictions in response to health emergencies or national security threats (WTO, 1994a, Articles XI, XX).

In a joint statement, WTO and the International Monetary Fund raised concerns about the use of export restrictions on food and medical products in response to the COVID-19 pandemic:

> Taken collectively, export restrictions can be dangerously counterproductive. What makes sense in an isolated emergency can be severely damaging in a global crisis. Such measures disrupt supply chains, depress production, and misdirect scarce, critical products and workers away from where they are most needed. Other governments counter with their own restrictions. The result is to prolong and exacerbate the health and economic crisis — with the most serious effects likely on the poorer and more vulnerable countries (IMF and WTO, 2020).

The committee concludes that *export restrictions may temporarily increase the availability of domestic supplies, but there are short- and long-term costs associated with such measures. Such measures disrupt supply chains, depress production, and misdirect scarce, critical products and workers away from where they are most needed.*

For example, in the European Union (EU), export bans on PPE coupled with demand surges early on in the pandemic led to shortages in non-EU countries in February and March 2020, resulting in hampered effective medical care in these countries (Bown, 2020; Keynes, 2020). Export bans can also have a long-term effect on global supply chains. For example, in response to the 2007-2008 global food crisis, temporary export bans and other trade restrictions implemented by major rice exporters contributed to record high global rice prices, which exacerbated hoarding, panic buying, food riots, and a breakdown of food supply chains (FAO, 2020).

The Need for International Cooperation

International cooperation can help minimize the effect of medical product shortages and strengthen supply chain resilience. The 1994 Agreement on Trade in Pharmaceutical Products (known as the Pharmaceutical Agreement) eliminates tariffs and other duties and charges on a number of pharmaceutical products and the substances used to produce them, permanently binding them at duty-free levels (WTO, 1994b). Canada, the EU, Japan, Norway, China, Switzerland, the United Kingdom, and the United States currently participate in this agreement (Hallak, 2020). Emerging markets, including Brazil, China, India, and Mexico, have increased imports along with their purchasing power (Donoghoe et al., 2012; Mariadoss, 2018). These countries have benefited from zero duties when importing from signatories of the Pharmaceutical Agreement. While this agreement has helped enable the growth of international trade in pharmaceutical products (European Commission, 2020a; Sunesen et al., 2016), additional cooperation is needed to curb export prohibitions or restrictions on medical products during public health crises.

Proposals to restrict export prohibitions and restrictions have been discussed among like-minded countries. In response to the ongoing trade response to the COVID-19 pandemic, a group of WTO members (Australia, Brazil, Canada, Chile, the EU, Japan, Kenya, South Korea, Mexico, New Zealand, Norway, Singapore, and Switzerland) called for restraint on the use of export restrictions, implementation of trade-facilitating measures, and improved transparency (European Commission, 2020b). This proposal was circulated among WTO members for consideration in May 2021 as a draft declaration, "COVID-19 and Beyond: Trade and Health" (WTO, 2021). In June 2021, the EU submitted a WTO proposal for a multilateral trade response to the COVID-19 pandemic. Among other commitments, the proposal called on WTO members to "subscribe to the G20 commitment to ensure that any export restrictive measures relating to health products are targeted, transparent, proportionate, and temporary, and consistent with WTO obligations" (European Union, 2021).

Industry trade associations and trade policy experts have voiced their support for such proposals. On the industry side there is the Association for Accessible Medicines (AAM), a trade association representing manufacturers and distributors of generic pharmaceutical products; it has called for an international pharmaceutical supply chain agreement:

> To promote the benefits of a globally diverse supply chain, the United States Trade Representative, working with the U.S. Department of Health and Human Services (HHS), should negotiate a plurilateral[1] agreement with U.S. allies to promote a cooperative approach to securing the U.S. supply chain, ensuring diversity of supply and responding to global health care challenges and natural disasters, without resorting to export controls or other trade barriers. In addition, coordinating the expansion of pharmaceutical manufacturing with U.S. allies will allow for economies of scale and a coordinated approach to global pandemics. Possible signatories would include U.S. allies such as Canada, Europe, India, Israel, Japan, Jordan, and Mexico. (AAM, 2020)

Trade experts have argued for proactive international cooperation to boost global surge capacity for PPE, encourage supply chain transparency, and prevent knee-jerk export restrictions in response to public health emergencies (Bown, 2021).

As discussed in Chapter 6, publicly available medical product supply chain data would enable stakeholders to proactively detect and respond to supply chain disruptions, improve coordination on a national and global level, and enhance situational awareness. Furthermore, previous National Academies' work acknowledges how information sharing among regulatory authorities is critical to ensure that patients and health care providers receive quality-assured, safe, and effective medical products (see Box 9-1) (IOM, 2013).

The health and well-being of the U.S. population is inextricably linked to the health and well-being of populations in other countries around the world. Public health crises, such as the current COVID-19 pandemic, are not restricted by country borders. As described in previous chapters, market forces, stockpiling, and on-shoring may resolve some barriers, but they are not a one-size-fits-all solution. For example, short-term medical product shortages may be managed through stockpiling, but this may not address the need for longer-term production capacity (Finkenstadt et al., 2020). Shifting

---

[1] WTO member countries are given the choice to agree to new rules in a plurilateral agreement on a voluntary basis (WTO, n.d.).

BOX 9-1
Summary of Recommendations from *Regulating Medicines in a Globalized World*

Recommendation 1: Leveraging key opportunities to overcome medicines regulatory challenges. All regulatory authorities and other key stakeholders (industry, patient advocates, consumer groups, etc.) should demonstrate support for formal and informal information sharing regarding medicines and medical technology.

Recommendation 2: Improving public health through better designed mutual recognition agreements (MRAs). Policy makers, including lawmakers, should explore empowering regulators to expand the scope and substance of future MRAs that address issues related to the safety, efficacy, and manufacturing quality of medicines, and to ensure that these MRAs are designed, developed, and implemented primarily by medicines regulators.

Recommendation 3: Responding to evolving science and technology. Increasing the current scope of both formal and less formal regulatory reliance arrangements, including MRAs, and that policy makers encourage regulatory authorities to explore formal and informal opportunities for reliance arrangements with other trusted regulatory authorities that give regulators greater flexibility in responding to challenges that affect their responsibility in overseeing the quality, safety, and efficacy of medicines throughout the medicines' life cycle.

Recommendation 4: Better utilization of the European Union-United States (EU-US) MRA. Regulatory authorities in the United States and the EU should immediately implement provisions included in the current EU-US MRA. Regulatory authorities also should begin considering the potential for expanding the EU-US MRA to include reliance in areas beyond good manufacturing practice (GMP) and a broader scope of products under the current GMP provisions.

Recommendation 5: Facilitating information sharing among international medicines regulators. Regulatory authorities should determine whether current limitations on sharing regulatory work products with other regulatory authorities are still fit-for-purpose to help protect and promote public health; reduce the burden of regulatory redundancy on patients, industry, and regulators; allow regulators globally to best utilize the limited technical and financial resources currently available to them to meet their public health mandates; and to bring needed quality medicines to patients domestically and globally as efficiently as possible.

Recommendation 6: Evaluating public health impacts of recognition and reliance arrangements for medicines. Regulatory authorities involved in formal and informal recognition and reliance arrangements should co-create a results framework with clear indicators/metrics and processes for monitoring and measuring the arrangements' results and impacts to enhance understanding of their public health and other benefits and associated regulatory efficiencies, and enable benefit/risk and cost/benefit analysis of the arrangements over time.

SOURCE: NASEM, 2020b.

toward more domestic manufacturing capabilities may offer some relief for aspects of medical product supply chain vulnerabilities, but would likely be insufficient to meet the demand if and when the next pandemic arises. Furthermore, it would be unrealistic for the United States to shift to a fully self-reliant domestic medical product supply chain given the significant time, cost, and complexity of drug and device inputs and manufacturing. For these reasons, international cooperation to faciliate global trade in medical products remains essential for maintaining the health and security of the United States.

Establishing an International Trade Agreement

To address the need for international cooperation, inside and outside of public health crises, there should be agreement among the major exporters of medical products to refrain from export bans or other interventions that would fragment or limit the global supply response, and to cooperate to avoid excessive concentration of key products or components in a single location or from a single producer. Such an agreement would also serve to strengthen supply chain resilience in the absence of a public health emergency by facilitating the manufacturing and distribution of lifesaving drugs and devices.

To ensure cooperation, this agreement would have to be binding and should include reputational and legal sanctions. Any country that violates the terms of the agreement would be subject to sanctions by other signatories of the agreement. Providing incentives for countries to uphold commitments and cooperate in the event of another public health crisis and disincentives for violating the terms of the agreement would help ensure that the treaty is self-enforcing.

Chapter 6 highlights the benefits of information sharing in supply chain management and provides recommendations for U.S. government actions to collect and publicly share data. Given the globalization of U.S. medical supply chains, information sharing across international borders will also be essential for stakeholders—including government and the private sector—to mount effective response measures to future supply chain disruptions. Therefore, in addition to constraining export bans in the face of global health emergencies, negotiators of this treaty could consider adding provisions to facilitate the sharing of relevant information regarding global supply chains, such as information on demand, inventory, capacity, and supply.

Trade policy experts have suggested that another important component of effective international policy coordination is a mechanism to enable U.S. investment in the production capacity of suppliers located abroad (Bown and Bollyky, 2021). While the DPA enabled the United States to invest in nation-wide coordinated expansion of medical product production capicity during the COVID-19 pandemic (GAO, 2020), similar investments in global manufacturing in response to future public health emergencies would benefit the United States as well as other countries. Such a concept merits further exploration and could be considered as an added provision within an international trade agreement.

It is important to recognize that multilateral trade agreements are complex, difficult to negotiate, and often take years to implement (Moser and Rose, 2012). Recent analysis finds that negotiations of trade agreements may take additional time when the United States, the EU, or Japan is a signatory (Arroyo and Castillo-Ponce, 2019; Moser and Rose, 2012). Additionally, the effect of the COVID-19 pandemic on international trade as described above coupled with the recent rise in nationalist economic policies on the part of advanced and emerging-market economies may make it more challenging for countries to pursue multilateral agreements, which depend on global cooperation.

Given the duration and considerable negotiations required to establish multilateral agreements within WTO, one approach for advancing this concept could be for a subset of WTO members comprising the major exporters of medical products—United States, EU, China, and India—to negotiate a plurilateral agreement (Statista Research Department, 2016). For example, the Information Technology Agreement, which eliminated tariffs on information technology products covered by the agreement, was first negotiated in 1996 and included 29 participants. As of October 2021 there were 82 participants in the Information Technology Agreement, and in December 2015, over 50 members expanded the agreement to cover an additional 201 products (WTO, n.d.).

The U.S. government must take on the task of better managing and reducing these risks, while maximizing the benefits of globalization. Recommendation 6 (international treaty) advocates a plurilateral agreement by major exporters of medical products, including the United States, under the WTO that prohibits export bans on components of critical medical products. Although such an agreement cannot prevent a worldwide shortage from occurring, it can limit the risk to any individual country by "spreading the pain" across the global economy. Furthermore, if such an agreement increases the collective trust in global supply chains during an emergency, then that can be used to strengthen Recommendation 5 (Capacity Buffering). It is almost certainly more cost-efficient to build virtual capacity globally than locally. Hence, using the treaty as the basis for collaboration, major medical product exporting countries could further cooperate on providing capacity buffering for medical products likely to be in short supply during global emergencies.

RESPONSE MEASURES FOR LAST-MILE DELIVERY AND END USERS

At a global level, supply chains focus on matching total supply to total demand. The awareness, mitigation, and preparedness recommendations of this report are predominantly aimed at enabling medical product supply chains to accomplish this in normal and emergency conditions. At the local level—often termed the "last mile"—supply chains focus on getting products to the individuals who need them. As the COVID-19 pandemic highlighted, supply shortages, whether the result of global disruptions or local imbalances such as hoarding or misallocation, present enormous challenges to end users, including public health workers, health care providers, and pharmacists. In the chaos of a crisis, these key personnel may not know what supplies exist or when they are coming. They may lack clear guidelines on how to allocate limited supplies to those who need them most. And, they may be unaware of best practices for protecting health in the face of medical supply shortages.

As described in Chapter 5, response measures can either close the gap between supply and demand or protect people from harm due to the gap (i.e., via prophylaxis measures). Both of these can be addressed by those managing the last mile of medical product supply chains. For example, an effective response by hospitals and clinics across the United States to reduce the serious shortage of N95 masks was to reuse masks with multiple patients (CDC, 2021; Chaudhuri, 2020; Hufford, 2020). Although reuse entailed some risk, it allowed the American health care system to function while dramatically reducing the required number of N95 masks. This provided a large and necessary "cushion" while global supply chains struggled to increase production. As this example illustrates, end users of medical supplies such as hospitals, clinicians, pharmacies, and patients have important roles to play in addressing disruptions to medical product supply chains. Although workarounds like this do not solve the larger supply shortage, they can alleviate the impact of shortages and provide much needed time for supply chains to catch up.

Protecting patient health through careful management of the last mile so that much needed medical products reach those who most need them, the end users need information, evidence-based best practices, and training. This section discusses ways to provide these types of last-mile support through resource sharing, development of a national framework for scarce medical product allocation, and the engagement of end users in planning and training for medical product shortages.

Mechanisms to Increase the Sharing of Critical Supplies

Resource sharing is a fundamental way to ensure that limited medical supplies go to those who need them most. This involves transferring supplies from one locality, state, or region to another. A key prerequisite for resource sharing is the transparency of critical supply availability across organizations (Devereaux et al., 2020).

Other key elements of a resource sharing system are mechanisms that facilitate (or require) the transfer of supplies and other resources when necessary. These can be established through the collaboration of local, state, and federal public health officials and clinicians, as well as public–private partnerships. For example, during the COVID-19 pandemic, regions developed innovative systems such as transfer centers to ensure patients and supplies were optimally matched (NRCC Healthcare Resilience Task Force and FEMA, 2020; Valin et al., 2020), but these systems typically required a voluntary willingness to share information with competitors about the presence or absence of critical supplies. Early in the COVID-19 pandemic such voluntary cooperation was relatively common, but in many less dire supply shortages it is not.

Recent experience suggests that regional and national multidisciplinary teams that proactively plan ahead for alternatives and prepare recommendations for substitution or conservation strategies prior to supplies becoming exhausted are more robust than single-center efforts (Devereaux et al., 2020; Tosh and Burry, 2020). When each facility creates its own strategies for responding to shortages, and when shortages are unevenly distributed among facilities, there is a significant risk of inequitable effects. For instance, in the last few decades, health care coalitions (HCCs) have become core components of regional emergency and disaster response, facilitating transparency about resource shortages and the sharing of scarce resources (Barnett et al., 2020). Additionally, some well-formed and well-organized HCCs play fundamental roles in the health of their communities during nonemergency times. HCCs like this could also play a role in developing standardized plans for responding to routine medical product shortages, including strategies for moving resources to where they are most needed, to help balance the disparate effects of shortages on different facilities. Indeed, HHS's Office of the Assistant Secretary for Preparedness and Response (ASPR) has already created several regional disaster response coalitions, which provide important opportunities to explore the possibility of sharing disaster response capabilities across multiple states (ASPR, 2018). Regional and national dashboards that include drug quantities available could provide valuable information when drug shortages arise and can facilitate moving drugs to areas of greatest need (Tosh and Burry, 2020).

A National Framework for Scarce Medical Product Allocation

Local resource sharing can work if the end users know and trust one another, but sharing resources on a larger scale, where personal relationships cannot be relied on, is extremely challenging. Even deciding who is most deserving of a scarce medical product presents a difficult question. Clinical need, age, equity, and a wide range of other factors can enter into this question. The COVID-19 pandemic highlighted an alarming number of inequities and challenges in the resource allocation process.

The allocation problem is well known to clinicians and has been the subject of a great deal of work at the National Academies of Science, Engineering, and Medicine (the National Academies) (NASEM, 2020a, 2021). However, even with this body of research, health care and public health officials were left without clear guidance on the best frameworks to use when allocating scarce medical products, resulting in inconsistent, and at times inequitable, use between and within states and within health care systems. For example, some implemented the Centers for Disease Control and Prevention's recommended Social Vulnerability Index and Area Deprivation Index frameworks (Ndugga et al., 2021; Schmidt et al., 2021) while others used different approaches for allocating medial products like the Fair Priority Model (Emanuel et al., 2020), all without a clear consensus on whether one worked better or more effectively than the other. It may also be that different frameworks are needed for different medical products.

Given the variety of frameworks to choose from and the lack of guidance around which one to use and when, it is clear that a standard ethical framework for scarce medical product allocation is needed at the national level if outcomes like those seen during COVID-19 are to be avoided. Such a framework must be designed in a way that is acceptable to all major actors—distributors, producers, end users—without undue burden placed on any one entity, and it must be flexible enough to provide guidance for decision making and deliberation within and across health sectors, health institutions, and health professionals in response to medical product shortages (Gibson et al., 2012). It must reconcile the actors' competing values and be accepted as ethical, not just seen as an assertion of power (Emanuel et al., 2020). In an ideal setting, use of this common ethical framework for scarce medical product allocation would have a cascading effect: producing less product waste would increase producer confidence that medical products will be fairly allocated to benefit people, which would in turn motivate an increase in production for continued distribution (Emanuel et al., 2020).

Furthermore, because of the vital role local health care professionals play in enabling the efficient delivery of medical products to the end user, it is essential that they be involved in the development of allocation frameworks. They can offer perspectives on how the framework would or would not be useful based on their clinical experiences (Gibson et al., 2012). Although training for disaster response preparedness is common for health care professionals, it is less common for it to include instruction regarding their potential roles in addressing population health concerns, such as health disparities, health inequities, and hesitancy receiving medical treatment (Aruru et al., 2021; Ducatman et al., 2020; Jacobsen et al., 2020; Johnson et al., 2020; Thibault, 2020). These elements should be included in trainings to address inequitable resource distribution during supply shortages so medical professionals can more effectively treat and advocate for their patients.

Engaging End Users in Last-Mile Planning

There is a close relationship between the virtual preparedness measures (Chapter 8) and response measures. Contingency planning and readiness activities taken prior to a disruptive event can improve the speed and accuracy of response activities. For instance, a contingency plan that identifies supplemental producers for specific supply chain critical medical products and readiness steps, such as sharing supplier and bill-of-material information with these producers, would make ramping up capacity in an emergency faster and more reliable.

Yet beyond a narrow role in devising a framework for scarce medical product allocation, end users must be involved more broadly in planning for medical product shortages. The reason for this is that, in order to respond more effectively to the next public health crisis, end users need a number of institutional capabilities, particularly those related to managing medical product shortages. These include clearly defined roles, standardized crisis standards and contingency operations, better communication channels, standards of practice that provide documentation of such things, and training of medical personnel to equip them to act more effectively when they are without the standard level of routine supplies. An end-user perspective is absolutely vital to develop guidelines and tools for building these capabilities.

An essential element of last-mile planning is clearly articulating who has authority and responsibility for coordinating health care systems and suppliers, particularly during an emergency or crisis situation. As discussed in Chapter 8, the National Academies has explored and developed systems for ethically addressing circumstances where usual care is unattainable due to resource shortages and crisis standards of care (CSC) are required (IOM, 2009), including resources and tools for implementing and executing CSC. A group, or appropriate set of teams, needs to have command and control responsibility for the last-mile response system when there is a medical product shortage and resource allocation is unbalanced. The recent development of ASPR-funded regional disaster response systems serving multiple states in geographic proximity presents opportunities for the exploration of systems to improve cross-state sharing of information on supply levels and resources (ASPR, 2021). This could help alleviate implicit rationing and hoarding of medical products during a crisis. Additional resources on CSC can be found in Chapter 8 in Box 8-4.

Building the institutional capabilities to support last-mile, contingency, and crisis planning will require extensive training. Because of their knowledge of both the institutions and the challenges of managing the last mile, health care professionals must be involved in the development and execution of training to prepare for medical product shortages. Although such resources are limited at present, there is an emerging trend in health professional education toward teaching students and trainees about the importance of medical ethics during emergency situations, including medical product shortages (Aruru et al., 2021; Ducatman et al., 2020; Jacobsen et al., 2020; Johnson et al., 2020; Thibault, 2020). This trend should be encouraged and could be used to improve workforce readiness and coordination to address supply shortages and problems of inequitable resource distribution.

Practicing clinicians and the leaders of health care delivery organizations can and should be encouraged to participate in planning for disruptions of medical product supply chains. This can be achieved in part by recognizing that supply chain disruptions, unlike pandemics and most other public health emergencies, are remarkably common. In fact, many health systems operate in a state of chronic contingency, with various supplies routinely being conserved, reused, and repurposed due to persistent shortages of critical resources (NASEM, 2018). However, these chronic contingency situations can provide health systems with opportunities to practice using CSC frameworks during less severe shortages and at much lower risk and cost to their operations and patient lives. As such, there is an ongoing need to establish platforms to facilitate communication during disruptions and platforms for sharing best practices among clinical end users facing supply shortages.

RECOMMENDATIONS

A critical component of supply chain resilience is the ability to recover from disruptions quickly and effectively. While disruptions at the global and end-user levels appear disparate and can be complex to manage, the key to the solution for both sets of problems is effective communication and cooperation. The specific and actionable recommendations listed below are intended to help stakeholders better manage and reduce the risks associated with the globalization of medical product supply chains and disruptions at the last mile of delivery. Recommendation 6 (International Treaty) does this at the global level by promoting open communication and cooperative efforts by medical exporting nations. Recommendation 7 (Last-Mile Management) does this at the local level by establishing a working group to detail and develop the tools needed by medical professionals to manage medical product shortages.

Recommendation 6 (International Treaty). Major exporters of medical products, including the United States, should negotiate a plurilateral

treaty under the World Trade Organization that prohibits export bans and restrictions on key components of global medical product supply chains. Any country that violates the terms of this agreement should be subject to sanctions by other signatories of the agreement. Specifically,

    a. The treaty should provide incentives for countries to uphold commitments and cooperate in the event of a public health crisis.

    b. The treaty should provide disincentives or sanctions, such as reputational, economic, and legal sanctions, for violating the terms of the agreement.

    c. Treaty negotiators could consider adding provisions to this treaty that facilitate information sharing, particularly during medical emergencies.

Recommendation 7 (Last-Mile Management). The Office of the Assistant Secretary for Preparedness and Response, in collaboration with the Centers for Disease Control and Prevention, should convene a working group of key stakeholders to examine and identify effective last-mile strategies to ensure end users are able to respond in the event of medical product shortages. The working group should

    a. Determine what information needs to be shared, with whom and in what form, in order for end users to be able to execute resource sharing, supply redistribution, substitution, adaptation, and other strategies for responding to medical product shortages at the local level.

    b. Develop a standard national ethical framework for allocating scarce medical products, building in previous crisis standards of care work, including attention to equity, efficiency, and additional ethical values.

    c. Develop and incorporate response plans and training for medical product shortages into public health and health care professional capabilities.

REFERENCES

AAM (Association for Accessible Medicines). 2020. *A blueprint for enhancing the security of the U.S. pharmaceutical supply chain* (2nd edition). https://accessiblemeds.org/sites/default/files/2020-04/AAM-Blueprint-US-Pharma-Supply-Chain.pdf (accessed October 20, 2021).

Arroyo, L., and R. A. Castillo-Ponce. 2019. The duration of trade agreement negotiations. *Applied Econometrics and International Development* 19(2):19-36.

Aruru, M., H.-A. Truong, and S. Clark. 2021. Pharmacy emergency preparedness and response (PEPR): A proposed framework for expanding pharmacy professionals' roles and contributions to emergency preparedness and response during the COVID-19 pandemic and beyond. *Research in Social and Administrative Pharmacy* 17(1):1967-1977.

ASPR (Assistant Secretary for Preparedness and Response). 2018. *HHS selects pilot projects to demonstrate better approach to disaster medical care.* HHS (U.S. Department of Health and Human Services). https://public3.pagefreezer.com/browse/HHS.gov/31-12-2020T08:51/https://www.hhs.gov/about/news/2018/09/27/hhs-selects-pilot-projects-demonstrate-better-approach-disaster-medical-care.html (accessed October 21, 2021).

ASPR. 2021. *Partnership for disaster health response cooperative agreement.* HHS. https://www.phe.gov/Preparedness/planning/PDHRCA-FOA/Pages/default.aspx (accessed February 17, 2021).

Barnett, D. J., L. Knieser, N. A. Errett, A. J. Rosenblum, M. Seshamani, and T. D. Kirsch. 2020. Reexamining health-care coalitions in light of COVID-19. *Disaster Medicine and Public Health Preparedness* 1-5.

Bown, C. 2020. E.U. limits on medical gear exports put poor countries and Europeans at risk. In *Trade and investment policy watch.* Peterson Institute for International Economics. https://www.piie.com/blogs/trade-and-investment-policy-watch/eu-limits-medical-gear-exports-put-poor-countries-and (accessed December 20, 2021).

Bown, C., and T. Bollyky. 2021. The world needs a COVID-19 vaccine investment and trade agreement. In *Trade and investment policy watch.* Peterson Institute for International Economics. https://www.piie.com/blogs/trade-and-investment-policy-watch/world-needs-covid-19-vaccine-investment-and-trade-agreement (accessed November 10, 2021).

Bown, C. P. 2021. How COVID 19 medical supply shortages led to extraordinary trade and industrial policy. *Asian Economic Policy Review* 17:114-135. https://doi.org/10.1111/aepr.12359.

CDC (Centers for Disease Control and Prevention). 2021. *Strategies for optimizing the supply of N95 respirators.* https://www.cdc.gov/coronavirus/2019-ncov/hcp/respirators-strategy/index.html (accessed October 26, 2021).

Chaudhuri, S. 2020. Coronavirus prompts hospitals to find ways to reuse masks amid shortage. *The Wall Street Journal*, March 31.

CRS (Congressional Research Service). 2021. *Export restrictions in response to the COVID-19 pandemic.* CRS. https://sgp.fas.org/crs/natsec/IF11551.pdf (accessed December 20, 2021).

Devereaux, A., H. Yang, G. Seda, V. Sankar, R. C. Maves, N. Karanjia, J. S. Parrish, C. Rosenberg, P. Goodman-Crews, L. Cederquist, F. M. Burkle, J. Tuteur, C. Leroy, and K. L. Koenig. 2020. Optimizing scarce resource allocation during COVID-19: Rapid creation of a regional health-care coalition and triage teams in San Diego County, California. *Disaster Medicine and Public Health Preparedness* 1-7.

Donoghoe, N., A. Gupta, R. Linden, P. Mitra, and I. Beyer von Morgenstern. 2012. Medical device growth in emerging markets: Lessons from other industries. *In Vivo: The Business and Medicine Report,* June 2012.

Ducatman, B. S., A. M. Ducatman, J. M. Crawford, M. Laposata, and F. Sanfilippo. 2020. The value proposition for pathologists: A population health approach. *Academic Pathology* 7:2374289519898857.

Emanuel, E. J., G. Persad, A. Kern, A. Buchanan, C. Fabre, D. Halliday, J. Heath, L. Herzog, R. J. Leland, E. T. Lemango, F. Luna, M. S. McCoy, O. F. Norheim, T. Ottersen, G. O. Schaefer, K. C. Tan, C. H. Wellman, J. Wolff, and H. S. Richardson. 2020. An ethical framework for global vaccine allocation. *Science* 369(6509):1309-1312.

European Commission. 2020a. *Communication from the European Commission to the European Parliament, the Council, the European Economic and Social Committee and the Committee of the Regions: Pharmaceutical strategy for Europe.* Brussels: European Commission. https://eur-lex.europa.eu/legal-content/EN/TXT/?uri=CELEX:52020DC0761 (accessed December 20, 2021).

European Commission. 2020b. *Ottawa group proposes a global trade and health initiative.* Brussels. https://trade.ec.europa.eu/doclib/press/index.cfm?id=2215 (accessed December 20, 2021).

European Union. 2021. *Communication from the European Union to the WTO general council: Urgent trade policy responses to the COVID-19 crisis.* Brussels. https://trade.ec.europa.eu/doclib/docs/2021/june/tradoc_159605.pdf (accessed December 20, 2021).

Finkenstadt, D., R. Handfield, and P. Guinto. 2020. Why the U.S. still has a severe shortage of medical supplies. *Harvard Business Review, September–October 2020*, September 17,.

FAO (Food and Agriculture Organization of the United Nations). 2020. *Why export restrictions should not be a response to COVID-19: Learning lessons from experience with rice in Asia and the Pacific.* https://www.fao.org/3/ca9362en/CA9362EN.pdf (accessed October 20, 2021).

GAO (Government Accountability Office). 2020. *Defense Production Act: Opportunities exist to increase transparency and identify future actions to mitigate medical supply chain issues.* https://www.gao.gov/assets/gao-21-108.pdf (accessed October 12, 2021).

Gibson, J. L., S. Bean, P. Chidwick, D. Godkin, R. W. Sibbald, and F. Wagner. 2012. Ethical framework for resource allocation during a drug supply shortage. *Healthcare Quarterly (Toronto, ON)* 15(3):26-35.

Hallak, I. 2020. *EU imports and exports of medical equipment.* European Parliamentary Research Service. https://www.europarl.europa.eu/RegData/etudes/BRIE/2020/649387/EPRS_BRI(2020)649387_EN.pdf (accessed December 20, 2021).

Hufford, A. 2020. Why are N95 masks so important? *The Wall Street Journal*, June 1.

IMF and WTO (International Monetary Fund and World Trade Organization). 2020. IMF and WTO heads call for lifting trade restrictions on medical supplies and food: World Trade Organization. https://www.wto.org/english/news_e/news20_e/igo_15apr20_e.htm (accessed December 20, 2021).

IOM (Institute of Medicine). 2009. *Guidance for establishing crisis standards of care for use in disaster situations: A letter report.* Washington, DC: The National Academies Press.

IOM. 2013. *International regulatory harmonization amid globalization of drug development: Workshop summary.* Washington, DC: The National Academies Press.

Jacobsen, K., M. Hay, J. Manske, and C. Waggett. 2020. Curricular models and learning objectives for undergraduate minors in global health. *Annals of Global Health* 86(1):102.

Johnson, S. B., M. A. Fair, L. D. Howley, J. Prunuske, S. B. Cashman, J. K. Carney, Y. S. Jarris, L. R. Deyton, D. Blumenthal, N. K. Krane, N. H. Fiebach, A. H. Strelnick, E. Morton-Eggleston, C. Nickens, and L. Ortega. 2020. Teaching public and population health in medical education: An evaluation framework. *Academic Medicine* 95(12):1853-1863.

Keynes, S. 2020. New trade barriers could hamper the supply of masks and medicines. *The Economist, March 7-13 2020*, March 11.

Mariadoss, B. J. 2018. Chapter 5: Emerging markets. In *Core principles of international marketing*. Vancouver, WA: Washington State University. https://opentext.wsu.edu/cpim/chapter/5-5-emerging-markets (accessed November 8, 2021).

Moser, C. and A. K. Rose. 2012. Why do trade negotiations take so long? *KOF Working Papers 295*. Zurich: KOF Swiss Economic Institute. http://dx.doi.org/10.3929/ethz-a-006844132.

NASEM (National Academies of Sciences, Engineering, and Medicine). 2018. *Medical product shortages during disasters: Opportunities to predict, prevent, and respond: Proceedings of a workshop—in brief.* Washington, DC: The National Academies Press. doi: https://doi.org/10.17226/25267.

NASEM. 2020a. A framework for equitable allocation of COVID-19 vaccine. In *Framework for equitable allocation of COVID-19 vaccine.* Washington, DC: The National Academies Press. Pp. 89-144.

NASEM. 2020b. *Regulating medicines in a globalized world: The need for increased reliance among regulators.* Washington, DC: The National Academies Press. https://doi.org/10.17226/25594.

NASEM. 2021. *Rapid expert consultation on allocating COVID-19 monoclonal antibody therapies and other novel therapeutics (January 29, 2021)*, edited by L. Brown, A. Downey, S. Wollek, C. Shore, E. Fine, and B. Kahn. Washington, DC: The National Academies Press.

Ndugga, N., S. Artiga, and O. Pham. 2021. *How are states addressing racial equity in COVID-19 vaccine efforts?* Kaiser Family Foundation. https://www.kff.org/racial-equity-and-health-policy/issue-brief/how-are-states-addressing-racial-equity-in-covid-19-vaccine-efforts/ (accessed August 27, 2021).

NRCC Healthcare Resilience Task Force, and the Federal Emergency Management Agency (FEMA). 2020. *Medical operations coordination cells toolkit: Department of Homeland Security (DHS)*. https://files.asprtracie.hhs.gov/documents/fema-mocc-toolkit.pdf (accessed October 14, 2021).

Schmidt, H., R. Weintraub, M. A. Williams, K. Miller, A. Buttenheim, E. Sadecki, H. Wu, A. Doiphode, N. Nagpal, L. O. Gostin, and A. A. Shen. 2021. Equitable allocation of COVID-19 vaccines in the United States. *Nature Medicine* 27(7):1298-1307.

Statista Research Department. 2016. *Main medical device exporters worldwide in 2015, by country*, edited by Statista. https://www.statista.com/statistics/619607/medical-device-exporters-worldwide-by-country/ (accessed Novemebr 10, 2021).

Sunesen, E., T. Jeppesen, and M. H. Thelle. 2016. *How a strong pharma chapter in TTIP will benefit the EU*. Copenhagen Economics. https://www.efpia.eu/media/25874/how_a_strong_pharmaceutical_chapter_in_ttip_will_benefit_the_eu_policy_brief.pdf (accessed Novemebr 8, 2021).

Thibault, G. E. 2020. The future of health professions education: Emerging trends in the United States. *Federation of American Societies for Experimental Biology (FASEB) BioAdvances* 2(12):685-694.

Tosh, P. K., and L. Burry. 2020. *Essential institutional supply chain management in the setting of COVID-19 pandemic*. The American College of Chest Physicians (CHEST). https://www.chestnet.org/resources/essential-institutional-supply-chain-management-in-the-setting-of-covid-19-pandemic (accessed October 14, 2021).

Valin, J. P., S. Gulley, B. Keidan, K. Perkins, C. Savor Price, W. Neff, G. Winfield, and D. Tad-y. 2020. Physician executives guide a successful COVID-19 response in Colorado. *New England Journal of Medicine Catalyst Innovations in Care Delivery* 1(5).

WTO (World Trade Organization). 1994a. *General agreement on tariffs and trade 1994*. Geneva, Switzerland: WTO. https://www.wto.org/english/docs_e/legal_e/06-gatt_e.htm (accessed December 8, 2021).

WTO. 1994b. The WTO's pharma agreement. In *Trade topics*. The World Trade Organization. https://www.wto.org/english/tratop_e/pharma_ag_e/pharma_agreement_e.htm (accessed October 20, 2021).

WTO. 2020. *Report on G20 trade measures (mid-October 2019 to mid-May 2020)*. WTO. https://www.wto.org/english/news_e/news20_e/report_trdev_jun20_e.pdf (accessed October 20, 2021).

WTO. 2021. *COVID-19 and beyond: Trade and health*. WTO. https://docs.wto.org/dol2fe/Pages/SS/directdoc.aspx?filename=q:/Jobs/GC/251R1.pdf&Open=True (accessed January, 21, 2022).

WTO. n.d. Information technology agreement. In *Trade topics*. The World Trade Organization. https://www.wto.org/english/tratop_e/inftec_e/inftec_e.htm (accessed October 21, 2021).

Appendix A

Study Methods and Public Agendas

At the request of the U.S. Congress, the National Academies of Sciences, Engineering, and Medicine (the National Academies) convened the Committee on Security of America's Medical Product Supply Chain to examine the security of America's medical product supply chains and provide recommendations to improve the resilience of medical product supply chains. The sponsor of this report was the U.S. Department of Health and Human Services (HHS) Office of the Assistant Secretary for Preparedness and Response (ASPR).

COMMITTEE EXPERTISE

The National Academies formed a committee of 13 experts to deliberate on and respond to the statement of task for the study (Box 1-1). The committee comprised members with expertise in crisis standards of care, emergency and critical care medicine, drug and device development and manufacturing, drug shortages, regulatory policy, health economics, medical logistics, supply chain management, risk and emergency management, operations research, public health preparedness and response, and state and local public health. Appendix E provides biographical information for each committee member.

MEETINGS AND INFORMATION-GATHERING ACTIVITIES

The committee held five virtual full committee meetings from September 2020 to September 2021. The committee held six meetings that included portions open to the public as well as one virtual, public workshop. A summary of this workshop is captured in a Proceedings of a Workshop—In Brief.[1] The agendas for these six open sessions are included at the end of this appendix.

To inform its deliberations, the committee gathered information through a variety of mechanisms including reviews of the literature on medical product supply chains and medical product shortages. Targeted literature reviews were conducted as novel issues arose throughout the committee's deliberations. All written information provided to the committee from external sources is available by request through the National Academies' Public Access Records Office.

Literature Search Strategy

Search Parameters:
- Date Parameters: All
- English only
- Peer-reviewed articles
- Trade publications
- Opinion publications
- Comments
- Editorial
- Reviews
- Proceedings
- Geographic region: International with a subset for the U.S.
- Humans research only

Databases:
- PubMed
- Cogress.gov
- Legistorm

Search Strategy:
Part I: Essential drugs/equipment AND supply chains

Database: PubMed

Date of Search: 09/08/2020

Filters: Humans, English

---

[1] See https://www.nap.edu/catalog/26137/the-security-of-americas-medical-product-supply-chain-considerations-for.

APPENDIX A   241

Results before deduplication:
International: 98
U.S.: 21

#	Query
1	"critical devices"[Title/Abstract] OR "critical drugs"[Title/Abstract] OR "critical medication"[Title/Abstract] OR "critical medicine"[Title/Abstract] OR "priority medical devices"[Title/Abstract]
2	"drugs, essential"[MeSH Terms]
3	"active pharmaceutical ingredient"[Title/Abstract] OR "finished dosage form"[Title/Abstract] OR "health commodities"[Title/Abstract] OR "medical commodities"[Title/Abstract] OR "medical devices"[Title/Abstract] OR "medical products"[Title/Abstract] OR "drug products"[Title/Abstract]
4	#3 AND #2
5	#1 OR #2 OR #4
6	"equipment and supplies/supply and distribution"[MeSH Terms] OR "prescription drugs/supply and distribution"[MeSH Terms]
7	"domestic manufacturing"[Title/Abstract] OR "supply chain"[Title/Abstract] OR "supply chain capacity"[Title/Abstract] OR "supply chain contingency planning"[Title/Abstract] OR "supply chain information gaps"[Title/Abstract] OR "supply chain redundancy"[Title/Abstract] OR "supply chain sustainability"[Title/Abstract] OR "drug industry/organization and administration"[MeSH Terms]
8	"drug shortage"[Title/Abstract] OR "manufacturing disruption"[Title/Abstract] OR "supply chain disruption"[Title/Abstract] OR "supply chain information gaps"[Title/Abstract] OR "supply chain vulnerability"[Title/Abstract]
9	#6 OR #7 OR #8
10	#9 AND #5
11	"economic impact"[Title/Abstract] OR "trade impact"[Title/Abstract] OR "socioeconomic factors"[MeSH Terms]
12	#11 AND #9
13	#12 AND #5
14	"disease outbreaks"[MeSH Terms] OR "epidemics"[MeSH Terms] OR "pandemics"[MeSH Terms] OR "public health"[MeSH Terms] OR "health security"[Title/Abstract] OR "national security"[Title/Abstract]
15	"disaster medicine/organization and administration"[MeSH Terms] OR "disaster planning/organization and administration"[MeSH Terms] OR "disaster planning/trends"[MeSH Terms] OR "emergency medicine/organization and administration"[MeSH Terms] OR "emergency medicine/standards"[MeSH Terms] OR "emergency medicine/trends"[MeSH Terms] OR "risk management/organization and administration"[MeSH Terms]
16	#14 OR #15
17	#16 AND #5

18	("united states"[MeSH Terms] OR "united states"[Title] OR "u.s."[Title] OR "american"[Title] OR "america"[Title] OR "united states"[Title/Abstract] OR "u.s."[Title/Abstract] OR "u.s.a."[Title/Abstract]) NOT ("americas"[Title/Abstract] OR "latin america"[Title/Abstract] OR "south america"[Title/Abstract] OR "central america"[Title/Abstract] OR "latin america"[MeSH Terms] OR "south america"[MeSH Terms] OR "central america"[MeSH Terms])
19	#10 OR #13 OR #17
20	#19 AND #18
21	"ambulatory"[Title] OR "animal model"[Title] OR "biological assay"[Title] OR "blood"[Title] OR "cbrn exposure"[Title] OR "dose-response"[Title] OR "drills"[Title] OR "eye care"[Title] OR "gain of function"[Title] OR "glucose"[Title] OR "licensure"[Title] OR "liver injury"[Title] OR "mass dispensing"[Title] OR "mass vaccination"[Title] OR "meter"[Title] OR "mice"[Title] OR "mouse"[Title] OR "neglected disease"[Title] OR "one health"[Title] OR "pathophysiology"[Title] OR "points of dispensing"[Title] OR "post-exposure"[Title] OR "schools"[Title] OR "transfusion"[Title] OR "veterinary"[Title]
22	#20 NOT #21
23	#10 OR #17
24	#23 NOT #21

Part II: Essential drugs/equipment AND Standards of care

Database: PubMed

Date of Search: 09/08/2020

Filters: Humans, English

Results before deduplication:
  International: 21
  U.S.: 1

#	Query
1	"critical devices"[Title/Abstract] OR "critical drugs"[Title/Abstract] OR "critical medication"[Title/Abstract] OR "critical medicine"[Title/Abstract] OR "priority medical devices"[Title/Abstract]
2	"drugs, essential"[MeSH Terms]
3	"active pharmaceutical ingredient"[Title/Abstract] OR "finished dosage form"[Title/Abstract] OR "health commodities"[Title/Abstract] OR "medical commodities"[Title/Abstract] OR "medical devices"[Title/Abstract] OR "medical products"[Title/Abstract] OR "drug products"[Title/Abstract]

APPENDIX A

4	#3 AND #2
5	#1 OR #2 OR #4
6	("crisis"[Title/Abstract] OR "crises" [Title/Abstract]) AND "standards of care"[Title/Abstract]
7	"critical care"[Title/Abstract] OR "emergency care"[Title/Abstract] OR "emergency management"[Title/Abstract] OR "risk management"[Title/Abstract]
8	"standard of care"[MeSH Terms] OR "delivery of health care/standards"[MeSH Terms]
9	#6 OR #7 OR #8
10	#9 AND #5
11	("united states"[MeSH Terms] OR "united states"[Title] OR "u.s."[Title] OR "american"[Title] OR "america"[Title] OR "united states"[Title/Abstract] OR "u.s."[Title/Abstract] OR "u.s.a."[Title/Abstract]) NOT ("americas"[Title/Abstract] OR "latin america"[Title/Abstract] OR "south america"[Title/Abstract] OR "central america"[Title/Abstract] OR "latin america"[MeSH Terms] OR "south america"[MeSH Terms] OR "central america"[MeSH Terms])
12	#10 AND #11
13	"ambulatory"[Title] OR "animal model"[Title] OR "biological assay"[Title] OR "blood"[Title] OR "cbrn exposure"[Title] OR "dose-response"[Title] OR "drills"[Title] OR "eye care"[Title] OR "gain of function"[Title] OR "glucose"[Title] OR "licensure"[Title] OR "liver injury"[Title] OR "mass dispensing"[Title] OR "mass vaccination"[Title] OR "meter"[Title] OR "mice"[Title] OR "mouse"[Title] OR "neglected disease"[Title] OR "one health"[Title] OR "pathophysiology"[Title] OR "points of dispensing"[Title] OR "post-exposure"[Title] OR "schools"[Title] OR "transfusion"[Title] OR "veterinary"[Title]
14	#12 NOT #13
15	#10 NOT #13

Part III: Essential drugs/equipment AND Accessibility/Equity

Database: PubMed

Date of Search: 09/08/2020

Filters: Humans, English

Results before deduplication:
    International: 716
    U.S.: 72

#	Query
1	"critical devices"[Title/Abstract] OR "critical drugs"[Title/Abstract] OR "critical medication"[Title/Abstract] OR "critical medicine"[Title/Abstract] OR "essential medicines"[Title/Abstract] OR "medical countermeasures"[Title/Abstract] OR "priority medical devices"[Title/Abstract]
2	"drugs, essential"[MeSH Terms]
3	"active pharmaceutical ingredient"[Title/Abstract] OR "finished dosage form"[Title/Abstract] OR "health commodities"[Title/Abstract] OR "medical commodities"[Title/Abstract] OR "medical devices"[Title/Abstract] OR "medical products"[Title/Abstract] OR "drug products"[Title/Abstract]
4	#3 AND #2
5	#1 OR #2 OR #4
6	"access to health care"[Title/Abstract] OR "accessibility"[Title/Abstract] OR "accessibility of health services"[Title/Abstract] OR "distribution"[Title/Abstract] OR "equity"[Title/Abstract] OR "health care delivery"[Title/Abstract]
7	"delivery of health care"[MeSH Terms] OR "health equity"[MeSH Terms] OR "health services accessibility"[MeSH Terms]
8	#6 OR #7
9	#8 AND #5
10	("united states"[MeSH Terms] OR "united states"[Title] OR "u.s."[Title] OR "american"[Title] OR "america"[Title] OR "united states"[Title/Abstract] OR "u.s."[Title/Abstract] OR "u.s.a."[Title/Abstract]) NOT ("americas"[Title/Abstract] OR "latin america"[Title/Abstract] OR "south america"[Title/Abstract] OR "central america"[Title/Abstract] OR "latin america"[MeSH Terms] OR "south america"[MeSH Terms] OR "central america"[MeSH Terms])
11	#9 AND #10
12	"ambulatory"[Title] OR "animal model"[Title] OR "biological assay"[Title] OR "blood"[Title] OR "cbrn exposure"[Title] OR "dose-response"[Title] OR "drills"[Title] OR "eye care"[Title] OR "gain of function"[Title] OR "glucose"[Title] OR "licensure"[Title] OR "liver injury"[Title] OR "mass dispensing"[Title] OR "mass vaccination"[Title] OR "meter"[Title] OR "mice"[Title] OR "mouse"[Title] OR "neglected disease"[Title] OR "one health"[Title] OR "pathophysiology"[Title] OR "points of dispensing"[Title] OR "post-exposure"[Title] OR "schools"[Title] OR "transfusion"[Title] OR "veterinary"[Title]
13	#11 NOT #12
14	#9 NOT #12

APPENDIX A

Part IV: Medical countermeasure/Stockpile AND Supply

Database: PubMed

Date of Search: 09/08/2020

Filters: Humans, English

Results before deduplication:
  International: 19
  U.S.: 18

#	Query
1	"medical countermeasures"[Title/Abstract] OR "stockpile"[Title/Abstract] OR "strategic stockpile"[Title/Abstract]
2	"strategic stockpile"[MeSH Terms] OR "strategic stockpile/organization and administration"[MeSH Terms] OR "strategic stockpile/trends"[MeSH Terms]
3	#1 OR #2
4	"domestic manufacturing"[Title/Abstract] OR "supply chain"[Title/Abstract] OR "supply chain capacity"[Title/Abstract] OR "supply chain contingency planning"[Title/Abstract] OR "supply chain information gaps"[Title/Abstract] OR "supply chain redundancy"[Title/Abstract] OR "supply chain sustainability"[Title/Abstract] OR "drug industry/organization and administration"[MeSH Terms]
5	"equipment and supplies/supply and distribution"[MeSH Terms] OR "prescription drugs/supply and distribution"[MeSH Terms]
6	#4 OR #5
7	#3 AND #6
8	("united states"[MeSH Terms] OR "united states"[Title] OR "u.s."[Title] OR "american"[Title] OR "america"[Title] OR "united states"[Title/Abstract] OR "u.s."[Title/Abstract] OR "u.s.a."[Title/Abstract]) NOT ("americas"[Title/Abstract] OR "latin america"[Title/Abstract] OR "south america"[Title/Abstract] OR "central america"[Title/Abstract] OR "latin america"[MeSH Terms] OR "south america"[MeSH Terms] OR "central america"[MeSH Terms])
9	#7 AND #8
10	"ambulatory"[Title] OR "animal model"[Title] OR "biological assay"[Title] OR "blood"[Title] OR "cbrn exposure"[Title] OR "dose-response"[Title] OR "drills"[Title] OR "eye care"[Title] OR "gain of function"[Title] OR "glucose"[Title] OR "licensure"[Title] OR "liver injury"[Title] OR "mass dispensing"[Title] OR "mass vaccination"[Title] OR "meter"[Title] OR "mice"[Title] OR "mouse"[Title] OR "neglected disease"[Title] OR "one health"[Title] OR "pathophysiology"[Title] OR "points of dispensing"[Title] OR "post-exposure"[Title] OR "schools"[Title] OR "transfusion"[Title] OR "veterinary"[Title]
11	#9 NOT #10
12	#7 NOT #10

Part IV: Legislation from the U.S. Congress (both House and Senate), Government Accountability Office, the Executive Office (Executive Orders), and Congressional Research Service

Database: Congress.gov AND Legistorm

Date: April-May 2021

Results:
  U.S.:19

1	"medical" AND "supply chain"
2	"medical supply chain" AND "data sharing"
3	"medical supply chain" AND "medical devices"
4	"medical supply chain" AND "PPE"
5	"medical supply chain" AND "Personal Protective Equipment"
6	"medical supply chain" AND "drug shortages"

PUBLIC AGENDAS

AGENDA

Monday, September 21, 2020
Zoom Webinar

SESSION I   DISCUSSION ON THE SCOPE AND CONTEXT OF THE STUDY CHARGE

Session I Objective: To hear from the sponsor of the study regarding their perspectives on the charge to the committee

11:00 a.m.   Welcome and Introductions
  WALLACE HOPP, *Committee Chair*
  Distinguished University Professor of Business and
    Engineering
  The University of Michigan

11:10 a.m.   Sponsor Perspective on Charge to the Committee
  DAVID (CHRIS) HASSELL, *Study Sponsor*
  Acting Principal Deputy Assistant Secretary
  Office of the Assistant Secretary for Preparedness and
    Response
  U.S. Department of Health and Human Services

APPENDIX A   247

                    LAURA (KWINN) WOLF, Study Sponsor
                    Director, Division of Critical Infrastructure Protection
                    Office of the Assistant Secretary for Preparedness and
                       Response
                    U.S. Department of Health and Human Services

11:25 a.m.   Remarks from Congressional Staff
             MAX KANNER
             Health Policy Advisor
             Office of Sen. Dick Durbin (D-IL)

11:30 a.m.   Discussion with Committee

12:15 p.m.   Break (*30 mins*)

SESSION II   ADDITIONAL CONTEXT FOR THE STUDY

Session II Objective: To hear from the sponsor of the study regarding their perspectives on the charge to the committee

12:45 p.m. Stakeholder and Regulatory Perspectives Panel
             STELIOS C. TSINONTIDES
             Office of Pharmaceutical Manufacturing Assessment
             Office of Pharmaceutical Quality
             Center for Drug Evaluation and Research
             U.S. Food and Drug Administration

             LINDA RICCI
             Director
             Division of All Hazard Response, Science and Strategic
                Partnerships
             Office of Strategic Partnerships and Technology Innovation
             Center for Devices and Radiological Health
             U.S. Food and Drug Administration

             MARTIN VANTRIESTE
             President & CEO
             Civica Rx

             WILLIAM (BILL) HAWKINS
             Senior Advisor
             EW Healthcare Partners

1:15 p.m.   Discussion with Committee

2:00 p.m.   ADJOURN

AGENDA
Monday, December 1–2, 2020
Zoom Webinar

Workshop Objectives
- Discuss key considerations for the formulation of a unified list of critical medical products;
- Examine current lists of critical/essential medical products with attention to how these lists were developed and how they are used to inform decisions;
- Consider tactical approaches for improving supply chain resilience;
- Consider on-the-ground perspectives from end users of the medical supply chain (e.g., patients, clinicians, health systems) when it comes to:
  - what makes a medical product critical; and
  - outcome measures that matter to end users.

Day 1: December 1, 2020 (12:00 p.m.–3:30 p.m. ET)

12:00 p.m.   Welcome and Introductions
             WALLACE HOPP, *Committee Chair*
             Distinguished University Professor of Business and Engineering
             University of Michigan

SESSION I   KEY CONSIDERATIONS FOR ESTABLISHING A FRAMEWORK FOR CRITICAL MEDICAL PRODUCTS

Session I Objectives: To discuss key considerations for the formulation of a unified list of critical medical products as it relates to this study; discuss how these considerations relate to

- Demand surge and supply shocks;
- The severity of effects on an individual affected by a shortage versus the number of people potentially affected by a shortage;

APPENDIX A   249

- Outcome measures that matter to end users; and
- Products that are most at risk (e.g., difficulty of manufacturing).

12:15 p.m.   **Key Considerations for Establishing a Framework**
             STEPHEN SCHONDELMEYER
             Professor, Department of Pharmaceutical Care and Health
                Systems
             College of Pharmacy
             Co-Principal Investigator, Resilient Drug Supply Project
             Center for Infectious Disease Research and Policy
             University of Minnesota

             NATHANIEL HUPERT
             Associate Professor of Population Health Sciences and of
                Medicine
             Weill Medical College, Cornell University
             Co-Director, Cornell Institute for Disease and Disaster
                Preparedness

             KHATEREH CALLEJA
             President and CEO
             Healthcare Supply Chain Association

             JAMES LAWLER
             Associate Professor, Department of Internal Medicine
             Director, International Programs and Innovation, Global
                Center for Health Security
             Director, Clinical and Biodefense Research, National
                Strategic Research Institute
             University of Nebraska Medical Center

             CHRIS LIU
             Director, Department of Enterprise Services
             Washington State

12:45 p.m.   **Discussion with Committee**

1:30 p.m.   **Break (*45 minutes*)**

SESSION II	CRITICAL/ESSENTIAL MEDICAL PRODUCTS LISTS

Session II Objectives: To examine current lists of critical/essential medical products with attention to how these lists were developed and how they are currently being used to inform decisions; discuss lessons learned and/or generalizable approaches for the formulation of a unified list of critical medical products for purposes of this study.

2:15 p.m. Current Critical/Essential Medical Product Lists
FDA's List of Essential Medicines, Medical Countermeasures, and Critical Inputs
LINDA RICCI
Director, Division of All Hazard Response, Science and Strategic Partnerships
Office of Strategic Partnerships and Technology Innovation
Center for Devices and Radiological Health
U.S. Food and Drug Administration

DOUG THROCKMORTON
Deputy Director for Regulatory Programs
Center for Drug Evaluation and Research
U.S. Food and Drug Administration

Resilient Drug Supply Project—Critical Acute Drug List
STEPHEN SCHONDELMEYER
Professor, Department of Pharmaceutical Care & Health Systems
College of Pharmacy
Co-Principal Investigator, Resilient Drug Supply Project
Center for Infectious Disease Research and Policy
University of Minnesota
WHO Essential Medicines List

LISA HEDMAN
Group Lead, Supply and Access to Medicines
World Health Organization

PERNETTE BOURDILLION ESTEVE
Team Lead, Incidents and Substandard/Falsified Medical Products
World Health Organization

APPENDIX A   *251*

2:45 p.m.   Discussion with Committee

3:30 p.m.   ADJOURN WORKSHOP DAY 1

               DAY 2: DECEMBER 2, 2020 (11:30 A.M.–3:30 P.M. ET)

11:30 a.m.   Welcome and Debrief of Day 1
               WALLACE HOPP, *Committee Chair*
               Distinguished University Professor of Business and
                   Engineering
               University of Michigan

SESSION III	PRACTICAL AND TACTICAL APPROACHES FOR EXECUTING A FRAMEWORK FOR CRITICAL MEDICAL PRODUCTS

Session III Objectives: To discuss generalizable lessons learned when it comes to implementing a resilient supply chain for critical medical products; consider practical and tactical approaches for executing a framework for critical medical products.

11:45 a.m.   Lessons Learned and Practical/Tactical Approaches
               HEATHER WALL
               Chief Commercial Officer
               Civica Rx

               DAN KISTNER
               Group Senior Vice President of Pharmacy Service
               Vizient

               CRAIG KENNEDY
               Senior Vice President, Global Supply Chain Management
               Merck

               BILL MURRAY
               Medical Device Specialist Executive
               Deloitte Consulting

NICOLE LURIE
Strategic Advisor to the CEO and Response Lead
Coalition for Epidemic Preparedness Innovations
Senior Lecturer, Harvard Medical School
Former Assistant Secretary for Preparedness and Response
U.S. Department of Health and Human Services

12:15 p.m. Discussion with Committee

1:00 p.m. Break (*45 minutes*)

| SESSION IV | END USER PERSPECTIVES: WHAT MAKES A MEDICAL PRODUCT CRITICAL? |

Session IV Objective: Consider on-the-ground perspectives from end users of the medical supply chain (e.g., patients, clinicians, health systems) when it comes to

- What makes a medical product critical;
- Outcome measures that matter to end users when it comes to supply chain resilience and success.

1:45 p.m. End User Perspectives Panel
SUZANNE SCHRANDT
Founder and CEO
ExPPect

CHRISTOPHER NEWTON
Director, Trauma Care
Co-Director, Neuroscience Center
UCSF Benioff Children's Hospital Oakland

RYAN MAVES
Faculty Physician
Naval Medical Center San Diego

SALLY WATKINS
Executive Director
Washington State Nurses Association

MICHAEL GANIO
Director, Pharmacy Practice and Quality
American Society of Hospital Pharmacists

APPENDIX A   253

      MICHAEL SCHILLER
      Senior Director
      Association for Health Care Resource and Materials
      Management
      American Hospital Association

2:30 p.m. Discussion with Committee

3:15 p.m. Concluding Remarks
      WALLACE HOPP, *Committee Chair*
      Distinguished University Professor of Business and
       Engineering
      University of Michigan

3:30 p.m. ADJOURN WORKSHOP DAY

AGENDA

Monday, April 23, 2020
Zoom Webinar

Meeting Objective

- To gather information on issues related to improving the resilience of medical product supply chains including: innovation and technology; geopolitical risks and national security; and on-shoring

---

12:30 p.m. Welcome and Introductions
      WALLACE HOPP, *Committee Chair*
      Distinguished University Professor of Business and
       Engineering
      University of Michigan

SESSION I	INNOVATION AND TECHNOLOGY CONSIDERATIONS

Session I Objective: To gather information on innovation and technology (e.g., blockchain, artificial intelligence, continuous manufacturing) applications that can improve transparency, risk assessments, and manufacturing capacity, and ultimately improve the resilience of medical product supply chains.

12:45 p.m.   Innovation and Technology Considerations
(*5–7 minutes each*)

BLOCKCHAIN
JOHN POLOWCZYK
Managing Director
Ernst and Young

JAMES CANTERBURY
Principal
Ernst and Young

ARTIFICIAL INTELLIGENCE
PETER SWARTZ
Chief Technology Officer
Altana

MANUFACTURING PROCESSES OF THE FUTURE
RYAN FURNELL
Vice President
Anklesaria Group, Inc.

1:05 p.m.   Discussion with Committee

1:45 p.m.   Break (*15 minutes*)

APPENDIX A

SESSION II	GEOPOLITICAL, NATIONAL SECURITY, AND ON-SHORING CONSIDERATIONS

Session II Objective: To gather information on the totality of geopolitical and national security risks to U.S. medical product supply chains and whether on-shoring manufacturing of critical drugs and devices would protect U.S. medical product supply chains.

2:00 p.m.   Geopolitical Risks and National Security Considerations
            (*5–7 minutes each*)

   GEOPOLITICAL CONSIDERATIONS
   YANZHONG HUANG
   Senior Fellow for Global Health
   Council on Foreign Relations
   Professor and Director of Global Health Studies
   School of Diplomacy and International Relations
   Seton Hall University

   DAMIEN BRUCKARD
   Deputy Director, Trade and Investment
   International Chamber of Commerce

   NATIONAL SECURITY CONSIDERATIONS
   COLIN CHINN
   Rear Admiral, U.S. Navy (Retired)
   Former Joint Staff Surgeon
   Former U.S. Pacific Command Surgeon

2:15 p.m.   Brief Discussion with Committee

2:30 p.m.   On-Shoring Considerations (*5–7 minutes each*)
   ROSEMARY GIBSON
   Senior Advisor
   The Hastings Center

   CHAD BOWN
   Reginald Jones Senior Fellow
   Peterson Institute for International Economics

2:45 p.m.   Full Discussion with Committee Regarding Geopolitical Risks, National Security, and On-Shoring

4:00 p.m.   ADJOURN OPEN SESSION

AGENDA

Wednesday, June 9, 2021
2:30 p.m.–5:00 p.m. ET
Zoom Webinar

Meeting Objective

- To gather information on issues related to medical device supply chains

2:30 p.m.   Welcome and Introductions
           WALLACE HOPP, *Committee Chair*
           Distinguished University Professor of Business and Engineering
           University of Michigan

SESSION I   MEDICAL DEVICE SUPPLY CHAIN CONSIDERATIONS

Objective:

- To gather information on medical device supply chains including, the current landscape, issues related to resilience (e.g., characteristics of device shortages, the management of device shortages, the effects of device shortages, tools for preventing device shortages), and similarities and differences between the drug and device supply chains.

2:45 p.m.   Medical Device Supply Chain Considerations
           (*5–7 minutes each*)
           MARK RUTKIEWICZ
           Vice President of Quality
           Innovize

APPENDIX A 257

                NOEL COLON
                Senior Vice President, Chief Quality Officer
                Medtronic

                GREG SMITH
                Executive Vice President, Supply Chain and Operations
                Medtronic

3:00 p.m.   Discussion with Committee

4:00 p.m.   Break (*15 minutes*)

SESSION II   UPDATE ON COMMISSIONED ECONOMIC ANALYSIS

4:15 p.m.   Progress Update and Discussion on Commissioned Economic Analysis
                PHILIP ELLIS
                Ellis Health Policy

4:30 p.m.   Discussion with Committee

5:00 p.m.   **ADJOURN OPEN SESSION**

AGENDA

Wednesday, August 18, 2021
1:30 p.m.–2:30 p.m. ET
Zoom Webinar

Meeting Objective

- To gather information on current FDA and ASPR activities related to increasing the resilience of medical product supply chains

1:30 p.m.   Welcome and Introductions
                WALLACE HOPP, *Committee Chair*
                Distinguished University Professor of Business and Engineering
                University of Michigan

SESSION I	FEDERAL UPDATES

Objective: To gather information on current FDA and ASPR activities related to increasing the resilience of medical product supply chains

1:35 p.m. **FDA Updates**
TAMMY BECKHAM
Associate Director for Resilient Supply Chain
Office of Strategic Partnerships and Technology Innovation
Center for Devices and Radiological Health
U.S. Food and Drug Administration

1:45 p.m. **ASPR Updates**
JOSEPH HAMEL
Director, ASPR Program Office for Innovation and Industrial Base Expansion (IBx)
HHS Office of the Assistant Secretary for Preparedness and Response

1:55 p.m. Discussion with Committee

2:30 p.m. **ADJOURN OPEN SESSION**

AGENDA

Wednesday, October 6, 2021
1:00 p.m.–3:00 p.m. ET
Zoom Webinar

Meeting Objectives

• Open session to gather additional information on trade policy as it relates to
   o Restrictions on export bans of medical products; and
   o International information sharing on the details of medical product supply chains

1:00 p.m. **Welcome and Opening Remarks**
LEE BRANSTETTER, *Committee Member*
Professor of Economics and Public Policy
Carnegie Mellon University

APPENDIX A   259

1:05 p.m.   **Speaker Presentations and Q&A Discussion with Committee**
               MONICA GORMAN
               Deputy Assistant Secretary for Manufacturing, Industry and
                   Analysis
               International Trade Administration
               U.S. Department of Commerce

               CARTER WILBUR
               Economic Officer
               Office of Multilateral Trade Affairs
               U.S. Department of State

1:50 p.m.   **Speaker Presentations and Q&A Discussion with Committee**
               JONATHAN KIMBALL
               Vice President, Trade and International Affairs
               Association for Accessible Medicines

               SCOTT KOMINERS
               MBA Class of 1960 Associate Professor of Business
                   Administration
               Entrepreneurial Management Unit, Harvard Business School

               CHAD BOWN
               Reginald Jones Senior Fellow
               Peterson Institute for International Economics

3:00 p.m.   **Adjourn Meeting**

Appendix B

Summary of Recommendations from Contemporary Reports

NATIONAL STRATEGY FOR A RESILIENT PUBLIC HEALTH SUPPLY CHAIN[1]

Robustness and Industry Sustainment

- Drive bold investments and incentives for the American industrial base
  - Make significant investments to sustain the U.S. public health industrial base
  - Expand Buy American and Berry Amendment rules to all agencies and grantees
  - Support the use of American-made public health supplies in the U.S. health care sector
  - Use trade tools to counter unfair trade practices and strengthen the public health industrial base needed for national security
  - Sustain a supply chain workforce with the people and skills needed for pandemic preparedness

Agility and Innovation

- Build a more capable and robust Strategic National Stockpile and expand state, local, tribal, and territorial stockpiling

---

[1] For more information on these recommendations and to read the full report, see https://www.phe.gov/Preparedness/legal/Documents/National-Strategy-for-Resilient-Public-Health-Supply-Chain.pdf (accessed October 7, 2021).

- Develop preemptive supply chain demand management capabilities to modulate demand before shortages occur
- Launch a new public health supplies innovation center and product standardization task force

Visibility and Engagement

- Maintain end-to-end supply chain visibility through expanded and continuous supply chain surveillance
- Streamline U.S. government–private sector coordination for sustained public health supply chain private-sector engagement
- Institute an annual resilience report card

Governance and Management

- Bolster interagency oversight of the public health supply chain, and sustain a strong U.S. government public health supply chain workforce
- Revise Executive Order 13603 on National Defense Resources Preparedness
- Establish a national framework for allocation of constrained resources
- Revamp global governance of the public health supply chain

BUILDING RESILIENT SUPPLY CHAINS, REVITALIZING AMERICAN MANUFACTURING, AND FOSTERING BROAD-BASED GROWTH[2]

Boost Local Production and Fostering International Cooperation

- Investment and Financial Incentives to Boost Production
  - Leverage the DPA and Current Public–Private Partnerships (PPPs) to Establish a Consortium for Advanced Manufacturing and On-shoring of Domestic Essential Medicines Production
  - Near-Term Next Steps:
    - HHS and the White House will host a high-level summit on drug supply chain resilience to kick off this new initiative.
    - The administration will assemble a consortium of public health experts (including emergency medicine and critical care) in the government, nonprofit, and private sectors to

---

[2] For more information on these recommendations and to read the full report, see https://www.whitehouse.gov/wp-content/uploads/2021/06/100-day-supply-chain-review-report.pdf (accessed October 7, 2021).

review the Essential Medicines List and recommend 50–100 drugs that are most critical to have available at all times for U.S. patients because of their clinical need and lack of therapeutic redundancy (Critical Drug List), and determine a potential volume that could be needed, using the surges during COVID-19 pandemic as one metric for that analysis.
- HHS will conduct an analysis of the Essential Medicines List that went into shortage in the past year to determine major drivers, including mapping their supply chains to characterize their redundancy, diversity, and manufacturing quality.
- HHS will leverage the DPA process to determine the financial incentives needed to on-shore or near-shore the production capacity needed for the global supply chain.
- Medium-Term Next Steps:
    - HHS will use the 708 process to assemble a group of pharmaceutical supply chain experts to develop a resilience framework, based on the above analysis, that details the characteristics of a high-quality, diverse, and redundant supply chain for pharmaceutical products.
    - HHS will map the supply chains for the Critical Drug List to the resilience framework for a robust supply chain and identify those for which on-shoring or near-shoring may be advisable.
    - HHS will determine if there is a need to increase production or stockpile APIs for the Critical Drug List, and if so, identify the amounts needed in such a stockpile, the benefit and risk of a virtual stockpile, and the ability to use platform technologies to provide surge production in crises.
    - Additionally, HHS will explore stockpiling strategies to reduce API supply risk, including an analysis of KSMs.
    - The U.S. government will review reimbursement models for key essential medicines to determine whether changes to reimbursement models could improve the resilience of key essential medicines without unduly affecting U.S. costs.
- Use Incentives to Create Redundancy for Sterile Injectable Production
    - To increase the resilience of the sterile injectable supply chain, three actions should be pursued to reduce risk:
    - Financial incentives to spur investment:
        - The United States will continue using the Biomedical Advanced Research and Development Authority and other incentive-based tools to invest in specialized equipment and updates to mature quality manufacturing processes, includ-

ing advanced manufacturing techniques, for these products. This will help reduce the barrier to entry for new manufacturers or reduce the cost to existing manufacturers looking to upgrade their facilities.
- Update reimbursement models:
  - For lower-cost drugs, profit margins from federal payers may play a role in ensuring that sterile injectables are at least at risk of being in short supply. Accordingly, to reduce the likelihood that these products will go into shortage because of low margins, the U.S. government will review reimbursement models to determine updates that may improve supply chain resilience.
- Procurement guarantees:
  - While incentives for establishing production and competitive reimbursement models are needed, manufacturers have indicated they also require consistent demand to justify investments for new production. Procurement guarantees, combined with using acquisition flexibilities, can be used to signal commitment to and demand for products from domestic and small firms. These will need to be established in a careful and nuanced manner to ensure that they serve the needs of agencies, including DoD and the Department of Veterans Affairs (VA), and to ensure consistency with U.S. procurement laws and obligations.
- Near-Term Next Steps:
  - HHS will convene a working group to analyze how reimbursement policies contribute to the lack of resilience for sterile injectables identified in the previous proposal as well as chemotherapeutics that have been in shortage in the past 5 years.
  - HHS will evaluate whether certain sterile injectables that are identified as being at significant risk of shortage but are not part of the Critical Drug List medicines identified above, such as sterile pediatric oncology drugs, should also be the subject of improved supply chain resilience work in addition to drugs on the Critical Drug List.

- Invest in Research and Development
  - Establish Novel Platform Production Technologies as Mainstream
  - Near-Term Next Steps:
    - Using funding from the American Rescue Plan, in June 2021, the Department of Commerce–sponsored National Institute for Innovation in Manufacturing Biopharmaceu-

ticals (NIIMBL) will launch a whole-of-industry effort to develop fully integrated and smaller footprint platforms that will reduce supply chain demands for raw materials, increase domestic biomanufacturing surge capacity, and more broadly improve technological capabilities that can lead to the biomanufacturing of APIs.
- HHS will create an internal task force with experts from FDA and ASPR to increase capacity for supporting development, evaluation, and, if possible, implementation of novel manufacturing technologies and processes. The task force will visit existing facilities and form partnerships with domestic manufacturers or universities to study advanced manufacturing technologies. It will develop a strategy for the secretary on how to facilitate a wider adoption of novel methods for commercial production of pharmaceuticals and biologics.

- Create Quality Transparency
  - Create a Rating System to Incentivize Drug Manufacturers to Invest in Achieving Quality Management Maturity
  - FDA should lead the development of a framework to measure and provide transparency regarding a facility's quality management maturity with engagement from industry, academia, and other stakeholders. The development and adoption of this rating would
    - Communicate the value of quality management maturity so it can be adopted by manufacturers and priced into contracts by purchasers;
    - Promote the adoption of better tools to measure manufacturing performance to allow earlier detection of potential problems that could lead to shortage; and
    - Incentivize improvements to manufacturing infrastructure that enhance reliability of manufacturing and thus supply.
  - Next steps:
    - Establishing a quality rating system for drug and API production is a long-term initiative that will have to be developed in collaboration with business partners and with stakeholders.
    - As a next step, FDA could begin consultations with stakeholders to develop a framework for rating quality management maturity.
    - Over time, FDA will consider whether to establish a new PPP with industry to develop and support use of such a rating system. PPPs have proven effective for other federal

- programs, such as the Pharmacy Quality Alliance, a PPP that develops quality measures for use of pharmaceuticals, some of which have been adopted under Medicare.
- Improve Information and Data Collection
  - Use Commercial Data to Improve the Resilience of Supply Chains:
    - Commercial data providers have begun to collect information on the drug and API supply chains. FDA and HHS should encourage stakeholders throughout supply chains to increase their use of commercial data to identify and mitigate supply chain risks while the U.S. government stands up a more comprehensive initiative to collect data and to improve surveillance and oversight of drug and API supply chains.
  - Seek Additional Authority Through Which FDA Can Collect Additional Data and Take Action to Improve Surveillance, Oversight, and Resilience of Supply Chains:
    - Over the longer term, the U.S. government should establish a new initiative to collect additional supply chain data to improve surveillance, oversight, and supply chain resilience.
    - The following are several critical sources of new data necessary to support such surveillance work:
      - Drug manufacturing volume information and reporting;
      - Complete registration and listing requirements;
      - Distribution data on prescription drugs and certain biological products;
      - Requiring manufacturers to notify FDA of an increase in demand; and
      - Requiring that the labeling of API and finished product labeling include original manufacturers.
  - Next Steps:
    - HHS will convene industry and other nongovernmental stakeholders to share insight on commercial data sources and to encourage stakeholders across the supply chains to increase their use of commercial data to improve supply chain resilience.
    - HHS will develop and make recommendations to Congress seeking statutory authorization to increase FDA and HHS ability to collect information and to require that API and finish drug labels identify original manufacturers.

Build Emergency Capacity

- Explore the Creation/Expansion of a Virtual Strategic Stockpile of API Reserve and Other Critical Materials Managed by the Strategic National Stockpile, Including Finished Doses
  - The United States should create a virtual stockpile of APIs and other critical materials necessary to produce the identified Essential Medicines, with prioritization of the Critical Drug List and reliance to the extent possible on domestic suppliers, especially small and small disadvantaged businesses.
  - Next Steps:
    - HHS will determine specific API and finished drugs that need to be stockpiled, and identify the amounts needed in such a stockpile, the benefit and risk of a virtual stockpile, and the ability to use on-demand manufacturing to provide surge production in crises.
    - As part of this analysis, HHS will explore stockpiling strategies to reduce API supply risk, including an analysis of KSMs.

Promote International Cooperation and Partner with Allies

- Ensure International Harmonization for Reviewing and Responding to Supply Chain Risk with Partnering Nations
  - The U.S. government should work through already established international regulatory collaboration and harmonization organizations, including but not limited to the International Coalition of Medicines Regulatory Authorities, the International Council for Harmonisation of Technical Requirements for Pharmaceuticals for Human Use, and the Pharmaceutical Inspection Cooperation Scheme to strengthen cooperation with allies and partners. The U.S. government should also use other bilateral and multilateral fora and engagements to strengthen drug and API supply chain cooperation.
  - Specifically, the U.S. government should use the criteria established in the first recommendation regarding the optimum geographic diversity and redundancy in a supply chain in collaborations with our major regulatory partners, who are already aligned on the need for more robust and stable supply chains and are beginning their own evaluations regarding the need for domestic manufacturing together with supply chains that are integrated with allies.

- Next Steps:
  - For the Critical Drug List identified in the first recommendation, engage with international partners to map a global supply chain where redundancy and diversity includes sufficient on-shoring, production in geographically accessible locations, and production by allies.

DRUG SHORTAGES: ROOT CAUSES AND POTENTIAL SOLUTIONS[3]

Recommendation 1: Create a Shared Understanding of the Impact of Drug Shortages and the Contracting Practices That May Contribute to Them

- Among the areas most needing attention are
  - Quantification of the harms of drug shortages, particularly those that lead to worsened health outcomes for patients:
    - Previous efforts to assess the costs of drug shortages have generally been limited in scope and depth, but nevertheless suggest that the total national effect of shortages may be very large. Given that FDA has recognized and posted on its website more than 100 shortages at a single point in time, it is especially important to have additional research to assess the full effect of shortages on patient outcomes and, more generally, on health care delivery and health care system costs. Previous estimates, at hundreds of millions of dollars annually, may have drastically underestimated the harms of drug shortages.
  - Better characterization of shortages:
    - Currently, public- and private-sector stakeholders have limited information to quantitatively characterize shortages in terms of their frequency, persistence, intensity, and effect on available treatments in specific therapeutic categories. Having this information would help improve stakeholders' understanding of the effect shortages have on the nation's health care.
      - Several stakeholders maintain information sources that, if combined, could shed more light on the extent of drug shortages and their potential effects on the health system.

---

[3] For more information on these recommendations and to read the full report, see https://www.fda.gov/media/131130/download (accessed October 7, 2021).

For example, wholesalers track order fill rates and inventory changes, and manufacturers oversee proprietary data on production capacity and production volume by facility. Combining these data could enable better measurement of the frequency, persistence, and intensity of shortages and of their effects.
- ○ Greater transparency in private-sector contracting practices:
  - Generic drug manufacturers have cited contracting practices as a source of business uncertainty and "race to the bottom" pricing dynamics. FDA heard from stakeholders that some contracts currently include "low-price clauses" that allow GPOs to unilaterally walk away from a contract if a competing manufacturer is willing to supply the same product or bundle of products for a lower price. FDA also reviewed evidence that "failure-to-supply clauses" in contracts are sometimes relatively weak, requiring that an alternative source of the drug is available and typically recovering just 10 percent of the lost value. More systematic study of current contracting practices is needed and could support development of a model contract designed to promote reliable access to safe and effective drugs.

Recommendation 2: Create a Rating System to Incentivize Drug Manufacturers to Invest in Achieving Quality Management System Maturity

- This proposal aims to rectify this failure by suggesting the development of a system to measure and rate the quality management maturity of individual manufacturing facilities based on specific objective indicators. A rating would evaluate the robustness of a manufacturing facility's quality system and could be used to inform purchasers and GPOs about the state of, and commitment to, the quality management of the facility making the drugs they are buying. Pharmaceutical companies could, at their discretion, disclose the rating of the facilities where their drugs are manufactured. GPOs and purchasers could require disclosure of the rating in their contracts with manufacturers. This effort would introduce transparency into the market, and provide top-rated producers with a competitive advantage, potentially enabling them to obtain sustainable prices as well as grow market share.

Recommendation 3: Promote Sustainable Private-Sector Contracts

- FDA believes that the private sector should establish contracts that address the first and second root causes of shortages by
    - Providing Financial Incentives:
        - Contracts should ensure that manufacturers earn sustainable risk-adjusted returns on their investment in launching or continuing to market prescription drugs, especially older generic drugs that remain important elements of the medical armamentarium.
    - Rewarding Manufacturers for Mature Quality Management:
        - Similarly, contracts should recognize and reward manufacturing quality maturity. This could be done through a number of different mechanisms, such as paying higher prices for drugs manufactured at top-rated facilities, requiring a certain quality maturity rating as a condition of contracting, or guaranteeing purchase of a set volume of products from sites achieving a certain maturity rating. By offering escalating premiums for drugs from more highly rated facilities, where the rating system recognizes different levels of achievement, purchasers could provide the incentives and means for manufacturers to move up the quality management maturity spectrum.

DRUG SHORTAGES: A REPORT FROM THE PEW CHARITABLE TRUSTS AND THE INTERNATIONAL SOCIETY FOR PHARMACEUTICAL ENGINEERING[4]

- The report recommends that the pharmaceutical industry should
    - Develop systems to proactively identify and resolve quality issues:
        - It was apparent from the interviews as well as a review of the 29 product examples that quality remains a primary driver behind shortages—one that the industry must address.
        - Improvement opportunities should focus on strengthening quality and also development and implementation of systems that proactively identify, measure, and monitor risks across the manufacturer's overall supply chain. This includes CGMP compliance risks as well as issues that may develop when there are less than robust development and/or

---

[4] For more information on these recommendations and to read the full report, see https://www.pewtrusts.org/-/media/assets/2017/01/drug_shortages.pdf (accessed October 7, 2021).

manufacturing processes in place. Manufacturers should be diligent in selecting suppliers and, when necessary, partner with them to help improve their quality systems.
- Understand the risks across the supply chain:
  - Despite uncertain market demands, companies should have (1) systematic approaches in place for evaluating the risks across their supply chains and (2) the ability to predict the amount of product needed. That would help them understand and apply the right mitigations across their portfolios by product type. These risk evaluations should look beyond a mere understanding of the compliance and specific individual product risks and instead be broadened to include a review across multiple dimensions. For example, ISPE's Drug Shortages Prevention Plan identified the following dimensions that should be reviewed to understand the risk of a potential shortage: corporate culture, quality systems, metrics, business continuity planning, communication with authorities, and building capabilities.
- Improve market forecasts:
  - Industry, regulators, and purchasers must begin working together to improve the accuracy of the information related to the risk of a shortage that they collect and communicate. Without these market insights, companies are not making the investments necessary to expand facilities or upgrade equipment to create the additional manufacturing capacity that would protect against future shortages. The ability to predict a drug's expected demand is especially important since having multiple replacements for a product does not protect it from experiencing a shortage. Although companies will not share specific market strategy information with their competitors, purchasers, or even regulators, they need a system to improve the accuracy of volume predictions for annual manufacturing, especially when it comes to low-volume drugs that have multiple replacements and variable annual demand cycles. Companies would be more likely to build the mitigations they need to reduce the risk of shortages if levels of confidence in the information provided were to increase.
- Improve overall incentives between purchasers and manufacturers:
  - Purchasing groups should offer incentives such as long-term, exclusive contracts or guaranteed orders to motivate companies to invest in backup manufacturing facilities. The

investments needed to build such facilities or develop dual sources can be significant, and incentives would help companies reduce the risk of building capacity they would not use.
- Improve collaboration with regulators:
  - While the companies said that relationships with regulators had improved, they also cited the need to continue identifying ways of addressing disconnections that limit the ability of the manufacturer—because of the time needed to obtain approval and implement changes—to expand capacity or invest in new equipment. In addition, a solution that enables a more effective way to update market authorizations for legacy products is needed. Putting such a solution in place would make it easier for manufacturers of these products to update their market authorizations and create the capacity needed to protect against shortages.

DRUG SHORTAGES AS A MATTER OF NATIONAL SECURITY: IMPROVING THE RESILIENCE OF THE NATION'S HEALTH CARE CRITICAL INFRASTRUCTURE SUMMIT[5,6]

Regulatory

- Develop a list of critical drugs. Use the WHO Model Lists of Essential Medicines and other existing resources as a starting point to define what a shortage is and develop a list of critical drugs needed for (1) emergency response and (2) saving and preserving life. Using historical data and manufacturing input, address why these drugs have been on the shortage list. The critical list can be used to
  - Stabilize the availability of critical drugs by working with manufacturers and the Food and Drug Administration (FDA) to create redundant product in multiple locations in anticipation of natural disasters and other supply chain threats.
  - Assess the quality of pharmaceutical manufacturers measured against the importance of drugs on the critical list.
  - Work with the private sector for greater transparency surrounding the source of raw materials and manufacturing locations so providers can more easily assess pharmaceutical product qual-

---

[5] These recommendations represent the thoughts of individual attendees of the summit and are not consensus recommendations.

[6] For more information on these recommendations and to read the full report, see https://www.ashp.org/-/media/assets/advocacy-issues/docs/Recommendations-Drug-Shortages-as-Matter-of-Natl-security.ashx (accessed October 7, 2021).

ity. FDA has proposed a star rating system for pharmaceutical manufacturers, which could increase transparency.
- Create a multistakeholder advisory panel with FDA to address key issues, such as the possibility of creating a stockpile of critical drugs, the logistics of warehousing such excess pharmaceutical inventory, and where the excess inventory should be stored.
- Improve communication with the entire drug supply chain, including health care providers during, or in advance of, a public health emergency or other event that may create a drug shortage. FDA should provide the health care community with information simultaneously on the type of products that may be affected and the expected duration of the effect. To prevent hoarding of inventory that could result from such communication, manufacturers could put product on allocation to ensure that remaining supply is distributed equitably.
- Streamline regulations to incentivize increased manufacturing production.
  ○ Compounding regulations: 503(b) outsourcers need incentives to make drugs in short supply; it is costly to ramp up for only a short duration.
  ○ Global regulatory environment: there are multiple agencies internationally, all with competing requirements for manufacturers.
  ○ Align with FDA's initiative to harmonize international technical standards for approval of generic drugs.
- Engage CMS to discuss the practice of citing hospitals that use medications after the guaranteed stability period in product labeling. This may, for example, address a powder after it is solubilized, which can contribute to unnecessary medical waste.
  ○ There are situations where evidence exists in the literature that stability goes well beyond the period of time listed in product labeling. However, CMS/TJC will cite a hospital even though the organization has evaluated this evidence and revised the date based on that. This warrants further discussion with CMS to see what might be needed to avoid or address drug shortage situations.
- Encourage FDA to consider how reducing the number of unapproved (pre-1938 FD&C) drugs on the market might affect shortages.
  ○ FDA has been assisting companies with finding opportunities to legally market older "grandfathered" products that are currently marketed without the required FDA approval. While the FDA approval process ensures that marketed drugs

meet current FDA standards for safety, efficacy, quality, and labeling—there have been concerns that these efforts to bring widely used but unapproved drugs into compliance with current FDA requirements have resulted in drug shortages.

Legislative

- Enact legislation that requires a notification requirement for medical product devices and equipment needed to administer medications, similar to the legislation enacted in 2012 that requires drug manufacturers to notify the Food and Drug Administration "of any changes in production that is reasonably likely to lead to reduction in supply" of a covered drug in the United States.
    - For example, fluid containers to dilute medications for infusion.
- Enact legislation requiring a risk assessment of foreign source active pharmaceutical ingredients (APIs).
    - Relying predominantly on other countries for the necessary ingredients to manufacture crucial drugs puts the United States at risk.
- Require federal government authorities with jurisdiction over national security to conduct an analysis of domestic drug and medical device manufacturing capability and capacity for critical products to assess whether a threat to national security exists.
- Require a GAO study to examine all aspects of the drug supply chain to see if there are any new issues exacerbating drug shortages.

Legislative and Regulatory

- Develop incentives for drug manufacturers to have contingency or redundant production plans for their pharmaceutical products on the critical drug list. The backup plan should include prioritizing the most medically necessary products, qualifying third-party suppliers across their network, and increasing production and inventory for API and finished goods.
- Investigate developing a system of paying suppliers to hold inventory, perhaps similar to the system employed by the DoD/Defense Logistics Agency. Consider partnering with the DoD to create contractual leverage with drug manufacturers for civilian hospitals.
- Incentivize manufacturers and work with the FDA to repackage pharmaceuticals according to the amount of medication commonly used to reduce waste (e.g., only a 30 mL vial of a drug is available when most common volume needed is 5 mL).

- Create an Office of Clinical Affairs within the Drug Enforcement Agency (DEA), so DEA personnel will be available to address the clinical side of medication shortages of controlled substances, rather than just the diversion enforcement aspect.

Market/Nonlegislative or Regulatory

- Standardize medical concentration, containers, and sizes to stabilize pharmaceutical supply and reduce the probability of patient harm caused by constantly needing to change concentrations and associated technology. Standardizing products reduces the risk of adverse drug events when shortage products are substituted. Standardizing the concentration of compounded products within organizations also helps provide a critical mass for industry to consider making previously unavailable products available.
- Identify tools that address supply access, such as Pfizer's web access tool, which provides information about happenings at Pfizer's facilities, latest product updates, and a Q&A forum.
- Ensure hospital staff, health care providers, and pharmacies have capacity to manage drug shortages.
    - Ensure early notification of predictable medication shortages and medication substitutes so staff can build necessary information into communication efforts.
    - Work with medical and specialty organizations to ensure necessary information is built into educational efforts, such as national guidelines and continuing education.
- Examine how changes in United States Pharmacopeia (USP) standards for drugs with a solid historical safety record can affect supply, and whether these changes are necessary.
    - Consult with USP representatives about pharmaceutical regulations that may lack an evidence base.
- Request that electronic health record (EHR) vendors make changes to their systems to ease the burden of making drug product changes when a shortage occurs. An example would be some sort of tool that makes changes to various integrated technology databases at the same time (like EHR and smart pump drug libraries, or automated dispensing cabinets and pharmacy inventory systems).

Appendix C

Determining Risk Values When Evaluating Medical Product Supply Chain Resilience

As described in Chapter 5, one way to think of the resilience of medical product supply chains is in terms of reducing the Total Expected Harm (Equation 5-1), which is the sum of expected harm to individual people. To compute Total Expected Harm, estimate the patient harm from a unit of shortage of product i (H_i) and the expected supply shortage of product i in any given year (S_i), and multiply them to compute product risk level ($R_i = H_i \times S_i$). Total patient harm is the sum of the risks from all medical products. To reduce it in an efficient manner, products with high expected risk levels (R_i) warrant increased attention. However, as pointed out in Chapter 5, equity and risk of events must be considered, which requires thinking beyond products with high expected risk levels. Reducing the likelihood or severity of shortages of some products may be needed to protect small populations (e.g., patients with a rare condition) from extreme harm, or to protect the public against unlikely but catastrophic events (e.g., nuclear attacks). Supply chain critical refers to products for which enhancing supply chain resilience is important to mitigate Total Expected Harm or specialized risks.

For each product on the supply chain critical list, appropriate targets must be determined for how much to enhance supply chain resilience. The reason for this is to achieve a balanced resilience strategy that allocates resources where they will do the most good. Adding protections should be avoided for one product that provides little added benefit when the resources could have yielded more benefit if spent protecting another product. This appendix describes the procedures for estimating expected risks and setting protection targets for medical products.

DETERMINING EXPECTED RISK VALUES

Assigning values to H_i and S_i for a given product can be done with simple, subjective surveys and/or sophisticated, analytical evaluations. An example of a simple process would be to survey appropriate experts for categorical (e.g., low, medium, high) estimates. For example, to estimate H_i, medical experts could be asked to evaluate the health consequences of a single patient being deprived of product i because of a shortage. To do this, the experts should consider the alternative treatment strategy (e.g., crisis standards of care) and the difference in the clinical outcome with and without product i. Knowledgeable professionals can probably give qualitative (low, medium, high) estimates with relative ease. Analogously, supply chain experts could be polled to estimate the likelihood of small (e.g., <10% of annual demand), medium (10-50% of annual demand) or large (>50% of annual demand). Averaging expert estimates would constitute a form of crowd sourcing to estimate H_i and S_i.

Subjective estimates by experts could be complemented or replaced by more detailed analytic evaluations. For example, one could estimate H_i by evaluating the impact on quality adjusted life years (QALYs) of forcing patients in different categories (e.g., age groups or severity levels) to substitute the next best treatment alternative for product i and averaging across categories. Similarly, analytic estimates of S_i could be made by evaluating shortages caused by various trigger events. Analytics techniques, such as machine learning, might be helpful in leveraging past data to estimate event probabilities and shortage levels.

However, because it is impossible to identify every possible trigger event, such estimates will always be subject to error. The uncertainty in estimates will be relatively small for routine events, such as shortages caused by manufacturing quality events or firm exit from the market. But they will be large for rare emergency events, such as global pandemics. To consider these, each trigger should be evaluated to generate a reasonably comprehensive range of scenarios. For example, the triggers might suggest scenarios that cause partial and full shutdowns of production, brief and lengthy disruptions, demand surges, and combinations of these (e.g., a scenario in which supply is constrained while demand surges, as happened with N95 masks in the early months of the COVID-19 pandemic). Clearly, such detailed scenario analysis is not needed to make reasonable choices about what products to include on the supply chain critical list. However, the data from such an analysis can be useful in determining supply chain resilience targets, which is the subject of the next section.

SETTING SUPPLY CHAIN RESILIENCE TARGETS

Knowing that a product presents a supply chain risk, the challenge then becomes how to reduce this risk to a socially acceptable level. To guide the risk reduction process, a target should be set for the amount of shortage protection needed for the product. Such a protection target can be thought of in terms of the number of units, X_i for product i, or equivalently in terms of the "weeks of supply," labeled T_i. These are equivalent because if D_i represents the average weekly demand for product i, then one can compute the time X_i units will last as follows:

$$T_i \text{ weeks} = X_i \text{ units} \div D_i \text{ units/week} \qquad \text{(Equation C-1)}$$

That is, a supply of X_i units will cover a shortage event that cuts off 100 percent of production for T_i weeks.

It is standard practice in inventory and supply chain management to refer to inventory levels in units of time because it highlights the level of protection much more clearly than does referring to inventory in units of items. For instance, holding 10,000 units of inventory in a stockpile provides a much higher level of protection for a product with weekly demand of 1,000 units than for a product with weekly demand of 100,000 units. This inventory level represents a 10-week supply in the first case, but only a 1/10-week supply in the second case.

However, the conversion between time and inventory needs to be adjusted when the disruption rate does not equal the normal demand rate. For example, if a product has multiple suppliers, it might be the case that almost all plausible disruptions would cut off only a fraction of the supply. If it were estimated that a disruption is likely not to exceed F_i times the demand, where F_i is an adjustment factor (unitless), the "weeks of supply" target T_i can be converted into inventory units as follows:

$$X_i \text{ units} = T_i \text{ weeks} \times D_i \text{ units/week} \times F_i \qquad \text{(Equation C-2)}$$

For many products, such as insulin for diabetics or chemotherapy drugs for cancer patients, the underlying demand D_i is very stable. For such products, the value of adjustment factor F_i will be less than or equal to 1 (≤ 1) and will depend on the diversification of the supply chain. However, some medical products, such as personal protective equipment (PPE) and blood plasma, are part of the emergency response and therefore can experience substantial demand surges. For these, it is possible for F_i to be greater than 1 (>1). Therefore, F_i must be accounted for when setting a protection target X_i, which may be more easily done by dividing the list of supply chain critical products into two subgroups, those for which demand is independent of an emergency and those for which demand may be amplified by an emergency.

Protection Volume and Time Targets

The protection volume target (X_i) for product i is the amount of supply shortfall that product i should be able to accommodate without harming people, while the protection time target (T_i) for product i is the duration of a disruption that creates a supply shortfall equal to a fraction (F_i) of the normal demand rate (D_i). The two targets are equivalent because they are related by Equation C-2.

Setting an appropriate protection volume target of X_i or a protection time target of T_i requires consideration of the profile of possible shortages. For example, if a detailed scenario analysis was performed to compute the expected shortage amount S_i, one could use the data shortage probabilities and magnitudes to generate a cumulative probability distribution like those shown in Figure C-2. In these histograms, the bars represent that the total shortage of supply in the upcoming year will be less than or equal to x for various values of x. The first bar on the left of each graph indicates the probability of a shortage of less than or equal to zero (i.e., equal to zero, since negative shortages do not occur), and hence all bars include the probability of no shortage at all.

The two graphs in Figure C-1 represent two very different types of products. The left graph, labeled "Short, Frequent," characterizes a product where shortages are likely, as indicated by the fact that the first bar in the histogram (which represents the probability of zero shortage) is substantially less than 1. However, the likelihood that the shortage will be small is high, as indicated by the fact that the bars approach 1 for a modest level of x. In contrast, the right graph, labeled "Long, Infrequent," characterizes a product where shortages are very unlikely, as indicated by the fact that the first bar is almost 1. But there is a small probability of a very large shortage (indicated by the slightly taller bar toward the far right of the graph).

It is possible that the two scenarios depicted in Figure C-1 have the same expected shortage (S_i). As such, if they both have high patient harm scores (H_i), they may both warrant inclusion on the supply chain critical list. Nevertheless, both present very different situations for setting and achieving a supply chain resilience target. The short, frequent shortage product might be virtually prevented by holding a relatively modest amount of inventory, which would be used often. This is why high-margin products generally have such protections built into their supply chains, since the revenue and reputation preservation value of maintaining continuity of supply outweighs

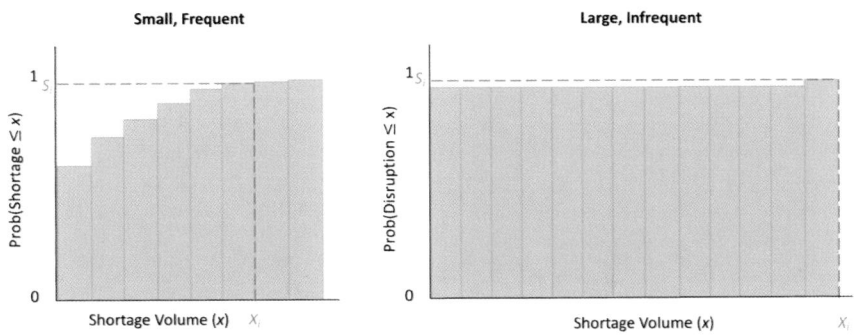

FIGURE C-1 Cumulative probability distributions of shortage volume.

the cost of holding extra inventory. However, as noted in Chapter 5, products with low margins, such as generic drugs, are much less likely to have protections against short, frequent shortages built into their supply chains.

In contrast, providing almost certain protection against long, infrequent shortages would require holding a massive amount of inventory, which is unlikely to be used. In general, regardless of margin, private industry will not find it economical to provide such protection. However, these scenarios will occur and may require public intervention to address. Since holding large amounts of rarely used inventory is expensive, there is strong incentive to consider alternative resilience interventions. The medical product supply chain resiliency framework in Chapter 5 provides a tool for identifying options.

Returning to the quantitative question of how much protection is appropriate for product i, suppose (for the sake of building intuition) that the bars in the Small, Frequent case of Figure C-1 are only one unit wide. That is, a massively detailed set of scenarios has been generated to estimate the probabilities of a shortage of 1 unit, 2 units, 3 units, and so forth. The Prob(Shortage ≤ x) for any integer value of x can be computed, which allows one to express the probability of needing the xth unit of protection in any given year as Prob(Shortage ≥ x) = 1 − Prob(Shortage ≤ x−1). Therefore, if H_i is expressed in QALYs, the expected benefit (in units of expected QALYs) of having the xth unit of protection is H_i [1 − Prob(Shortage ≤ x−1)]. Therefore, if H_i is expressed in QALYs, the expected benefit (in units of expected QALYs) of having the xth unit of protection is H_i [1 − Prob(Shortage ≤ x−1)]. If that protection is provided by inventory, then the cost of this extra inventory is simply the cost to hold one unit of inventory for one year, which is conventionally expressed by h_i. This would imply one is paying

$$\frac{h_i}{H_i\left[1 - Prob(Shortage \leq x-1)\right]} \qquad \text{(Equation C-3)}$$

dollars per QALY saved.

If the objective is to save as many QALYs as possible for a given investment budget, then protection targets should be set for the various products on the supply chain critical list so that the cost per QALY is roughly the same. If not, then the implication is that shifting investment from one product to another can increase the reduction in total harm. Deliberate overspending on some products may occur to avoid inequitable risk to certain populations or to provide protection against rare but catastrophic outcomes. Furthermore, it is clear that probability data at a granular level in the real world will almost never be possible. Nevertheless, this technical dive into the analytics of setting protection targets highlights the need for alignment of risks and rewards. For example, if the Strategic National Stockpile holds inventory for two products with similar H_i values but holds an amount equivalent to the 99.9th percentile of the shortage distribution for one product and inventory equivalent to the 50th percentile of the shortage distribution for the other, then there is probably an opportunity to make better use of resources.

An approximate or qualitative version of the above calculation can be useful for products subject to short, frequent shortages. But for products with long, infrequent shortages, even a heuristic version of this calculation is impractical because we must deal with tiny probabilities of major events, where the tiny probabilities are subject to considerable uncertainty. Because of this, it makes sense to approach products with a very low risk of a major disruption by focusing on a single reference event that represents a major emergency, such as a global pandemic. One rationale for this is that whatever measures used to attain a given service level for this major reference event will provide even higher service levels for smaller events. Furthermore, considering a single scenario allows for the disruption factor (F_i) to be fixed, for instance to account for a demand surge that is part of the scenario. This in turn will allow for considering the protection target in terms of the more intuitive weeks of supply (T_i) instead of in terms of volume (X_i).

With a single major reference event in mind, a more narrowly focused risk analysis of the possible outcomes can be made, from best case to worst case, and generate a conditional cumulative probability distribution like that shown in Figure C-2. This distribution is conditional because it assumes the event has happened. Hence, the histogram bars represent the probability that the reference shortage event results in a shortage of t weeks or less (at an adjusted demand level of $F_i D_i$) *given that the trigger event has occurred*. If the event is presumed to have occurred, there is no chance of zero shortage (and hence no histogram bar at the origin). Furthermore, the probabilities represented by the histogram bars will rise steadily to 1 as the values of t traverse the possible durations of the shortage event. The choice

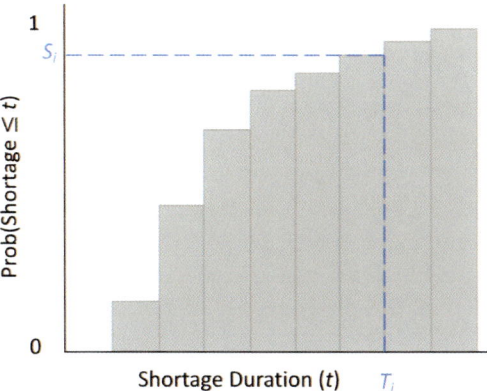

FIGURE C-2 Conditional cumulative probability distributions of shortage duration for a reference scenario.

of a protection time target (T_i) will boil down to deciding the length of a disruption to the supply chain for product i that can be endured without harm to humans.

Note that the histogram bars in any conditional cumulative probability distribution like that depicted in Figure C-2 will equal 1 for all values of t above some level. The reason is that, given sufficient lead time, new production capacity can be brought online. For example, suppose a massive natural disaster destroys a large percentage of the world's capacity for producing N95 masks at the same time a global biological event spikes worldwide demand for masks. Surging demand means the demand fraction adjustment factor (F_i) will be greater than 1, and hence weekly shortfall may well exceed the pre-emergency demand rate. Hence, a very large protection volume target (X_i) will be needed to provide protection for several weeks or months. Nevertheless, if X_i is sized to cover a time period long enough to repair and expand the existing production facilities or to construct new ones, the service level will be 1 (100 percent).

This implies the need to consider existing capabilities for capacity expansion or restoration when deciding on a volume or time protection level for a given product. For example, a trigger event should not be considered a shortage until it exceeds readily available capacity, which includes that from working overtime or scheduling extra shifts. Intermediate lead time capacity must also be accounted for, such as that achieved by hiring and training new workers or repurposing existing facilities to expand capacity, when estimating shortage magnitudes in the risk assessment process. Finally, the time to bring entirely new capacity online as an upper limit on the protection time target must also be accounted for. The framework in Chapter 5 provides a structure for thinking through options for generating capacity that will limit the need to store excessive amounts of inventory as protection against a rare but extreme emergency.

Appendix D

Commissioned Economic Analysis

The committee commissioned one white paper to further their understanding in the economic considerations for enhancing the resilience of medical product supply chains: Ellis, P. 2021. *Where There's a Will: Economic Considerations in Reforming America's Medical Product Supply Chains.* Paper commissioned by the Committee on Security of America's Medical Product Supply Chain.

WHERE THERE'S A WILL: ECONOMIC CONSIDERATIONS IN REFORMING AMERICA'S MEDICAL PRODUCT SUPPLY CHAINS

Philip Ellis, Ph.D.
Consultant to the Committee

November 10, 2021

EXECUTIVE SUMMARY

- For a range of reasons, it is useful to distinguish rather sharply between the issues raised by the shortages of personal protective equipment (PPE) and other supplies that arose during the COVID-19 pandemic, and the issues involved in the persistent supply problems for generic drugs. Simply put, they have different causes, involve different orders of magnitude, and will likely require different solutions.

- Another very important distinction to draw is between the desired level of supply that is needed and the location of the production facilities used to generate that supply. In short, total supply can be increased and supply chains can be made more robust by either domestic or foreign production, so increasing the level of supply does not require moving production to the United States. In general, foreign production will be the less expensive option.
- To help size up the problem, total purchases of PPE in the United States during 2019 were about $5 billion. But PPE use rose 10-fold or more in 2020, and would have increased further except for the PPE shortages that emerged. N95 masks are a useful example, with their use increasing from about 50 million in 2019 to about 600 million in 2020. Firm figures are harder to come by for the generic drugs involved in ongoing shortages, but total demand for these at preshortage prices is probably in the range of $700 million to $1 billion per year; sterile injectable drugs account for a substantial share of the shortage problem. It is worth noting that these are often produced in this country.
- In effect, the benefits of having ample medical supplies can be seen in the cost of not having them. Credible estimates indicate that the lack of adequate PPE in 2020 may have caused between 1,000 and 2,000 deaths from COVID-19 nationwide among health care staff and other essential workers, imposing costs of $5 billion to $10 billion. Other costs, such as those for avoidable hospitalizations, are much smaller, around $300 million. These figures likely understate the costs of PPE shortages. Drug shortages also impose costs but the effects are often harder to quantify.
- Although estimates vary widely, domestically produced PPE and generic drugs would probably cost 20 to 50 percent more than supplies produced abroad. At nonpandemic levels of demand for PPE, that would increase total spending in the United States by $1 billion to $2.5 billion per year. To provide pandemic-level quantities of supplies, spending might have to rise from $50 billion, a 10-fold increase in quantities at prepandemic prices, to between $60 billion and $75 billion when purchased domestically. The incremental cost of domestic production in this scenario could be as much as $10 billion to $25 billion per year, or $5 billion to $12.5 billion for a 6-month supply.
- Maintaining the capacity to meet pandemic levels of demand from domestic suppliers would also seem to present daunting challenges since it is not economical for producers to maintain that capacity absent extensive subsidies or other federal interventions. These same issues arise regarding the option to have a domestic surge capacity that is available to make a substantial contribution to out-

- put in a pandemic. It is also worth remembering that a pandemic that strikes the United States could significantly inhibit domestic production, as could a natural disaster.
- One conclusion I draw is that pandemic-level demand for medical supplies would be met most efficiently by stockpiling large quantities of these supplies. That approach should provide more certainty that the supplies will be available when needed, and will allow those products to be purchased at prices close to nonpandemic levels from less expensive foreign suppliers. Models exist for rotating supplies through storage so that the stockpiled supplies do not become stale or ineffective.
- To address the ongoing problems with shortages of generic drugs, hospitals are already incurring costs because of inefficient workarounds and patchwork efforts undertaken at the last minute. Those costs have been credibly estimated at about $360 million per year, which is about 35 to 50 percent of the annual costs of the shortage of the drugs themselves. It follows that purchasers should be willing to pay prices that are 35 to 50 percent higher in order to ensure a reliable supply of these drugs.
- However, most hospitals and other purchasers have shown, by revealed preference, that they are largely unwilling to pay the extra costs involved in producing more reliable supplies. The federal government will most likely need to take steps to change that behavior, but the optimal approach is unclear, partly owing to limited data.
- To bring about changes in medical product supply chains more generally, the federal government would need to take steps that actually change the incentives facing suppliers and purchasers, through some combination of subsidies for preferred activities or outcomes, penalties for the opposite, or regulations designed to achieve those goals, which in turn will often impose costs on suppliers, purchasers, or both.
- The federal government can also facilitate changes in medical product supply chains by generating more information about the ultimate sources of production for many items, the quality of those products, and the status of existing stockpiles across the country, but by themselves, those steps will not incentivize changes in medical product supply chains.
- Absent such steps, purchasers will gravitate back toward the cheapest sources of supply that provide prepandemic levels of quality and reliability. If that were to happen, our country would be back in the same boat when the next pandemic occurs, which is a matter of when, not if. However, these problems are tractable and another truism also applies: where there is a will, there is a way.

INTRODUCTION

The COVID-19 pandemic has stressed the U.S. health care system in many ways, not least in its ability to provide the medical supplies needed to treat and care for patients in hospitals, doctors' offices, and other settings. Policy makers understandably want to address those problems so that the country is better prepared for the next pandemic, whenever it happens, and for other unexpected events. That focus has also drawn more attention to long-standing problems with the supply of various drugs, mostly generic, which are usually made overseas. A general goal is to make the medical product supply chains that yield those products more reliable and secure.

In both cases, the basic options under discussion include moving more production of medical supplies to domestic sources, an approach known as on-shoring production, or at least creating more capacity to surge domestic production in a crisis. Other primary options are stockpiling more supplies to address shortages when they arise, or continuing to rely on global medical product supply chains but work to make them more robust and less vulnerable to disruption. Still other options may yet emerge in the debate.

When considering the available options, the field of economics, which at root is the study of how scarce resources are allocated, has much to contribute. Each of the options will have its own costs and benefits, and choices among them will often involve trade-offs that policy makers might prefer to avoid confronting. Some costs are easier to identify, such as federal subsidy payments to cover the added costs of buying more reliable supplies or of stockpiling supplies. Other costs are harder to observe, such as those stemming from regulations of suppliers or purchasers that raise their costs, but those are economic costs nonetheless. The goal of this analysis is to spell out as well as possible the key costs, benefits, and trade-offs among the basic options available for making America's medical product supply chains more reliable and secure with quantitative information, if possible.

Economics also tells us that, in general, market forces provide powerful incentives that must be understood and harnessed in the pursuit of policy goals, and not simply ignored. In particular, it stands to reason that current procurement practices are roughly optimal for private buyers and sellers in light of the objectives they have, the incentives they face, and the information available to them. However, those choices may not be socially optimal because buyers and sellers may not take into account costs their actions impose on others or benefits that accrue to others, such as health improvements or reductions in risks to the overall economy or national security. Another lesson from economics is that the last increments of risk reduction are likely to be the most expensive, and that people generally do accept some risks in their daily lives, so seeking to reduce risks is more feasible than trying to eliminate them.

Perhaps the central point economists make is that changing behavior will require changes in the incentives that buyers and sellers face and improving the information available to them, with the incentives being the most important factor. In general, economists would also argue for using market mechanisms to the greatest extent feasible, so that producers can devise the most efficient means of meeting the objectives, whatever they may be. But this statement is not an endorsement of laissez-faire economics; that is, some set of government interventions is needed if we hope to avoid ending up with roughly the same medical product supply chains that we had before the COVID-19 pandemic.

The remainder of this analysis proceeds as follows: the next section reviews key background points about the shortages and supply problems that have emerged both in the COVID-19 pandemic and before it. I then examine the benefits that are likely to accrue from having more reliable medical supplies, benefits that would be common to all of the options, to the extent they achieve that goal. Next, I turn to consider in greater detail the four options mentioned above for changing medical product supply chains, including any quantitative information that is available to help think about the costs of the options and the trade-offs among them. Finally, I examine the economics surrounding the options that policy makers could employ to bring about desired changes in medical product supply chains, including regulations, subsidies, and penalties, as well as improvements in information.

BACKGROUND: THE PROBLEM

The COVID-19 pandemic has highlighted two broad types of problems or challenges with the country's supply chains for medical goods:

- First and foremost, the demand for some products that was needed to address the pandemic itself soared, just as the supply of those products fell because of pandemic-related shutdowns of economic activity around the globe and the associated disruptions of international trade. Shortages of PPE were perhaps the most obvious examples of the gap between demand and supply, but basic and needed drugs such as antibiotics were also scarce.
- Second, the pandemic also shed new light on ongoing problems with certain supplies which both predated that outbreak and are likely to continue into the future unless new policies are implemented to address them. The most notable cases involve generic drugs, some of which are key components of chemotherapy treatments for cancer patients.

In many but not all cases, the problems have involved products that are primarily made overseas. Most of the world, for example, relies heavily on China for supplies of many types of PPE; by some estimates, about 70 percent of U.S. masks and more than half of all its PPE come from China.[1] Most generic drugs are made abroad as well, although important information about their production is simply not available. Before exploring the options for addressing these concerns, it is first necessary to review the problem or problems these options are supposed to solve in order to arrive at an accurate diagnosis. The recent experience with COVID-19 and PPE is fairly familiar, and can be reviewed briefly, whereas the background on shortages of generic drugs is longer and more complex.

A. PPE Shortages and the COVID-19 Pandemic

The pandemic highlighted an important characteristic of current medical product supply chains—a high reliance on foreign producers, especially China. This focus arose in part because the pandemic started in China, so shutdowns of production there had global consequences. But China and other countries also started to hoard their own supplies, in ways both overt and subtle. As a result, just when the demand for PPE started to spike, supplies were actually becoming scarce. This is not to suggest, however, that domestic production of PPE would have prevented the shortages that arose, which were driven more by a sharp increase in demand than by the limits on foreign supplies.

In the ensuing months, shortages worsened, prices for PPE spiked, bidding wars broke out, and the environment was chaotic. Reports abounded of medical personnel reusing their masks and gowns, or even turning to makeshift substitutes, including garbage bags.[2] The Associated Press found that no imports of N95 masks had arrived anywhere in the United States during the month of March 2020.[3]

Rather quickly, the federal government relaxed regulations around PPE use and reuse, and also made it easier to use telehealth as an alternative to in-person visits in order to reduce the need for PPE. The federal government

---

[1] See page 15 of Congressional Research Service, *COVID-19: China Medical Supply Chains and Broader Trade Issues* (updated December 23, 2020), https://crsreports.congress.gov/product/pdf/R/R46304; and "Chinese Share Among Selected U.S. Imports of Medical Supplies and Equipment in 2019," *Statista* (July 20, 2020), https://www.statista.com/statistics/1122414/select-us-imports-from-china-medical-supplies-under-tariff-exclusions/.

[2] Susan Glaser, "How Did the United States End Up with Nurses Wearing Garbage Bags?" *The New Yorker* (April 9, 2020). https://www.newyorker.com/news/letter-from-trumps-washington/the-coronavirus-and-how-the-united-states-ended-up-with-nurses-wearing-garbage-bags.

[3] Juliet Linderman and Martha Mendoza, "First N95 Medical Mask Imports Finally Reaching US," *Associated Press* (March 31, 2020). https://apnews.com/article/health-global-trade-asia-ca-state-wire-virus-outbreak-1d5aff5e3a3970fac857e3ae01e9d321.

also established a "control tower" within the Department of Health and Human Services (HHS). This entity worked with the major U.S. wholesalers through which nearly all PPE are purchased to establish daily monitoring of the demand for—and supply of—these supplies. By the summer of 2020, Chinese supplies had become broadly available again.[4] However, shortages of PPE in the United States persisted for the remainder of 2020 and seem to have extended well into 2021.[5]

In considering the options for dealing more effectively with future pandemics, data on the amount of spending involved are crucial. Some information is available to help size up the U.S. market for PPE and for some specific products, but it is sparse. For N95 masks, publicly available estimates of their use in 2020 vary quite widely, but more reliable information seems to come from the Defense Department, which through its Defense Logistics Agency effectively provided oversight for the market once the pandemic got going. According to those reports, the United States had been using about 50 million N95 masks *per year* prior to the pandemic, but use soared to about 47 million *per month* in the spring of 2020.[6] On an annual basis, that would amount to about 560 million masks. This figure is likely to understate what the demand was in the pandemic because it reflects only the units that were actually sold and delivered at the higher prices which prevailed at the time, not the amounts that hospitals and other purchasers would have wanted to use at the more moderate prices that would have been charged if supplies had been more plentiful.

What were those prices? Public reports on pricing also vary but tend to indicate that N95 masks were going for about $1 each before the pandemic. Thus, total spending in the United States on N95 masks prepandemic was about $50 million. During the pandemic, however, prices reportedly rose to about $7 or $8 per mask. At those prices, 560 million masks would have cost about $4 billion, an 80-fold increase in spending.[7]

More broadly, estimates indicate that total worldwide spending on PPE prior to the pandemic was on the order of $13 billion. The United States

---

[4] Ken Roberts, "China More Dominant Than Ever In Covid-Related 'PPE' — And U.S. Flags," *Forbes* (September 19, 2020). https://www.forbes.com/sites/kenroberts/2020/09/19/china-more-dominant-than-ever-in-covid-related-ppe---and-us-flags/?sh=8f5df4f17f71.

[5] Andrew Jacobs, "Health Care Workers Still Face Daunting Shortages of Masks and Other P.P.E.," *The New York Times* (December 20, 2020). https://www.nytimes.com/2020/12/20/health/covid-ppe-shortages.html.

[6] See Jared Serbu, "Pentagon Says it Needs Billions to Repay Contractors for Employee Leave," *Federal News Network* (June 11, 2020). https://federalnewsnetwork.com/defense-main/2020/06/pentagon-says-it-needs-billions-to-repay-contractors-for-employee-leave/.

[7] Data on PPE prices and spending in this paragraph and the next one drawn from this report: *2020 HIDA Personal Protective Equipment Market Report*, Health Industry Distributors Association (December 2020). https://www.hida.org/distribution/research/market-reports/PPE-Market-Report.aspx.

represents about 40 percent of global spending on all medical care, which would imply that total U.S. spending on PPE was about $5 billion in 2019. Of that total, hospitals spent about $2 billion and doctors' offices and other entities spent about $3 billion. Ideally, more precise figures would be available, but for the time being, these data may have to suffice.

B. Ongoing Problems with Supplies of Generic Drugs

A second set of issues arises around the ongoing problems with medical product supply chains, ones that predated the COVID-19 pandemic and are likely to continue afterwards unless they are addressed in a new way. Those problems primarily involve generic drugs, particularly sterile, injectable drugs. As Figure 1 shows, the number of new drug shortages has generally been higher since 2006, with the average number more than doubling from 81 over the 2001–2006 period to 173 over the 2007–2019 period.[8] The figure also shows that a substantial share of the new shortages in any year involve sterile injectable drugs, even though those drugs constitute a small share of total drug spending.

Observers have identified several factors that contribute to these shortages. Generic drugs generally have very thin profit margins, meaning that producers do not suffer extensive losses during a shortage, and so have limited incentives to avoid them. Indeed, establishing robust supply lines would be more costly, and thus would put a company at a cost disadvantage against its competitors. To minimize costs, production processes for generic drugs are typically very lean, with little margin for error or unexpected events. By contrast, brand-name drugs with patent protection gener-

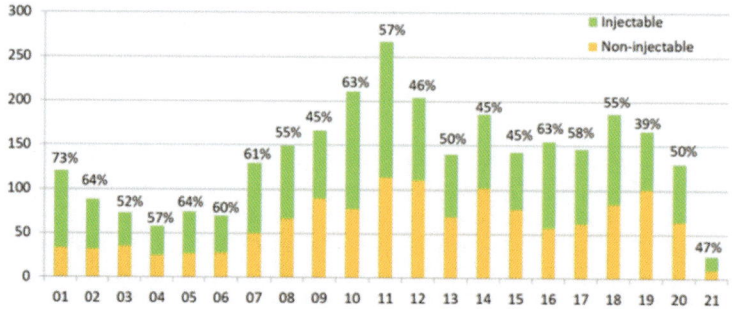

FIGURE 1 National Drug Shortages: New Shortages by Year – Percent Injectable

---

[8] Data and figure drawn from American Society of Health-System Pharmacists, "Drug Shortages Statistics," available at https://www.ashp.org/drug-shortages/shortage-resources/drug-shortages-statistics.

ally have high margins on their unit sales, giving their manufacturers strong incentives to avoid shortages in order to continue making those sales.

Roughly 90 percent of prescriptions filled in the United States are for generic drugs, so these pills account for the vast majority of drug production. As Table 1 shows, the production of both active pharmaceutical ingredients (APIs) and final dosage forms (FDFs) for the U.S. market is usually done overseas. APIs are the key ingredients of drugs, which are then combined with other ingredients and shaped into pills or other forms to be used by patients. An important limitation of those figures, however, is that the U.S. Food and Drug Administration (FDA) has information on where facilities are located, but not on how much is produced at each facility. With that proviso in mind, the United States, Canada, and the European Union collectively account for 43 percent of the facilities for production of APIs and 59 percent of the facilities for production of FDFs.[9]

The same FDA report found the following:

> the number of ongoing drug shortages has recently been increasing after declining from a peak in 2011, and drug shortages have been lasting longer, in some cases more than 8 years. FDA analyzed 163 drugs that went into shortage in the 5-year period between 2013 and 2017. Of the 163 drugs in the sample, 63 percent (103) were drugs administered by injection (sterile injectables) and 67 percent (109) were drugs that have a generic version on the market.[10]

Table 1 Regional Distribution of Facilities Manufacturing Finished Dosage Forms and Active Pharmaceutical Ingredients in 2018

County/Region	Active Pharmaceutical Ingredient	Final Dosage Form
U.S.	12%	37%
Canada	0%	4%
European Union	31%	18%
China	14%	8%
India	31%	24%
Latin America	2%	0%
Rest of World	11%	10%
TOTAL	100%	100%

---

[9] Data in this paragraph and Table 1 drawn from Food and Drug Administration, *Drug Shortages: Root Causes and Potential Solutions* (October 2019; updated February 2020). https://www.fda.gov/drugs/drug-shortages/report-drug-shortages-root-causes-and-potential-solutions.

[10] See page 5 of FDA, Drug Shortages: Root Causes and Potential Solutions.

To an economist, the idea that a true economic shortage could continue for several years, much less 8 years, is hard to believe.[11] One would expect that prices would rise and that existing producers would thus have incentives to resume production and that other companies would find it attractive to start making the product that's in short supply. If the drug is essential for care, demand for the drug should be "inelastic," meaning that purchasers should be willing to pay substantially higher prices in order to bring the quantity supplied close to the preshortage level. As economists say, the cure for high prices is high prices.

But according to FDA's own analysis, that typically does not happen for prescription drugs. Specifically, the agency conducted a study of drugs in shortage and found the following:

- Only 18 percent had a sustained price increase (i.e., an increase of 50 percent or more that began during the shortage and lasted for 6 months).
- Only 42 percent had significant production increases; either new suppliers were entering the market or existing suppliers were increasing production during the shortage to restore at least 50 percent of the unavailable quantity.
- Only 30 percent had the quantity of the drug sold restored to at least 100 percent of its amount prior to the shortage (i.e., after 12 months of being in shortage, or at the end of the shortage if it had already been resolved within 12 months).[12]

These findings would seem to indicate rather modest responses to the shortages, in contrast to the price spikes and production increases that might have been expected. One possible explanation is that doctors and hospitals are able to use other drugs instead when one is in short supply. Certainly, some efforts in that regard go on, and by some estimates those activities costs hospitals about $360 million per year.[13] But in other cases,

---

[11] The term *shortage* can be defined in various ways, and is typically meant to describe a situation in which the quantity demanded exceeds the quantity supplied. This definition is adequate, so long as the quantity demanded truly reflects the most that buyers are willing to pay and not just an abstract expression that buyers would like more supplies, but not if they cost more. For economists, a more precise definition of a shortage is that buyers are willing to pay more than the current cost of production for an item but are unable to purchase that item. If buyers would like to have more, but are not willing to pay more for it, then the correct term is *scarcity*.

[12] See pages 36-37 of FDA, Drug Shortages: Root Causes and Potential Solutions.

[13] Alex Kacik, "Drug Shortages Drain at Least $359M from Health Systems," *Modern Healthcare* (June 26, 2019). https://www.modernhealthcare.com/finance/drug-shortages-drain-least-359m-health-systems.

treatments must be delayed. Data on the extent of those substitutions and delays would be quite useful.

The FDA report itself concludes that, taken together, "these findings lead to the hypothesis that drugs that go into shortage are products that companies may not have a strong financial incentive to market or to produce using mature manufacturing quality management." This finding simply begs the question of why producers lack these financial incentives, and why the drugs go into shortage in the first place. The report states that the market does not foster a reliable supply of generic drugs. But markets are simply made up of people and companies, the buyers and suppliers, and reflect their choices and preferences. To quote Shakespeare, "the fault, dear Brutus, is not in our stars, but in ourselves." For these reasons, I find it difficult to avoid the conclusion that markets do not reward these things because most of the providers that purchase the drugs involved are not actually willing to pay much more for those drugs, at least not enough to cover what it would cost to produce the drugs with substantially fewer quality problems and supply disruptions.

Certainly, there are ways of changing the incentives for drug makers, if the requisite willingness to pay more on the part of buyers exists. An HHS report on drug shortages from 2011 stated the following:

> Private organizations that purchase drugs and vaccines…can help alleviate future shortages by strengthening the failure-to-supply requirements in their contracts in exchange for increases in price. Such contract changes are likely to lead manufacturers to invest in extra capacity of both production lines and API.[14]

Evidently, that approach has gained little traction.

Alternatively, an intermediary company could come forth to serve as a reliable supplier and take on the responsibility of establishing more reliable lines of supply. Such a company was formed in 2018, called Civica Rx, with funding from some major hospitals and health systems as well as three health-focused foundations, which provided about 30 percent of the start-up funding.[15] The company's stated focus is on making generic drugs generally and sterile injectable drugs particularly. To date, that company has been approved to market about 40 different drugs. Precise information on their prices and sales is not available, although industry sources indicate

---

[14] Office of the Assistant Secretary for Planning and Evaluation (ASPE), "Economic Analysis of the Causes of Drug Shortages" (October 2011). https://aspe.hhs.gov/sites/default/files/migrated_legacy_files//57791/ib.pdf.

[15] The Editorial Board, "Pharma Disrupter: Nonprofit Drugmaker Targets Supply, Costs," Pittsburgh Post-Gazette (January 13, 2019). https://www.post-gazette.com/opinion/editorials/2019/01/13/Pharma-disrupter-Nonprofit-drugmaker-targets-supply-costs/stories/201901130087.

that Civica Rx's products are more expensive than those of traditional suppliers of generic drugs. While a promising development, it remains to be seen how well or sustained these efforts or similar initiatives will succeed at reducing shortages.

More broadly, some information is available to try to size up the markets for generic drugs during shortages and for generic sterile injectable drugs; this information should be helpful in thinking about the costs of addressing the supply problems. The HHS report cited above indicates that drugs in shortage typically account for about one-half of 1 percent of all drugs, but did not indicate how much was typically spent on those drugs prior to the shortage. However, if we focus on generic drugs and assume that generic drugs in shortage accounted for the same share of spending as they do for all drugs, we can derive some rough figures. On the basis of my own analysis, I estimate that total outpatient spending in 2019 on all generic drugs (including physician-administered drugs) was about $135 billion. One-half of 1 percent of that amount would be less than $1 billion, or to provide a more precise point estimate, $675 million in that year.

As for sterile injectables that are available in generic form, Medicare enrollees used about $725 million worth of these drugs in 2019. Since Medicare accounts for about 25 or 30 percent of health care spending in the United States, a reasonable extrapolation is that total spending in the United States on these drugs was three to four times Medicare's spending, between $2 billion and $3 billion. Reports have not been clear on what percentage of sterile injectables are in shortage at any one time, but if that were 10 percent then preshortage spending on those drugs would have been around $200 million or $300 million per year, or roughly half of all spending on generic drugs in shortage.

It is worth noting that some additional use of drugs occurs in an inpatient setting, but this spending is difficult to identify because it is generally included in a broader bundled payment to the hospital. At the same time, physician-administered drugs, including those for chemotherapy, are typically given in an outpatient setting and providers receive a separate payment for those drugs that usually exceeds their acquisition cost, at least on average. As a result, more data are available for such spending. These arrangements also mean that hospitals are often *not* required to finance any extra costs for drugs in shortage out of a fixed payment per admission.

THE BENEFITS OF MORE RELIABLE MEDICAL PRODUCT SUPPLY CHAINS

As we consider the benefits of different options for improving the reliability and security of America's medical product supply chains, it is useful and important to distinguish between benefits that may be unique to each of those options on the one hand and benefits associated with improved supply chains generally on the other. The first category is discussed in the next section, where we examine these distinct options. Here we review the benefits that are likely to stem from any of the options. The costs of the options can then be evaluated relative to those benefits, taking into account the likelihood that the option, with sufficient funding in the cost column, will achieve the desired goals.

Some of the benefits of having reliable and robust medical product supply chains will be difficult to quantify. In particular, there may be benefits to national security that stem from being less dependent on or beholden to a given country, but such benefits are inherently hard to measure. Even so, it can be useful to quantify those benefits that can be quantified so an assessment can be made about whether the intangible benefits are likely to be large enough to warrant the costs involved. Even some tangible benefits can be hard to quantify. As discussed above, the COVID-19 pandemic gave rise to shortages of PPE as well as many key drugs, including antibiotics. Because some data were available regarding PPE, I focused on that case rather than the pandemic-related shortages of drugs.

In the case of PPE, the benefits of having reliable supplies were amply illustrated in the spring of 2020 when the opposite occurred, and demand for PPE greatly outstripped supply. Focusing on items such as masks, gloves, and gowns, and their use by health care workers and other essential personnel, one can envision the following principal risks that arose as a result of inadequate supplies:

- Greater risk of transmitting the virus to hospital patients who were *not* admitted with COVID-19, increasing their risk of developing a serious case and risk of death
- Greater risk of transmitting the virus among hospital staff, which not only poses health risks for those people but also makes them more likely to miss work, which in turn reduces the capacity of the health care system to exacerbate bottlenecks in patient care
- Greater perception of risk among the general public about seeking medical care, which may lead them to forego other necessary services. For example, a particularly troubling statistic from early in the pandemic was that the number of emergency room visits for strokes or heart attacks declined by roughly 40 percent.[16] There is no reason to believe those underlying medical events happened less often.

---

[16] Lenny Bernstein and Frances Stead Sellers, "Patients with Heart Attacks, Strokes and Even Appendicitis Vanish from Hospitals," *The Washington Post* (April 19, 2020). https://www.washingtonpost.com/health/patients-with-heart-attacks-strokes-and-even-appendicitis-vanish-from-hospitals/2020/04/19/9ca3ef24-7eb4-11ea-9040-68981f488eed_story.html.

A study from 2020 provides some data with which to quantify some of the benefits. The government of California tracked COVID-19 infections and deaths among health care workers, allowing some calculations to be made regarding the effect of limited PPE supplies, which I then extrapolated to the country as a whole.[17] Specifically, I applied the ratios from California to national data about the pandemic through the end of November 2020, which roughly corresponds to the period in which PPE supplies were most constrained. The figures indicate that about 600,000 cases of COVID-19 occurred among health care workers nationwide over that period, resulting in roughly 3,000 deaths.[18]

The authors of the study estimated that about one-third of those cases could have been prevented if PPE had been readily available. Thus, about 200,000 cases of COVID-19 among health care workers could arguably have been avoided, along with about 1,000 deaths. If the analysis were extended to other essential workers, who also lacked for supplies of PPE, those figures would roughly double to about 400,000 avoidable cases of COVID-19 and 2,000 avoidable deaths. Even if ample supplies of PPE would have prevented only half as many cases and deaths as the authors estimated, the effect would be substantial. Assuming that a statistical life for working-age people is worth $5 million, or about $125,000 per year, the cost to society of 1,000 deaths would be $5 billion and the cost of 2,000 deaths would be $10 billion.

In addition to avoiding deaths among essential workers, substantial costs for pandemic-induced hospitalizations also could have been averted with proper supplies of PPE. Based on the study of California cited above, I estimate that through November 2020 there were about 10,000 hospitalizations nationwide among health care workers and other essential workers that could have been avoided with plentiful supplies of PPE. In making that calculation, I estimated that the COVID-19 hospitalization rate among non-elderly adults was about 2.5 percent. Estimates of the average costs of hospitalizations for COVID-19 vary, but several analyses point to an average cost of about $20,000 per admission.[19] Using that figure yields an estimated national cost of about $200 million for avoidable hospitalizations among health care workers and other essential workers. Even if the actual number

---

[17] William Dow, Kevin Lee, and Laurel Lucia, *Economic and Health Benefits of a PPE Stockpile* (August 12, 2020). https://laborcenter.berkeley.edu/economic-and-health-benefits-of-a-ppe-stockpile/.

[18] See also https://www.theguardian.com/us-news/ng-interactive/2020/aug/11/lost-on-the-frontline-covid-19-coronavirus-us-healthcare-workers-deaths-database.

[19] See Krutika Amin and Cynthia Cox, "Unvaccinated COVID-19 Hospitalizations Cost Billions of Dollars," Peterson-KFF Health System Tracker (September 14, 2021), https://www.healthsystemtracker.org/brief/unvaccinated-covid-patients-cost-the-u-s-health-system-billions-of-dollars/; and FAIR Health, *Key Characteristics of COVID-19 Patients* (July 14,2020), https://www.fairhealth.org/article/fourth-covid-19-study-from-fair-health-examines-patient-characteristics.

were half of that estimate, the costs are considerable. And that analysis does not take into account the effect on hospital patients stemming from the spread of the coronavirus that is attributable to a supply shortage of PPE.

Less information is available to quantify the overall costs of ongoing supply problems involving generic drugs and the benefits of avoiding those problems, but some data points do exist. One study of a shortage of norepinephrine found that hospital death rates from septic shock increased by about 10 percent, or 3.7 percentage points, as a result.[20] The 2019 FDA report on drug shortages noted that affected patients "may experience treatment delays, receive alternative treatments that are not as effective or well tolerated, or may have to forgo treatment" and cited several specific examples. As noted earlier, a recent study estimated that costs to hospitals dealing with drug shortages were about $360 million per year.

These benefits would stem from any approach that achieves the objective of having reliable medical product supply chains, or at least, those that are substantially more reliable than the current arrangements. As a result, the key question in evaluating the options for strengthening these medical product supply chains is not what the benefits will be, but what are the chances that the option in question will yield the desired increase in reliability. Perhaps a better way to frame the issue is to say that each of the options below has *some* probability of making the supply chains "substantially" more reliable. The expected benefits of each option are, in the simplest terms, the benefits of that increase in reliability times the probability of achieving that increase via the option. Then those expected benefits can be weighed against the expected costs.

CHANGING MEDICAL PRODUCT SUPPLY CHAINS: A MENU OF OPTIONS AND TRADE-OFFS

The country has a number of options or approaches that it could pursue to improve the security and reliability of its medical product supply chains. At least for analytic purposes, it is useful to distinguish between the direct changes to the supply chains and the policies that are designed to bring about or encourage those changes. This section focuses on the direct changes. The subsequent section focuses on policy options to support those changes, which could include

- subsidies for purchasing supplies that have a more robust supply chain and penalties for failing to do so;

---

[20] Emily Vail and others, "Association Between US Norepinephrine Shortage and Mortality Among Patients with Septic Shock," Journal of the American Medical Association, vol. 317, no. 14 (April 11, 2017). https://jamanetwork.com/journals/jama/fullarticle/2612912.

- temporary or permanent changes in regulations affecting the supply of, demand for, and price of these products; and
- improvements to the information available to purchasers as well as suppliers.

However, I will defer discussion of these measures until the changes that they would be designed to encourage are examined more fully.

Direct changes to the supply chains can be arrayed on something of a continuum, as follows:

a. On-shoring of production;
b. Creating or arranging for domestic surge capacity;
c. Stockpiling supplies; and
d. Making global medical product supply chains more diverse and robust.

The differences across those options largely involve how much production capacity or supply would be shifted to domestic locations. On-shoring would obviously involve the highest shift of production locations, though even within that broad approach, there are a range of options regarding the extent to which medical product supply chains are made domestic. For example, on-shoring could occur only for the final assembly of supplies or could instead encompass all or most stages of the production process. At the other end of the spectrum, steps could be taken to make medical product supply chains more robust without moving any additional production capacity or supplies on-shore, for example, by spreading capacity across more global locations to limit the risk of specific bottlenecks or disruptions. The second and third options represent something of a middle ground, with steady levels of supply being provided largely as they have been, but with added measures taken to ensure that supplies are available domestically in case of a disruption or shortage.

Those options are not mutually exclusive; indeed, even for a given product, a combination of approaches could be used. For example, the United States could increase its stockpile of N95 masks at the same time that it takes steps to diversify its ongoing sources of supply. And depending on the particular mix of costs and benefits involved, different approaches may be more appropriate for different types of supplies. For example, some prescription drugs may expire or lose effectiveness rapidly enough that stockpiling would be useful only on a limited basis, if at all, while others may require raw materials or other input that would not be feasible to produce domestically. As a general rule, it may be best to think of all the real policy options as involving a combination of approaches in order to have a comprehensive approach for improving the robustness of medical product supply chains. Or, as the saying goes, don't put all of your eggs in one basket.

Another very important distinction to emphasize is to distinguish between the desired level of supply that is needed and the location of the production facilities that are used to generate that supply. Just because policy makers may conclude that more capacity is needed to produce more supplies in response to a pandemic-style spike in demand, it does not mean that such capacity has to be created domestically. In principle, global medical product supply chains could be made more diverse, primarily to guard against supply shocks, and at the same time more extensive, primarily to accommodate demand shocks.

Ideally, the choice of approaches used, and the particular policy levers employed to pursue those approaches, would be informed by a careful consideration of the costs and benefits involved. Some benefits, such as increased national security, may be difficult or impossible to quantify in any precise way. Potentially, those intangible benefits could still be compared to the economic effect that can be quantified to allow policy makers to make informed decisions about whether the net benefits of a given option are likely to be sufficient or not. Unfortunately, it has proven difficult to develop even rudimentary estimates of many of the costs or benefits involved because of the lack of data.

A. On-Shoring Production

The economic debate about on-shoring can essentially be reduced to two key questions. First, how much more would it cost to produce medical supplies domestically? Second, to what extent would on-shoring actually solve the problem of supply disruptions or shortages? Both sets of information are crucial for determining whether the costs of on-shoring will outweigh the benefits, but unfortunately very little information is publicly available about how costs compare between domestic and foreign production, or about the quantitative increase in reliability that would come from on-shoring. Obviously, the answers will depend mainly on the nature of the product itself, and on the extent of the production process that is brought on shore.

Costs of On-Shoring. The stages of the production process will vary by the type of product being produced, but a useful distinction can be seen in the process for making prescription drugs. In that process, the API may be produced in one location, but inactive ingredients may come from other sources, which are then combined into FDFs that have a particular shape, color, strength, form, and dosage. That latter step is sometimes referred to as the fill-and-finish stage of the production process.

Clearly the costs of any on-shoring efforts would depend on whether the entire production process, including the supply of raw materials, would be made domestic, but distressingly little information is available about the cost of the production of medical supplies, much less how these costs break down by stage. Naturally, it would be less costly to on-shore the fill-and-finish stage of production, but at the same time concerns about relying on foreign suppliers would be addressed only modestly by such a step; disruptions in the supply of APIs or other inputs could still create shortages. These issues would also be relevant for any proposals to require or encourage U.S. purchasers to "Buy American" because a reasonably precise definition would have to be established for what counts as domestic production of these medical supplies.

One limited exception to the rule of data scarcity about production costs for medical supplies concerns N95 masks, where at least some data are available. Discussions with industry experts indicate that domestically produced N95 masks might need to be priced only 20 to 30 percent higher than masks produced in China to be profitable. A recent press report also indicated that production costs for N95 masks are about 25 cents, on average, in China, but can be more than double that amount in the United States.[21] Despite indicating a wide range of possibilities, these two data points may actually be compatible, since masks produced in China will have additional costs for transportation to the United States that would make the aggregate costs of supply less disparate between the two countries than their respective costs of production might indicate.

Another helpful data point was provided in the Biden administration's recent report on building resilient medical product supply chains. The report, citing an FDA study from 2011, indicated that the production of APIs in India could reduce costs by 30 to 40 percent compared with production costs in the United States or Europe.[22] In other words, production of APIs in the United States would cost about 50 percent more than production in India. This explains why the production of most of these supplies has shifted overseas, given that purchasers seem to value low prices for medical supplies and have evidently found their associated levels of quality and reliability to be acceptable at those prices.

A related point worth noting about the economics of on-shoring is that the cost figures suggest a smaller role for differences in labor costs across the counties than might be anticipated. The Biden administration's report also noted, citing a 2009 study by the World Bank, that overall labor costs in China and India are about 8 and 10 percent, respectively, of labor costs

---

[21] Monika Evstatieva, "U.S. Companies Shifted to Make N95 Respirators During COVID. Now, They're Struggling," National Public Radio (June 25, 2021). https://www.npr.org/2021/06/25/1009858893/u-s-companies-shifted-to-make-n95-respirators-during-covid-now-theyre-struggling.

[22] See page 215 of *Building Resilient Supply Chains, Revitalizing American Manufacturing, And Fostering Broad-Based Growth* (June 2021). https://www.whitehouse.gov/wp-content/uploads/2021/06/100-day-supply-chain-review-report.pdf.

in typical Western countries.[23] Therefore, U.S. labor costs are about 10 times higher than those in China and India. U.S. production costs, on the other hand, at least for some products, are only two times higher, perhaps less. What accounts for the difference? Presumably, the manufacturing process in the United States uses much less labor and much more capital and equipment, including robots and other forms of automation. That inference makes perfect sense from an economic perspective, with U.S.-based production methods substituting relatively cheap machines for relatively expensive workers.

How much would those subsidies cost? As indicated above, the United States typically buys about 50 million N95 masks per year, at a total cost of about $50 million. Hypothetically, a 50 percent increase in those costs would raise spending on N95 masks by about $25 million per year. To subsidize the extra costs of pandemic-type levels of demand would necessarily be more expensive. Covering the added expenses for domestic production of 500 million masks would cost $250 million if the average incremental cost was 50 cents per mask. If that added cost were $1 per mask (a doubling of the price) and 1 billion masks were needed, then subsidies would run to $1 billion. An increase in average costs of 50 percent at nonpandemic levels of demand would thus increase nationwide spending on PPE by about $2.5 billion per year, with $1 billion attributable to hospitals and $1.5 billion to other purchasers.

Another point concerning on-shoring indicates that its costs are probably too high to be sustainable without some form of government subsidies. The economics of such subsidies are discussed in more detail in the next section. This inference is based on developments with the N95 mask, when the Defense Department contracted in mid-2020 to quickly increase domestic production to roughly one billion units per year. Companies responded and built capacity accordingly, but now that the total demand for masks has dropped and foreign supplies are available again, these very companies are having to lay off workers and close down production lines.[24] Absent federal financial support or other interventions that make it optimal for purchasers to obtain most or all of their supplies from domestic sources, the United States is likely headed back to the same situation that existed prior to the pandemic in fairly short order regarding medical supplies.

Some argue that new production methods, such as continuous production processes, will make domestic production more competitive or

---

[23] See pages 214-215 of *Building Resilient Supply Chains*. I have assumed that the underlying analysis controlled for average differences across the countries in skill levels – that is, in the mix of jobs.

[24] Timoth Aeppel, "America's Mask Makers Face Post-Pandemic Meltdown," *Reuters* (May 11, 2021). https://www.reuters.com/business/healthcare-pharmaceuticals/americas-mask-makers-face-post-pandemic-meltdown-2021-05-11/.

perhaps even less costly than foreign production. While that is theoretically possible, it would generally be more efficient to let the market work out the best way to produce a given quantity of medical supplies, given the incentives for such production. In my opinion, federal efforts to invest in specific new production technologies that are aimed at making domestic manufacturing more competitive are probably misguided, or are, at the least, an inefficient use of federal resources. As economist Larry Summers reportedly observed in 2011 when he was serving as the head of President Obama's National Economic Council, the government is generally not a very good venture capitalist.[25]

Benefits of On-Shoring. The second key consideration regarding on-shoring is to determine what the benefits would be. In particular, the central question is whether and to what extent on-shoring would actually solve the supply problems that exist, either with the ongoing issues concerning generic drugs or future pandemic-style spikes in demand and drops in supply.

An important point on this dimension was contained in the Biden administration's recent report highlighting the fact that domestic production is by no means a panacea. The report noted that the majority of drug shortages over the past decade have been for sterile injectable drugs, a relatively small subset of drugs. Furthermore, the report acknowledged that the problem "is not necessarily an issue of foreign manufacturing because much of the infrastructure for sterile injectable manufacturing is located in the United States owing to the high costs of transporting liquids that often require climate control."[26] In other words, natural disasters, pandemics, and other surprises can also disrupt a domestic medical product supply chain. Supply disruptions have happened often with sterile injectable drugs even though their production has been completed on shore.

Moreover, on-shoring may be a solution that is poorly suited in the case of a pandemic that is acutely affecting the United States, since that same pandemic could easily cause workforce or supply disruptions for domestic manufacturers just as domestic demand for medical supplies is increasing. By itself, on-shoring can create many of the same risks of having "all of your eggs in one basket" as exists currently by relying so extensively on China for many medical supplies. In that light, I will analyze other options for changing medical product supply chains.

---

[25] Roberta Rampton and Mark Hosenball, "In Solyndra Note, Summers Said Feds 'Crappy' Investor," *Reuters* (October 3, 2011). https://www.reuters.com/article/us-solyndra/in-solyndra-note-summers-said-feds-crappy-investor-idUSTRE7925C520111003.

[26] See page 223 of Building Resilient Supply Chains.

B. Creating Domestic Surge Capacity

An alternative to on-shoring all production of various medical supplies is to create surge capacity to produce them domestically only when a shortage or disruption arises. A historical analogy for this approach would be its role as "arsenal of democracy" that the United States played during World War II, with arms production ramping up over several years from practically nothing to high levels of output. In principle, this approach would be less expensive than on-shoring all production because typical levels of demand would still be met using lower-cost foreign sources of supply. The option to create or rely on surge capacity located in other countries is discussed below in the section on diversifying global medical product supply chains. Just how feasible a strategy it is, particularly if demand jumps 10-fold or more during a pandemic, and how costly it would be are unclear.

In economic terms, the two key questions about this option are first, how to maintain surge capacity during times of normal demand, and second, how to be confident that the surge capacity can actually surge when it is needed. On the second point, a further question is whether enough of the right types of labor and equipment would be available for a production surge. Some observers have noted that in the lead-up to World War II, the United States still had substantial numbers of workers who were unemployed or underemployed stemming from the Great Depression who could be put to work on defense production. Indeed, it was the wartime production surge that finally brought the Great Depression to an end. In the case of a pandemic, such an army of the unemployed may not be available. Also, the amount of labor needed to produce PPE would probably be limited as well, but as we saw in 2020, many workers of various skill levels became unemployed during the pandemic and might be available to make PPE.

Rather than wondering whether surge capacity can arise, a better way to frame that issue is to ask: how long would it take for any surge capacity to be available, given the need to assemble the necessary inputs, and how much could policy initiatives affect that timing? Experience from the COVID-19 pandemic sheds some light on those questions. A number of companies were able to start producing masks and other PPE within a few months of the pandemic's outbreak. In some cases, that added production was timely enough to help ameliorate the shortage, but in other cases the companies were not able to bring their capacity online in substantial amounts until other sources had largely filled the gap.

Importantly, one of the factors that helps bring forth surge capacity is the increase in prices that typically stems from a shortage. As noted above, prices for N95 masks grew from about $1 each to about $8 each at the peak of the shortage. But that phenomenon means that items bought during the surge will typically be substantially more expensive than items bought when demand is at normal levels. To a certain extent, surge capacity will occur naturally, at least for PPE. As prices rise, more companies will find it economically feasible to enter into production or they will shift existing production lines that make similar products as that of PPE. We have seen this to a certain extent during the COVID-19 pandemic. For drugs, however, the requirements for FDA approval of production facilities, intended to ensure that the drugs those facilities produce are safe, makes it very difficult to enter the market during a shortage or shift production from other types of drugs to those in that are in shortage.

A policy option to encourage or force such shifts is the Defense Production Act (DPA), which essentially allows the federal government to commandeer production facilities in times of national emergency.[27] According to many press reports, the Trump administration was somewhat reluctant to invoke the DPA, often preferring to work out voluntary arrangements with the appropriate firms. Even so, the threat of temporary nationalization presumably encouraged those companies to show flexibility. These experiences also suggest that at least 3 months, and more likely 6 to 9 months, may be needed to ramp up production of PPE by domestic sources.

In any event, all of these issues lead back to the central question of how to foster or support enough surge capacity in times of normal demand when that capacity is not needed. The closer to being ready these facilities are, the less time would be needed to ramp up production when needed, despite the higher the costs of maintaining that surge capacity in the interim. As an example, one option would be for companies to maintain excess capacity and run their plants at, say, 50 percent of their potential output. That would help to ensure that output could be expanded quickly when necessary.[28] However, this would obviously be costly, so producers would need to be paid extra to do so, roughly double, in this case. Even then, the question of how they would obtain twice the raw materials they would normally use in order to double their output would remain. If output were to increase 10-fold, the economics of maintaining surge capacity would become more daunting still. The same issues arise when considering surge capacity in locations overseas, but at a lower level of spending because production costs are lower overseas.

---

[27] The Defense Production Act became law in 1950. Rather famously, President Truman's effort in 1952 to seize control of domestic steel mills during the Korean War was rebuffed by the Supreme Court. See Steve Hendrix, "Truman Declared an Emergency When He Felt Thwarted. Trump Should Know: It Didn't End Well," *The Washington Post* (January 11, 2019). https://www.washingtonpost.com/history/2019/01/08/truman-declared-an-emergency-when-he-felt-thwarted-trump-should-know-it-didnt-end-well/.

[28] The United States and most other countries essentially do this with their militaries, maintaining much larger forces than are needed on a routine basis so as to have the ability to respond quickly to a crisis.

C. Stockpiling Supplies

Rather than maintaining surplus production capacity that could be surged, an obvious alternative would be to maintain actual surplus supplies that could be drawn upon in a shortage, particularly a large-scale one induced by a future pandemic. An analogy would be like saving for a rainy day, or perhaps a bird in the hand being worth two in the bush. A major advantage of this approach is that PPE and other supplies could be purchased from existing suppliers at roughly nonpandemic price levels. The obvious downsides of this approach, from an economic perspective, are the storage costs that have to be incurred in the interim, and the risk that the amounts stockpiled will either be too large, implying a waste of some resources, or too small, necessitating a surge in production or other measures. Even in these cases, however, addressing a given shortage would be easier than it would be in the absence of such a stockpile.

Background on Stockpiling. The federal government had already established a Strategic National Stockpile (SNS) containing PPE, certain drugs, and other supplies deemed essential. However, those stockpiles were drained early in the pandemic, and some of the products it contained were found to be ineffective or expired.[29] New targets have been set for the SNS, and these figures, along with the stockpiled inventories at recent points, are shown in Table 2. For reasons that are not clear, the most recent data on the contents of the stockpile that were available as of this writing is from May 21, 2021, nearly 6 months ago.[30]

TABLE 2 PPE in the Strategic National Stockpile (Millions of Items)

Product	Inventory on 2/26/21	Inventory on 5/21/21	Planned 90-day Inventory	5/21/21 as Percent of Planned
Surgical/Exam Gloves	227	516	4,500	11.5%
N95 Respirators	307	424	300	141.3%
Surgical/Face Masks	411	273	400	68.3%
Surgical Gowns & Coveralls	66	17	265	6.4%
Goggles & Face Shields	18	20	18	111.1%

---

[29] Nick Miroff, "Protective Gear in National Stockpile is Nearly Depleted, DHS Officials Say," *The Seattle Times* (April 1, 2020). https://www.seattletimes.com/nation-world/protective-gear-in-national-stockpile-is-nearly-depleted-dhs-officials-say/.

[30] See https://www.phe.gov/about/sns/COVID/Pages/personal-protective-equipment.aspx.

As the table shows, the SNS held more than the target amount of certain PPE items, particularly N95 masks, but far less than other targets, particularly for surgical gowns. Also, SNS holdings increased between February and May for some items and decreased for others. The budget to operate and maintain the SNS in 2020 and 2021 was about $700 million per year; the Biden administration has requested about $900 million for 2022.[31] Those budgetary figures do not include any additional appropriations that may have been provided through pandemic-related legislation in 2020 or 2021.

The target amounts for the SNS have been described as "90-day inventories," but I was not able to determine how these targets were set, and in particular, what use rate was assumed in setting those targets. The target of 300 million N95 masks corresponds to annual usage of 1.2 billion masks, which is in the range of the quantity that would probably have been demanded in 2020, absent major supply constraints. But that target appears to have been set as early as February 2020, before the pandemic really began in earnest.

One important consideration regarding the federal government's decisions about the extent of stockpiling is that state and local governments as well as medical providers themselves are likely to increase their stockpiles of PPE, at least for some period of time. Data on these activities are also hard to come by, but a survey by the National Governors Association in 2020 found that 9 out of 12 states surveyed indicated that they planned to increase their stockpiles, and 5 of those states intended to maintain a 90-day level of supply.[32] Importantly, those levels of supply would be based on use rates observed in the pandemic. Another source indicated that 18 states aimed to maintain at least a 90-day supply of PPE, and another 10 states aimed to maintain at least a 30-day supply.[33] Unfortunately, information was not available about the use rates used to develop the 90-day requirement for the level of those supplies.

Costs of Stockpiling. As stated previously, finding data on the costs involved in stockpiling PPE and other key medical supplies was difficult. Nevertheless, there are a few available data points that may be informative.

The first one is the budget of the SNS itself. As indicated above, the budget to maintain a 90-day supply of PPE at pandemic-level use rates is about $900 million per year. This implies that doubling the size of the SNS to hold a 6-month supply would cost roughly $1 billion per year, or

---

[31] Additional information about the SNS budget is here: https://www.phe.gov/about/aspr/Pages/Budget.aspx.

[32] National Governors Association, *Strategies to Address the Need for Personal Protective Equipment as States Gradually Reopen* (July 28, 2020). https://www.nga.org/center/publications/ppe-reopening-covid19/.

[33] See page 17 of the 2020 HIDA Personal Protective Equipment Market Report.

perhaps less, to the extent that the existing budget would reflect some fixed costs of simply having an SNS in the first place. Another data point comes from England, where press reports indicate that PPE storage is costing the government about £1 million per day.[34] Conversion to dollars and adjusting for the fact that the U.S. population is about five times larger, that translates into $2.5 billion per year in storage costs.

A third and somewhat more obscure data point comes from Taiwan, which, like many countries, has also maintained a stockpile of PPE and other supplies prior to the COVID pandemic. About 10 years ago, Taiwan adopted a replacement model for its reserves of supplies, in which the oldest stock is sold off on a continuing basis, thus keeping the stockpiled supplies fresh. According to one analysis of that model,

> The Taiwan CDC adopted a more economical and efficient way to refresh the stockpile, in which it pays the private contractors only a service fee instead of new products' purchase cost. The service fee includes the manual and the computational process the contractors need to refresh the stockpile, which is less than the original purchasing cost, because the contractors could further sell the replaced stockpile to domestic institutions through the joint e-purchasing platform or to other countries through their own channels of distribution.[35]

Specifically, the authors estimated that the service fee for surgical masks was only 27 percent of the purchase price for those items; for N95 respirators, the fee was 46 percent of the purchase price, and for surgical gowns, it was 34 percent of the original price.

A final economic consideration regarding the option to stockpile PPE and other supplies is that the costs of that option will largely be the same regardless of whether the federal government maintains the stockpile itself or imposes stockpiling requirements on states or on health care providers. While there could be some economies of scale that make federal control of the stockpile advantageous, as with the SNS model, there could also be some advantages to local control of stockpiles and associated innovations in stockpile management. At the same time, a stockpile that is federally controlled could more easily be directed to areas of the country where the need for supplies is most acute. From an economic standpoint, a combination of local and national stockpiles would be ideal, and the most efficient.

---

[34] Katherine Rushton, Sophie Barnes, and Laura Donnelly, "Government Paying £1M a Day to Store Mountain of PPE," *The Telegraph* (November 22, 2020). https://www.telegraph.co.uk/news/2020/11/22/government-paying-1m-day-store-mountain-ppe-nhs-staff-still/.

[35] Yu-Ju Chen and others, "Stockpile Model of Personal Protective Equipment in Taiwan," *Health Security*, vol. 15, no. 2 (April 2017). https://www.ncbi.nlm.nih.gov/pmc/articles/PMC5404251/.

C. Diversifying Global Medical Product Supply Chains

Probably the least expensive option for expanding the capacity and improving the reliability of medical product supply chains is to continue purchasing supplies from other countries, while diversifying the specific sources used in order to reduce the risk that a single disaster, breakdown, or political event could disrupt supplies. However, keeping track of these medical product supply chains to ensure they remain robust under various scenarios may be challenging. In principle, treaties or other agreements could be reached in advance so countries do not hoard supplies in a future pandemic, but these agreements could be difficult to enforce, and the parties may prefer to violate the agreements first and deal with the consequences afterwards.

Costs of Diversification. It is obvious that purchasing PPE and other medical supplies from foreign suppliers is less expensive than purchasing from domestic producers, which is why most PPE presently comes from abroad, where labor costs are lower. At the same time, diversifying medical product supply chains so supplies come from a broader set of companies, countries, or regions will cost somewhat more than current supplies; if it did not cost more, the supply chain would probably be more diversified already. In other words, the current suppliers and their supply chains are probably the least expensive sources of medical supplies at the quality and reliability levels observed today. If we were to want more suppliers or higher-quality supplies, or both, it would necessitate an increase in prices of at least a few percentage points. Unfortunately, data on the costs of such options are unavailable to me.

A related consideration is how to monitor the resiliency of medical product supply chains and to assess the costs of that monitoring. My understanding is that FDA has the theoretical obligation or right to inspect foreign production facilities used to make products bound for the U.S. market. In practice, however, the costs and challenges of sending inspectors abroad have proven to a barrier, so those inspections have been few and far between. Apparently, FDA cannot or does not hire local workers to carry out such inspections; the reason why is not clear. One option is simply to increase funding for those activities. As discussed in the next section, however, other options include having FDA move away from its focus on approving production facilities and instead focus on testing the products that are imported for quality, which will encourage producers to take steps to improve the quality and reliability of their supplies.

The Role of International Agreements. Another set of steps that could be taken to help improve the reliability of global medical product supply chains would be to establish agreements or treaties to help govern activities in the next pandemic and to manage ongoing medical product supply chains. Such agreements could include penalties that would raise the cost of hoarding supplies by allowing importers to apply tariffs. These pacts could also provide a structure for managing global production chains in an emergency.

However, arranging for international cooperation is easier said than done. Nations are essentially autonomous, acting largely in their perceived self-interest, and the ties between the developed countries that mostly buy medical supplies and the developing countries that mostly make them are weak. In a crisis, or when they perceive their national interests to be at odds with the interests of the larger group, nations have a strong tendency to put their own interests first, ahead of any treaty obligations that would obligate them to cooperate.

This challenge has been discussed extensively in other contexts, particularly in the area of international relations and security studies. Robert Jervis, a professor of political science at Columbia University, began his classic article entitled "Cooperation Under the Security Dilemma" in the following way:

> The lack of an international sovereign not only permits wars to occur, but also makes it difficult for states that are satisfied with the status quo to arrive at goals that they recognize as being in their common interest. Because there are no institutions or authorities that can make and enforce international laws, the policies of cooperation that will bring mutual rewards if others cooperate may bring disaster if they do not. Because states are aware of this, anarchy encourages behavior that leaves all concerned worse off than they could be, even in the extreme case in which all states would like to freeze the status quo.[36]

While Jervis was focused on a situation in which nations wanted to maintain the status quo—peace—with a focus on nuclear arms control, the same issues arise when trying to cooperate to improve upon the status quo with respect to global medical product supply chains.

For their part, economists will recognize these concerns as practical examples of the "prisoners' dilemma" scenario. In this scenario, two prisoners have been arrested for a crime they committed together. The prisoners involved would be better off if they could cooperate with each other and say nothing to the police. But each prisoner is tempted to cheat on the other by turning state's evidence in order to gain a short-term advantage or to hedge against cheating by the other prisoner. The equilibrium result is that they both fink on each other; a poor outcome, from the prisoners'

---

[36] Robert Jervis, "Cooperation Under the Security Dilemma," *World Politics*, vol. 30, no. 2 (January 1978). http://www.sfu.ca/~kawasaki/Jervis%20Cooperation.pdf.

perspective, with a longer sentence for both than they would have achieved if they had both stayed silent. In some versions, the prisoners are unable to communicate, but the same basic result holds if they are unable to credibly commit to keeping mum.

Of course, such situations are not hopeless, as shown by the substantial number and scope of international agreements, particularly regarding trade. In general, game theorists have shown that repeated interactions tend to increase the odds of cooperative outcomes. Even so, disputes can go unresolved for many years, as evident in many long-standing disagreements between China and other countries regarding unfair trading practices, currency manipulation, and the protection of intellectual property rights. Simply put, pandemics that may occur years apart could be too infrequent to prevent countries from focusing heavily on the crisis that is at hand and ignoring concerns about dealing with the next crisis at some future point; that is, myopia would prevail. In any event, agreements related to medical product supply chains are likely to take many years to hammer out.

D. Quantifying Some Comparisons Across Options

Although data limitations make it difficult to quantify many of the trade-offs between these options, some useful calculations can still be made. In particular, it is feasible to illustrate some of the break-even points that exist as well as the sensitivity of those findings to different values of the key economic factors involved. Probably the most useful cases to illustrate are those involving the country's preparedness for similar COVID-19 global pandemic. If the medical product supply chains were able to handle that set of circumstances, they would almost certainly be able to address less cataclysmic events such as natural disasters or regional health crises.

A specific question of interest is whether and under what circumstances it may be less expensive to stockpile supplies that are made abroad than to move production on shore. In the case of N95 masks, the information cited above indicates that domestic production would be about 50 percent more expensive. Stockpiling would allow the supplies themselves to be purchased at lower prices, but would also incur some ongoing costs for storage. Industry sources suggest that such costs are about 15 percent of the value of the inventory being stockpiled.

Now let us consider the costs of procuring a 6-month supply of N95 masks via on-shoring or stockpiling, that is, a 6-month supply to satisfy pandemic-type levels of demand. In the absence of major supply constraints, or equivalently at prices close to the prepandemic average price of $1 per mask, usage might be about 100 million masks per month, or 1.2 billion per year. A 6-month supply would be 600 million N95 masks, or double the current target level for the SNS. The cost of domestic production would be

(1) $1.50 per mask * 50 million masks = $75 million per year
(2) $1.50 per mask * 600 million masks = $900 million
(3) $Z = Annual cost of maintaining domestic surge capacity for 600 million masks

The first expression captures that annual cost of meeting nonpandemic demand levels at domestic prices; the second is the cost of buying the masks needed when the pandemic hits; the third term reflects the annual cost of maintaining domestic surge capacity so that supplies can be ramped up from 50 million per year to 100 million per month when the next pandemic hits.

If instead, masks were purchased from foreign sources and stockpiled, the three corresponding terms would be as follows, with the third term here representing storage costs:

(4) $1.00 per mask * 50 million masks = $50 million per year
(5) $1.00 per mask * 600 million masks = $600 million
(6) $1.00 per mask * 600 million masks * 15 percent = $90 million per year

Taking the differences between these three components yields expression (7) below, which captures the added costs (if any) of domestic production. The relative costs depend on how many years it will be until the next pandemic occurs, which is hard to predict. That unknown is represented by the variable X. The relative costs also depend on what $Z equals and how it compares to the annual costs of maintaining the stockpile.

(7) $25 million * X + $300 million + ($Z million − $90 million) * X

If $Z happened to equal $90 million, then expression 7 would always be positive, meaning that on-shoring would never be cheaper than stockpiling. Indeed, the expression would be positive for all values of X so long as $Z was greater than or equal to $65 million. Alternatively, if $Z was equal to $5 million, the added costs of domestic production would simplify to this:

(8) $300 million − $60 million * X

In this case, on-shoring would be cheaper than stockpiling if the stockpile had to be maintained for more than 5 years. If $Z were $45 million, or half of the annual costs of maintain the stockpile, then stockpiling would be cheaper as long as X is less than 15 years.

More generally, Figure 2 below shows the points at which on-shoring and stockpiling would have the same costs as a function of $Z and X. In

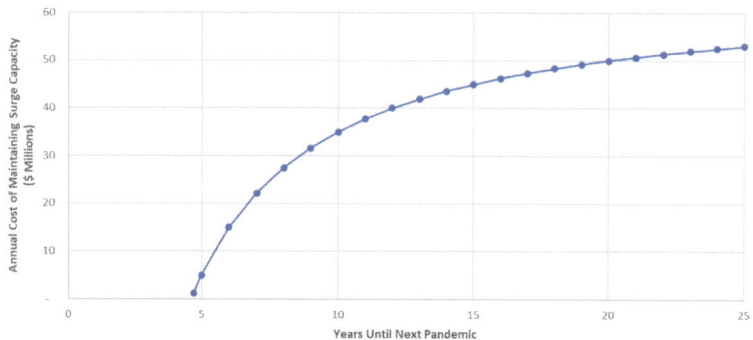

FIGURE 2 Cost Comparison of On-Shoring vs. Stockpiling (50% Price Premium)
Above the Line, Stockpiling Is Cheaper

this analysis, I have maintained the assumption that domestic production involves a 50 percent price premium. Above the blue line, stockpiling is the cheaper option, which happens when the next pandemic is expected to occur sooner, or when the annual costs of maintaining domestic surge capacity rise.

The same approach can be used to assess how sensitive the results are to other assumptions or estimates. In Figure 3 below, I hold X equal to 10 years and examine how the break-even points vary as a function of $Z and the domestic price premium. Here, the relationship is linear, with stockpiling being less costly when the domestic price premium is higher or the annual costs of maintaining domestic surge capacity increase.

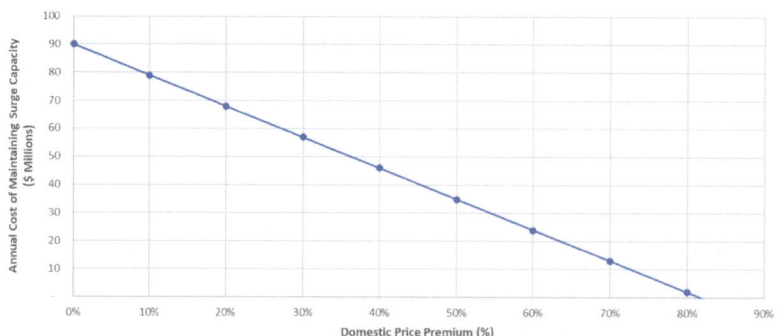

FIGURE 3 Cost Comparison of On-Shoring vs. Stockpiling (10-Year Horizon)
Above the Line, Stockpiling Is Cheaper

POLICY OPTIONS TO SPUR CHANGES IN MEDICAL PRODUCT SUPPLY CHAINS

In general, where the elements of medical product supply chains are located and how they operate are up to the private companies and organizations that produce and purchase these products. These private actors make choices in light of the incentives they face and the goals they seek to achieve. In order to change how medical product supply chains work, federal policies will have to influence those choices through some combination of regulations, subsidies, and penalties. In some cases, the distinction between subsidies and penalties on the one hand, and regulations on the other, can become blurred. Private actors may also lack the information they need to make the choices that achieve their goals and ideally, to also produce outcomes that are better for society as a whole. Thus, another role for government may be to improve the information available to them that concerns the medical product supply chains.

A. Improving Information

As noted throughout this analysis, the issues involved in supplying PPE and other materials during a pandemic and the issues involved in addressing ongoing problems with the supply of generic drugs are often sufficiently distinct as to warrant different solutions. Such is the case regarding the information that would be helpful in bringing about more reliable and secure medical product supply chains. Potentially, this information could be used in structuring subsidies for favorable actions or actors and penalties for the unfavorable ones, which would indeed provide incentives to improve behavior. However, in and of itself, the provision of information generally does not incentivize action.

Information on Pandemic-Related Supplies. One problem that quickly became evident at the start of the COVID-19 pandemic is that no clear and comprehensive picture was available regarding the status of PPE supplies and the demand for them, as expressed in orders. In the United States, the vast majority of those supplies are purchased from one of five large distributors. Rather quickly, HHS was able to establish agreements with those companies to receive continuous updates about their holdings and the orders and supplies that they had received. This repository of information was known, at least informally, as the "control tower."

Because the infrastructure for such a control tower can be difficult to erect at the onset of a pandemic, or may at least take up precious time, it makes sense to continue that activity after the COVID-19 pandemic subsides. How much it would cost to maintain that capability, however, and under what terms the companies involved would agree to do so, are not clear.

Information on Generic Drug Production. A prominent proposal in the recent FDA report on drug shortages was to improve the information available to purchasers about where and how the drugs they buy are made. Specifically, the report recommended "the development of a system to measure and rate the quality management maturity of individual manufacturing facilities based on specific objective indicators. The rating system would evaluate the robustness of a manufacturing facility's quality system" and could help identify manufacturers that maintain a robust medical product supply chain. Currently, purchasers and other observers have noted that they lack "line of sight" into where the drugs they buy are made, and do not have an easy way of assessing their quality. Toward that end, simply rating individual facilities might be insufficient; instead, a more fulsome assessment of the reliability of entire medical product supply chains may be necessary. The costs of establishing such a system, however, are hard to estimate.

Such a step would probably be helpful in improving the reliability of medical product supply chains, particularly for generic drugs. It is worth noting, however, that consumers often have little information about where or how the products they buy are made except for perhaps a "made in" label. Clearly, drugs are not average consumer goods and problems with their quality would cause substantial harm. Therefore, one might expect drug purchasers to be hypervigilant about product quality as a result. Although individual hospitals might well find it challenging to establish their own quality-control systems, additional private actors could fill the gap if there was indeed a willingness to pay the costs of these activities. Automobiles are another complex product with important safety dimensions. For these, the Insurance Institute for Highway Safety (IIHS) provides crash test information that is summarized in a user-friendly way, while J.D. Power and Associates provides quality awards.[37] The apparent lack of such mechanisms for generic drugs again suggests that there is not a sufficient willingness to pay for that information on the part of drug purchasers.

B. Relaxing or Strengthening Regulations

The choices of private actors that affect the structure and performance of medical product supply chains are themselves influenced by a wide range of regulations, many but not all of which are set at the federal level. In some cases, policy makers could seek to improve the reliability of sup-

---

[37] The federal government also provides crash test results, but the IIHS assessments may be more useful to consumers.

plies by relaxing certain safety regulations. For example, FDA could make it easier for new suppliers to enter a market if a drug shortage has arisen, or regulations governing reuse of PPE could be relaxed. These approaches, however, run the risk of reducing safety for patients and care providers, as well as generating additional adverse outcomes.

In other cases, policy makers may seek to impose more extensive regulations on suppliers or purchasers than those that exist today, but such approaches also tend to raise costs for suppliers and purchasers. For example, federal programs like Medicare and Medicaid could require providers to obtain their supplies from companies that can demonstrate they have robust supply chains, or FDA could even require such a demonstration as a condition of selling generic drugs in the U.S. market. In addition to regulations primarily affecting the supply or demand of medical products, federal and state regulations for price or payment rates for items under Medicare or Medicaid also have a ripple effect on medical product supply chains, and may need to be reconsidered in light of efforts to improve reliability.

Regulations Primarily Affecting Demand. The most obvious examples of regulations affecting the demand for medical supplies may be the ones governing how often PPE must be changed in the course of treatment. In general, the rule of "one patient, one unit" had applied to PPE prior to the pandemic. However, because of the PPE shortages that arose, FDA relaxed some of its regulations temporarily, and CDC issued guidance indicating that prolonged use or reuse of certain PPE should be allowed as needed to address shortages.[38]

Concerns about the effects of relaxing regulations on safety and disease transmission are certainly warranted, but in a crisis the alternatives may be worse. Even with time to plan in advance for what to do in another pandemic, the option of relaxing these regulations is still worth considering because its costs could also be less than those for other approaches. I presented some estimates above about the costs of relaxing those rules, particularly in terms of excess lives lost. But those estimates are based on limited information. A more extensive analysis of the risks involved and any excess transmissions that may have been caused by the emergency use authorizations related to COVID-19 should be undertaken as part of a broader assessment of the competing risks posed by all of the options for improving the reliability of medical product supply chains.

Regulations Primarily Affecting Supply. FDA regulations affect the supply of drugs in many ways. First and foremost is the requirement for drugs to have approval as being safe and effective, without which they cannot be supplied at all. FDA then regulates drug production processes in several

---

[38] Centers for Disease Control and Prevention, "Summary for Healthcare Facilities: Strategies for Optimizing the Supply of PPE During Shortages" (updated Dec. 29, 2020). https://www.cdc.gov/coronavirus/2019-ncov/hcp/ppe-strategy/strategies-optimize-ppe-shortages.html.

ways. As part of the application for a new drug, FDA assesses whether the manufacturing methods will be adequate to assure the drug's identity, strength, quality, and purity. Additionally, FDA seeks to ensure product integrity on a continuing basis "through product and facility registration; inspections; chain of custody documentation; and technologies to protect against counterfeit, diverted, subpotent, adulterated, misbranded, and expired drugs."[39] As a part of this process, FDA has established a set of Current Good Manufacturing Practices that drug makers are required to follow.

To an outside observer, it is somewhat surprising that FDA puts so much emphasis on what might be called process measure of quality, rather than on outcome measures. The agency requires some sampling and testing of in-process materials and drug products, and it does try to track adverse outcomes among patients through postmarket surveillance programs, but arguably a better approach would be to test the finished products extensively for purity and potency. To a certain extent, FDA's focus on production processes may be from the historical legacy of predecessor agencies going back to the early 1900s, for which "ensuring product integrity was the key task." Granted, the costs of testing a sufficient sample of each of the products under its purview may be greater than the costs of overseeing production processes, but the results might also be better. Both the costs of testing and the risks of shifting from one regulatory regime to another could be limited in two ways: one, if such testing were used as an added measure rather than a substitute measure, at least initially, and two, if the initial focus of the testing program was narrowed to the types or categories of drugs that have had repeated quality problems or shortages, such as generic sterile injectables.

Some observers argue for going further. In a recent piece, Dr. Rena Conti and Dr. Fiona Scott Morton, two widely recognized experts on prescription drugs, argue that drug companies should be required to report detailed information about their medical product supply chains in order to "receive annual approval to sell into the U.S. market, which would create a strong incentive for manufacturers to comply in a timely fashion."[40] Furthermore, they propose a new office should be created within the Department of Health and Human Services, but outside of FDA, that would be charged with analyzing and improving the reliability of pharmaceutical supply chains. Among the reasons they cite are that "FDA has been the agency responsible for supply chain disruptions for over a decade, includ-

---

[39] This discussion is drawn in part from Congressional Research Service, *How FDA Approves Drugs and Regulates Their Safety and Effectiveness* (May 8, 2018). https://sgp.fas.org/crs/misc/R41983.pdf.

[40] Rena M. Conti and Fiona Scott Morton, "Building a Resilient Rx Drug Supply: A New HHS Office and Other Steps," *Health Affairs Blog* (August 27, 2021). https://www.healthaffairs.org/do/10.1377/hblog20210824.559824/full/.

ing the sale of substandard products into the U.S. market that have harmed Americans."[41]

Regulations Governing Prices. While regulations affecting the demand for—or supply of—medical products obviously influence their prices as well, some federal regulations affect the prices of those goods more directly. In particular, recent studies indicate that laws and regulations reducing the payment rates for generic drugs under Medicare and Medicaid have played a role in causing shortages of these drugs. While the specifics differ, it stands to reason that a reduction in revenue for generic drug makers would put pressure on them to adopt lower-cost production methods and to use supply lines that are more vulnerable to disruptions, or at least to limit their investments in robust medical product supply chains.

Under Medicaid, the most relevant regulation may be one that was enacted recently. Medicaid has long required drug manufacturers to pay rebates on original, brand-name drugs when their prices rise faster than the general rate of inflation. Legislation enacted in 2015 extends that same requirement to generic drugs. While the desire to reduce spending on Medicaid is understandable, that requirement means that any price spikes stemming from a generic drug shortage will have to be rebated to that program.[42] As a result, generic drug makers gain less from a given price increase, and would therefore not increase supply as much, nor would they have to raise prices higher to bring supply and demand into alignment. Shortages are somewhat more difficult to address, and since Medicaid accounts for about one-eighth of all domestic spending on generic drugs, the effect may be substantial.

A similar trend has been observed for a price reduction in Medicare, and in that case the magnitude of the effect could be quantified. Specifically, a study looked at the effect of substantial reductions in Medicare's payment

---

[41] Having worked for the federal government for 2 decades, and having studied its operations, I respectfully disagree with their proposal to create a new agency outside of FDA that has overlapping responsibilities with it. I agree with their diagnosis that FDA has been slow to change and has not been effective enough in responding to ongoing shortages of drugs, but I believe that establishing a new center within FDA focused on issues involved in drug production, including the reliability of medical product supply chains, is more likely to succeed. That success is by no means guaranteed, however, and determined leadership over a period of many years will be needed to make a new center, and a new approach, take hold. (FDA's organizational chart is at https://www.fda.gov/about-fda/fda-organization-charts/fda-overview-organization-chart).

[42] See Richard Manning and Fred Selck, Penalizing Generic Drugs with the CPI Rebate Will Reduce Competition and Increase the Likelihood of Drug Shortages (Bates-White Economic Consulting: September 12, 2017). https://www.accessiblemeds.org/sites/default/files/2017-09/Bates-White-White-Paper-ReportCPI-Penalty-09-12-2017.pdf.

rates for physician-administered drugs that were implemented in 2005.[43] The resulting reductions in prices averaged about 50 percent. That change in policy was quite understandable, since by all accounts Medicare had previously been paying much higher prices, based on the drugs' list prices, than private insurers had paid. Nevertheless, a payment cut is a payment cut, and the study's authors estimated that this cut could account for a 25 percent increase in the expected number of shortage days per year for generic drugs. This change may have been an important factor behind the rise in shortages that has been observed over the past 15 years.

C. Providing Subsidies or Imposing Penalties

If it chose to do so, the federal government could subsidize the higher costs of domestically produced PPE or the higher cost of maintaining robust supply lines for generic drugs in a wide variety of ways:

- Medicare and Medicaid payments to hospitals could be increased to reward hospitals that purchase PPE domestically or that maintain robust supply lines.
- Tax credits or deductions could be used to reward companies that make improvements to their supply chain's reliability and security.
- The federal government could set up a program of direct outlays of subsidies to accomplish the same goals.

In each of these endeavors, the two key challenges will be defining what activities qualify for subsidies and determining the subsidy rate. Inevitably there will be some perverse compliance and some "buying out the base," a term budget analysts use when referring to payments to people or organizations for complying with program requirements when they would have complied anyway, without a payment.

Even so, economists often recommend providing subsidies or imposing penalties as a means of changing the behavior of private actors in a relatively efficient way. Examples include subsidies for clean forms of energy use, free vaccinations for communicable diseases, and "sin" taxes on cigarettes and alcohol. In general, the goals of such approaches include having private actors internalize the benefits or costs that their actions impose on others, as well as those which they might ordinarily fail to consider, plus yielding too much activity that can cause external harm and too little activity that could provide external benefits. Such policies effectively lower

---

[43] Ali Yurukoglu, Eli Liebman, and David B. Ridley, "The Role of Government Reimbursement in Drug Shortages," *American Economic Journal: Economic Policy*, vol. 9, no. 2 (May 2017). https://www.jstor.org/stable/26156409. See also: https://www.nber.org/system/files/working_papers/w17987/w17987.pdf.

the price of favored activities and raise the price of unfavored ones. The resulting quantities that are supplied depend on how responsive buyers and sellers are to the changes in prices.

Instead of adjusting prices, an alternative approach is to limit the quantity that can be produced of a product that is known to have had adverse effects. For example, certain forms of pollution are capped, with tradeable permits issued that allow polluters to buy and sell emission rights in a way that helps minimize the cost of achieving a given reduction in pollution. As a result, the market price of polluting will settle at the level needed to limit pollution to the prescribed amount. It might seem that imposing a tax on pollution and limiting the quantity of allowed pollution would be equally effective, but an important article in the field of regulatory economics found that in the face of uncertainty between optimal price and optimal quantity, the more efficient approach is to regulate the one which is less uncertain.[44]

How do these rather abstract considerations apply to medical product supply chains? In the case of PPE, the federal government could increase domestic production, either by subsidizing domestically produced items, or by ordering a certain quantity of domestically produced goods. If the government was omniscient, it could choose either target with equal precision. But in reality, we have only a rough idea of how much PPE we might need in a future pandemic, and an even rougher idea of what sort of subsidy domestic producers would need in order to be competitive with foreign sources of supply, nor do we know how much these domestic producers would supply.

We, as a polity, may be more certain about the quantity of PPE that we want rather than the price we should pay to get that quantity. In other words, setting a subsidy for PPE may require more trial and error than specifying an amount to stockpile and purchasing that amount, at whatever price emerges. Likewise, with generic drugs, we may have a better idea of what quantities we want to maintain in the event of a supply disruption than we do about the subsidies needed to yield the desired increase in reliability and reduction in shortages.

---

[44] Martin L. Weitzman, "Price vs. Quantities," *Review of Economic Studies*, vol. 41, no. 4 (October 1974). https://scholar.harvard.edu/weitzman/publications/prices-vs-quantities.

Appendix E

Committee and Staff Biosketches

COMMITTEE MEMBERS

Wallace J. Hopp, Ph.D. (Chair), studies the design, control, and management of operations systems, with emphasis on manufacturing and supply chain systems, innovation processes, and health care systems. His teaching and research in these areas has been recognized with a number of awards, including being named a Fellow of Institute of International Education, Institute for Operations Research and the Management Sciences, SME, Manufacturing & Service Operations Management, and the Production and Operations Management Society (POMS), and his election to the National Academy of Engineering. He has previously served as President of POMS, as Editor-in-Chief of the journal *Management Science*, and is currently a founding editor of the *Management and Business Review*. He is an active industry consultant whose clients have included many Fortune 500 firms.

Mahshid Abir, M.D., M.Sc., is an associate professor in emergency medicine at the University of Michigan (U-M) and a Senior Physician Policy Researcher at the RAND Corporation. She is the director of the Acute Care Research Unit at the U-M Institute for Healthcare Policy and Innovation. Her health services and policy research is focused on improving acute care delivery along the continuum of care during routine and catastrophic conditions, including in the ambulatory care, prehospital, emergency department, and inpatient settings. She has been an integral member of several teams of researchers at RAND, developing various aspects of the National Health Security Strategy funded by the Department of Health and Human Services, Office of the Assistant Secretary for Preparedness and Response; developing tools to measure hospital and health care coalition surge capacity in response to mass casualty incidents, including a tool designed to evaluate community disaster preparedness. More recently, Dr. Abir has led an internally funded RAND project evaluating strategies for critical care surge capacity in the United States in response to the COVID-19 pandemic, as well as a project funded by the Assistant Secretary for Planning and Evaluation comparing national and international approaches to pandemic-related outcome measurement.

George Ball, Ph.D., M.B.A., is an associate professor of operations and decision technologies and the Weimer Faculty Fellow at the Kelley School of Business, Indiana University, Bloomington. George's research focuses on medical devices and pharmaceutical supply chain quality, and in particular, medical product recalls. George has conducted several collaborative research projects with the Center for Device and Radiological Health and the Center for Drug Evaluation and Research at the Food and Drug Administration (FDA). In particular, George was a co-principal investigator for a large multiuniversity, multimillion-dollar federal contract with FDA to identify unique predictors of drug shortage and drug quality risks. George's research has been published in several top-tier journals including *Management Science*, *Manufacturing & Service Operations Management*, and the *Journal of Operations Management*. Prior to his time at Indiana University, George spent 11 years in various manager and director roles at two major medical device companies and 5 years on active duty as a U.S. Naval Officer. George received his Ph.D. in supply chain and operations, an M.B.A. from the Carlson School of Management at the University of Minnesota, and a B.S. in aerospace engineering from the U.S. Naval Academy.

Lee Branstetter, Ph.D., is a professor of economics and public policy at Carnegie Mellon University with a joint appointment to the Social and Decision Sciences Department. He joined the Heinz College faculty in 2006 as a tenured associate professor. Dr. Branstetter is also a research associate of the National Bureau of Economic Research and nonresident senior fellow at the Peterson Institute for International Economics. From 2011 to 2012, he served as the Senior Economist for International Trade and Investment for the President's Council of Economic Advisors. Prior to coming to Carnegie Mellon, he was the Daniel J. Stanton Associate Professor of Business and the Director of the International Business Program at Columbia Business School. Dr. Branstetter has also taught at the University of California, Davis, where he was the director of the East Asian Studies Program, and at Dartmouth College. He has served as a consultant to the Organisation for Economic Co-operation and Development Science and Technology

Directorate, the Advanced Technology Program of the U.S. Department of Commerce, and the World Bank. In recent years, Dr. Branstetter has been a research fellow of the Keio University Global Security Research Institute and a visiting fellow of the Research Institute of Economy, Trade, and Industry in Japan. Branstetter holds a B.A. in economics and mathematical methods in the social sciences from Northwestern University, and he earned his Ph.D. in economics at Harvard in 1996.

Robert Califf, M.D., MACC, is the Head of Clinical Policy and Strategy for Verily and Google Health. Previously, Dr. Califf was the vice chancellor for health data science for the Duke University School of Medicine, director of Duke Forge, Duke's Center for Health Data Science, and the Donald F. Fortin, M.D., Professor of Cardiology. He served as Deputy Commissioner for Medical Products and Tobacco in the U.S. Food and Drug Administration (FDA) from 2015 to 2016, and as Commissioner of Food and Drugs from 2016 to 2017. Prior to joining FDA, Dr. Califf was a professor of medicine and vice chancellor for clinical and translational research at Duke University. He was the founding director of the Duke Clinical Research Institute. As a nationally and internationally recognized expert in cardiovascular medicine, health outcomes research, health care quality, and clinical research, Dr. Califf has led many landmark clinical trials and is one of the most frequently cited authors in biomedical science, with 1,250 publications in peer-reviewed literature. Dr. Califf is also a member of the National Academy of Medicine (formerly the Institute of Medicine [IOM]). Dr. Califf has served on numerous IOM committees, and was a member of the FDA Cardiorenal Advisory Panel and FDA Science Board's Subcommittee on Science and Technology. Dr. Califf has also served on the Board of Scientific Counselors for the National Library of Medicine, as well as on advisory committees for the National Cancer Institute, the National Heart, Lung, and Blood Institute, the National Institute of Environmental Health Sciences, and the Council of the National Institute on Aging. He has led major initiatives aimed at improving methods and infrastructure for clinical research, including the Clinical Trials Transformation Initiative, a public–private partnership co-founded by FDA and Duke. He also has served as the principal investigator for Duke's Clinical and Translational Science Award, the National Institutes of Health Health Care Systems Research Collaboratory coordinating center, and as co-PI of the National Patient-Centered Clinical Research Network (PCORnet). He currently serves as chair of the board of the People-Centered Research Foundation, a not-for-profit organization that is supporting and extending the work of PCORnet.

Asha Devereaux, M.D., M.P.H., completed her medical degree in biology from the University of California, San Diego, followed by a M.D. and

M.P.H. from Tulane University School of Medicine and Public Health. Upon graduation, she served in the United States Navy achieving the rank of Commander while receiving board certification in internal medicine, pulmonology, and critical care. During her 11-year naval career, Dr. Devereaux served on the Navy Surgeon General's Panel for Tobacco Cessation, served as Head of Medicine at Beaufort Naval Hospital, served on numerous committees, and spent three years covering the USNS Mercy's Chem/Bio intensive care unit. She is currently on staff at Sharp-Coronado Hospital. In addition to her private practice of pulmonary medicine, she has co-chaired and remains on the Executive Committee of the American College of Chest Physicians (ACCP) Mass Critical Care Task Force, has served on National Academy of Medicine and Centers for Disease Control and Prevention panels for influenza, anthrax, and crisis care, is Past-Chairman of the ACCP Disaster Response Network, and is a former President of the California Thoracic Society. She has responded to natural disasters ranging from fires to hurricanes with the Medical Reserve Corps, the National Disaster Medical System, and as the Senior Medical Officer for San Diego CAL-MAT. She has provided care in Alternate Care Sites for COVID-19 throughout Southern California. Dr. Devereaux was selected as a Top Doctor in San Diego in 2009 and 2021 and was named the Outstanding Pulmonologist by the California Thoracic Society in 2017 by her peers.

Özlem Ergun, Ph.D., is a professor and associate chair for graduate affairs in mechanical and industrial engineering at Northeastern University. Dr. Ergun's research focuses on design and management of large-scale and decentralized networks. She has applied her work on network design, management, and resilience to problems arising in many critical systems including transportation, pharmaceuticals, and health care. She has worked with organizations that respond to emergencies and humanitarian crises around the world. She was the President of INFORMS Section on Public Programs, Service and Needs in 2013. She currently serves as the Area Editor at the *Operations Research* journal for policy modeling and the public sector area, and a Department Editor for the journal of Manufacturing & Service Operations Management within the Environment, Health and Society Department. Dr. Ergun is also a founding co-chair of the annual Health and Humanitarian Logistics Conference, held annually since 2009. In addition, Dr. Ergun was the Vice President of Membership and Professional Recognition on the INFORMS Board of Directors from 2011 to 2015. Prior to joining Northeastern, Dr. Ergun was the Coca-Cola Associate Professor in the School of Industrial and Systems Engineering at Georgia Institute of Technology, where she also co-founded and co-directed the Health and Humanitarian Systems Research Center at the Supply Chain and Logistics Institute. She received a B.S. in operations research and industrial engineering from Cornell University in 1996 and a Ph.D. in operations research from the Massachusetts Institute of Technology in 2001.

Erin Fox, Pharm.D, BCPS, FASHP, is senior pharmacy director of the Department of Pharmacy Services at University of Utah Health. Erin is also associate professor (adjunct), at the Department of Pharmacotherapy, University of Utah College of Pharmacy. The University of Utah Drug Information Service provides content for the American Society of Health-System Pharmacists (ASHP) Drug Shortage Resource Center and Erin serves as a media resource and advocate for changes to improve the ongoing drug shortage situation and rising drug costs. Erin is also active in both state and national pharmacy and health-related societies serving in a variety of volunteer and elected positions. Erin is recognized as an expert in drug shortages and has received the ISMP Cheers Award and ASHP Award of Excellence in recognition for her work on drug shortages. Erin has also been honored with the William A. Zellmer Lecture award for her advocacy efforts to address drug shortages and rising drug prices.

Larry M. Glasscock, B.A., is a businessperson who has been either at the helm of, or has provided executive leadership for, companies across a variety of segments. Presently, Mr. Glasscock holds the position of Chief Operating Officer of NFH, Inc. and serves in an executive advisory capacity for MNX Global Logistics. Mr. Glasscock serves on the Board of Kershaw's Challenge, a public charity founded by Ellen and Clayton Kershaw, and is a member of the Radiopharmaceutical Shippers and Carriers Conference. Mr. Glasscock has extensive experience in the development of unique, global supply chain solutions for health care and medical research companies of all types with specific leadership in nuclear medicine and immunotherapy. He is known to be particularly adept at forming partnerships and alliances for the benefit of manufacturers, researchers, treatment centers, and patients throughout the world.

Lewis Grossman, J.D., Ph.D., is professor of law at the Washington College of Law, where he has taught since 1997 and where he served as Associate Dean for Scholarship from 2008 to 2011. He teaches and writes in the areas of food and drug law, health law, American legal history, and civil procedure. He has also been a visiting professor of law at Cornell Law School and a Law and Public Affairs (LAPA) Fellow at Princeton University. Prior to joining the American University faculty, he was an associate at Covington & Burling LLP in Washington, D.C. Previously, he clerked for Chief Judge Abner Mikva of the U.S. Court of Appeals for the D.C. Circuit. Professor Grossman's scholarship has appeared in the *Cornell Law Review*, *Law and History Review*, *Yale Journal of Health Policy, Law*

& *Ethics*, and *Administrative Law Review*, among others. He has made recent contributions to volumes published by Oxford University Press and Columbia University Press. He is the co-author of *Food and Drug Law: Cases and Materials* (with Peter Barton Hutt and Richard A. Merrill), and of a widely used supplement to the first-year civil procedure course titled *A Documentary Companion to A Civil Action* (with Robert G. Vaughn). In 2021, Oxford University Press published Professor Grossman's book titled *Choose Your Medicine: Freedom of Therapeutic Choice in America*. He has served as a member or legal consultant on three previous committees of the Health and Medicine Division of the National Academies of Sciences, Engineering, and Medicine (formerly the Institute of Medicine). Professor Grossman earned his Ph.D. in history from Yale University, where he was awarded the George Washington Egleston Prize for Best Dissertation in the Field of American History. He received a J.D. magna cum laude from Harvard Law School and a B.A. summa cum laude from Yale University.

W. Craig Vanderwagen, M.D., RADM, USPHS, is a family physician who retired as a Rear Admiral in the United States Public Health Service in 2009. He served for 25 years in the Indian Health Service, the federal program of medical and public health services for American Indians and Alaska Natives. During this time, he also served as the lead health official at a number of disasters including medical care for Kosovar refugees (1999); advisor to the Afghan Ministry of Health (2002); director of public health and advisor to the Iraq Ministry of Health (2003-2004); the USNS Mercy's response to the 2004 tsunami; and commander of the public health and medical response to Hurricanes Katrina/Rita. Dr. Vanderwagen's last federal assignment (2006-2009) was as the Assistant Secretary for Preparedness and Response at the U.S. Department of Health and Human Services (HHS). He was responsible for leading all federal public health and medical assets in disaster response, as well as for guiding the $11 billion HHS medical countermeasure advanced development program to address chemical, biological, radiological and nuclear threats which now has over 100 products in the development pipeline. Dr. Vanderwagen is a Director and General Manager of East West Protection, a Potomac, Maryland, based firm he co-founded with Fuad El Hibri, specializing in public health and medical preparedness, detection, response, and command and control systems for CBRN threats and other disasters. He also has equity in a company that builds specialized vehicles (E-N-G Mobile Systems) and a company that builds long-endurance drones for commercial and other uses (ARS). He is Immediate Past Chairman of the Board at VIDO-Intervac, a Canadian vaccine research and development company. He is also a senior partner at Martin, Blanck, and Associates, a consulting firm of retired generals and flag officers specializing in military health matters. He is a frequent public speaker on biodefense, public health preparedness, and leadership.

Alastair Wood, M.D., was professor of both medicine and pharmacology at Vanderbilt University Medical School and served as both Assistant Vice Chancellor for Clinical Research and Associate Dean at Vanderbilt Medical School, before being appointed Emeritus Professor of Medicine and Emeritus Professor of Pharmacology in 2006. He served as the Drug Therapy Section Editor of the *New England Journal of Medicine* from 1985 to 2004. He was a Partner at Symphony Capital LLC, a private equity company investing in the clinical development of novel biopharmaceutical products from 2006 to 2018. Dr. Wood has been honored by being elected to the National Academy of Medicine (formerly the Institute of Medicine), the American Association of Physicians, the American Society for Clinical Investigation, Honorary Fellow in the American Gynecological and Obstetrical Society, Fellowship of the American College of Physicians, Fellowship of the Royal College of Physicians of London, and Fellowship of the Royal College of Physicians of Edinburgh. He was the 2005 recipient of the Rawls-Palmer Award and in 2008 received the honorary degree of Doctor of Laws, *honoris causa*, from the University of Dundee. Dr. Wood has served on a number of editorial boards including the *New England Journal of Medicine* editorial board and his research has resulted in over 300 articles, reviews, and editorials.

Matthew K. Wynia, M.D., M.P.H., has had a career that includes developing a research institute and training programs focusing on bioethics, professionalism and policy issues (the American Medical Association [AMA] Institute for Ethics), and founding the AMA's Center for Patient Safety. His research has focused on novel uses of survey data to inform and improve the practical management of ethical issues in health care and public policy. He has led projects on a wide variety of topics related to ethics and professionalism, including understanding and measuring the ethical climate of health care organizations and systems; ethics and quality improvement; communication, team-based care, and engaging patients as members of a team; defining physician professionalism; public health and disaster ethics; medicine and the Holocaust, with the United States Holocaust Memorial Museum; and inequities in health and health care. He has served on committees, expert panels, and as a reviewer for the National Academies, The Joint Commission, the Hastings Center, the American Board of Medical Specialties, federal agencies, and other organizations. Dr. Wynia is the author of more than 160 published articles, chapters, and essays, co-editor of several books, and co-author of a book on fairness in health care benefit design. His work has been published in *JAMA*, the *New England Journal of Medicine*, *Annals of Internal Medicine*, *Health Affairs*, and other leading medical and ethics journals, and he is a contributing editor for the *American Journal of Bioethics*. He has discussed his work as a guest on the BBC, ABC News, and National Public Radio, among others. Dr. Wynia is a past president of the American Society for Bioethics and Humanities, and has chaired both the Ethics Forum of the American Public Health Association and the Ethics Committee of the Society for General Internal Medicine.

STAFF

Lisa Brown, M.P.H. (*Study Codirector*), is a Senior Program Officer on the Board on Health Sciences Policy at the National Academies of Sciences, Engineering, and Medicine (the National Academies) and develops and manages projects at the National Academies related to solving the nation's most pressing health security issues. She currently serves as a director for the Standing Committee on Emerging Infectious Diseases and 21st Century Health Threats and the Security of America's Medical Product Supply Chain. She has directed several projects, including the Committee on Equitable Allocation of Vaccine for the Novel Coronavirus, the Committee on Data Needs to Monitor Evolution of SARS-CoV-2, the Committee on Evidence-Based Practices for Public Health Emergency Preparedness and Response, and the Committee on Strengthening the Disaster Resilience of Academic Research Communities. Prior to the National Academies, Lisa served as Senior Program Analyst for Public Health Preparedness and Environment Health at the National Association of County and City Health Officials (NACCHO). In this capacity, Lisa served as project lead for medical countermeasures and the Strategic National Stockpile, researched radiation preparedness issues, and was involved in high-level Centers for Disease Control and Prevention (CDC) initiatives for the development of clinical guidance for anthrax and botulism countermeasures in a mass casualty event. In 2015, Lisa was selected as a fellow in the Emerging Leaders in Biosecurity Initiative at the Center for Health Security, a highly competitive program to prepare the next generation of leaders in the field of biosecurity. Prior to her work at NACCHO, Lisa worked as an Environmental Public Health Scientist at Public Health England (PHE) in London, England. While at PHE, she focused on climate change, the recovery process following disasters, and the impact of droughts and floods on emerging infectious diseases. Lisa received her master of public health from King's College London in 2012 and her bachelor of science in biology from The University of Findlay in 2010.

Carolyn Shore, Ph.D. (*Study Codirector*), is director of the Forum on Drug Discovery, Development, and Translation and a senior program officer with the Board on Health Sciences Policy of the National Academies of Sciences, Engineering, and Medicine. Before joining the National Academies, Carolyn was an officer on Pew's antibiotic resistance project, leading work on research and policies to spur the discovery and development of urgently needed antibacterial therapies. She previously served as a foreign affairs officer at the U.S. Department of State, where she led an initiative on open data and innovation-based solutions to global challenges. She also served as the State Department's representative to intergovernmental organizations focusing on food safety, plant and animal health, biosecurity, and agricultural trade policy. Carolyn was an American Society for Microbiology congressional fellow, working on science-based policy related to antibiotic stewardship and other public health issues. She holds a doctoral degree in microbiology and molecular genetics from Harvard University. As a graduate student, she studied anti-malarial drug resistance in Senegal and worked jointly between the Medicines for Malaria Venture, Genzyme Corporation, and the Broad Institute of Harvard and MIT to discover new anti-malarial compounds. Carolyn was awarded a Fulbright Fellowship for work at the University of Queensland in Brisbane, Australia, and a National Institutes of Health Training Grant for postdoctoral work at the University of Iowa.

Kelsey R. Babik, M.P.H., is an Associate Program Officer in the Health Medicine Division at the National Academies of Sciences, Engineering, and Medicine. In addition to this study, she works on projects initiated by the Committee on Personal Protective Equipment for Workplace Safety and Health. This is a standing committee at the National Academies of Sciences, Engineering, and Medicine sponsored by the National Personal Protective Technology Laboratory of the National Institute for Occupational Safety and Health, to provide a forum for discussion of scientific and technical issues relevant to the development, certification, deployment, and use of personal protective equipment, standards, and related systems to ensure workplace safety and health. Previously, at the Risk Sciences and Public Policy Institute of the Johns Hopkins Bloomberg School of Public Health, she worked on occupational health risk assessments for first responders. She has a B.S. in molecular biology from the University of Pittsburgh and an M.P.H. from the University of Maryland.

Leah Cairns, Ph.D., is a Program Officer on the Board on Health Sciences Policy. Her primary interests include health policy and biomedical research. Prior to joining the National Academies, she served as a Science and Technology Policy Fellow for the Association for the Advancement of Science working as legislative staff for a member of Congress focusing on health policy and appropriations. Dr. Cairns also previously served as a Christine Mirzayan Science & Technology Policy Fellow at the National Academies in the Policy and Global Affairs Division. Dr. Cairns received her Ph.D. in biophysics from the Johns Hopkins University School of Medicine and a B.A. in biochemistry and molecular biology from Hamilton College.

Melvin Joppy, B.S., is a Senior Program Assistant on the Board on Health Sciences Policy, with the Forum on Drug Discovery, Development, and Translation. He was recently a Program Assistant at the Department of Energy (DOE) working in the Office of Basic Energy Sciences. Prior to DOE, Melvin served as the Committee Manager for the Presidential Advisory Council on HIV/AIDS within the U.S. Department of Health and Human Services. Melvin received his B.S. in communications from Bowie State University.

Andrew March, M.P.H., is an Associate Program Officer on the Board on Health Sciences Policy, with the Forum on Drug Discovery, Development, and Translation. Andrew joined the National Academies in 2018. His previous work at the Academies includes consensus studies on dementia care interventions, and the safety and effectiveness of compounded drug preparations. Prior to coming to the National Academies, he performed research on sickness absence in working women at the Center for Research in Occupational Health, and worked in the Epidemiology Department at the Hospital de la Santa Creu i Sant Pau. Andrew obtained his M.P.H. at the Universitat Pompeu Fabra and his B.S. degree in biology and Spanish from Roanoke College.

Margaret McCarthy, M.Sc., is a Research Associate with the Board on Health Sciences Policy. She is currently working with the Committee on the Security of America's Medical Product Supply Chain and the Standing Committee for CDC Preparedness and Response. In 2018, Margaret interned with Committee on Human Rights and Office of News and Public Information, where she collaborated with fellow colleagues to organize the Second International Summit on Human Genome Editing. Before rejoining the National Academies as a Research Associate, she previously worked at Brigham and Women's Hospital in Boston, Massachusetts, as an infectious diseases research assistant. Her interests include migration, biosecurity, and European politics. Margaret received her B.A. in international studies from American University and her M.Sc. in global health and development from University College, London.

Shalini Singaravelu, M.Sc., is an Associate Program Officer on the Board on Health Sciences Policy and works on the Standing Committee on Emerging Infectious Diseases and 21st Century Health Threats. Prior to joining the National Academies, Shalini managed a portfolio of digital health tools as a Program Manager at IBM. From 2015 to 2019, she was a consultant for the World Health Organization Health Emergencies Programme in Geneva. In this role, she supported preparedness and response to emerging infectious disease epidemics with a focus on operational data systems, risk communication, and community engagement. Before this, she worked on psychosocial support programming for HIV-affected orphans and vulnerable children in South Africa. Shalini has a graduate certificate in risk sciences and public policy from Johns Hopkins Bloomberg School of Public Health (2021), where she is currently a part-time doctor of public health (Dr.P.H.) student in health security. She received her M.Sc. in global mental health from London School of Hygiene and Tropical Medicine (2014) and her B.A. in anthropology from Union College (2012).

Appendix F

Disclosure of Unavoidable Conflict of Interest

The conflict of interest policy of the National Academies of Sciences, Engineering, and Medicine (http://www.nationalacademies.org/coi) prohibits the appointment of an individual to a committee authoring a Consensus Study Report if the individual has a conflict of interest that is relevant to the task to be performed. An exception to this prohibition is permitted if the National Academies determines that the conflict is unavoidable and the conflict is publicly disclosed. A determination of a conflict of interest for an individual is not an assessment of that individual's actual behavior or character or ability to act objectively despite the conflicting interest.

Robert M. Califf has a conflict of interest in relation to his service on the Committee on Security of America's Medical Product Supply Chain because he is employed by Verily Life Sciences and has current relationships with Google Health and Cytokinetics.

The National Academies has concluded that for this committee to accomplish the tasks for which it was established, its membership must include at least one person who has substantial relevant experience in FDA regulatory policy, drug and device development, drug and device manufacturing, and drug shortages. As described in his biographical summary, Dr. Califf has extensive current experience as Head of Clinical Policy and Strategy for Verily Life Sciences and Google Health in FDA regulatory policy, drug and device development and manufacturing. As Commissioner of the U.S. Food and Drug Administration (FDA), and as Deputy Commissioner for Medical Products and Tobacco, Dr. Califf gained valuable expertise and perspective on the entirety of the health care ecosystem, including companies, hospitals, and health systems. Additionally, Dr. Califf has led clinical research studies and clinical trials and previously served as vice chancellor of clinical and translational research and the director of the Duke Translational Medicine Institute.

The National Academies has determined that the experience and expertise of Dr. Califf is needed for the committee to accomplish the task for which it has been established. The National Academies could not find another available individual with the equivalent experience and expertise who does not have a conflict of interest. Therefore, the National Academies has concluded that the conflict is unavoidable.

The National Academies believes that Dr. Califf can serve effectively as a member of the committee, and the committee can produce an objective report, taking into account the composition of the committee, the work to be performed, and the procedures to be followed in completing the study.